PLANT BASED COOKING FOR EVERYONE

Reader's Digest

New York | Montreal

A READER'S DIGEST BOOK

44 South Broadway
White Plains, NY 10601

ISBN 978-1-62145-577-6 (ppb)
ISBN 978-1-62145-578-3 (e-pub)

We are committed to both the quality of our products and the service we provide to our customers. We value your comments, so please feel free to contact us at TMBBookTeam@TrustedMediaBrands.com.

For more Reader's Digest products and information, visit our website:
www.rd.com (in the United States)
www.readersdigest.ca (in Canada)

Printed in China
10 9 8 7 6 5 4 3 2

Pictured on the cover are the Salsa Black Bean Burger (p. 103) and Arugula & Brown Rice Salad (p. 116).

NOTE TO OUR READERS

The information in this book should not be substituted for, or used to alter, medical therapy without your doctor's advice. For a specific health problem, consult your physician for guidance.

Eating eggs or egg whites that are not completely cooked poses the possibility of salmonella food poisoning. The risk is greater for pregnant women, the elderly, the very young and persons with impaired immune systems. If you are concerned about salmonella, you can use reconstituted powdered egg whites or pasteurized eggs.

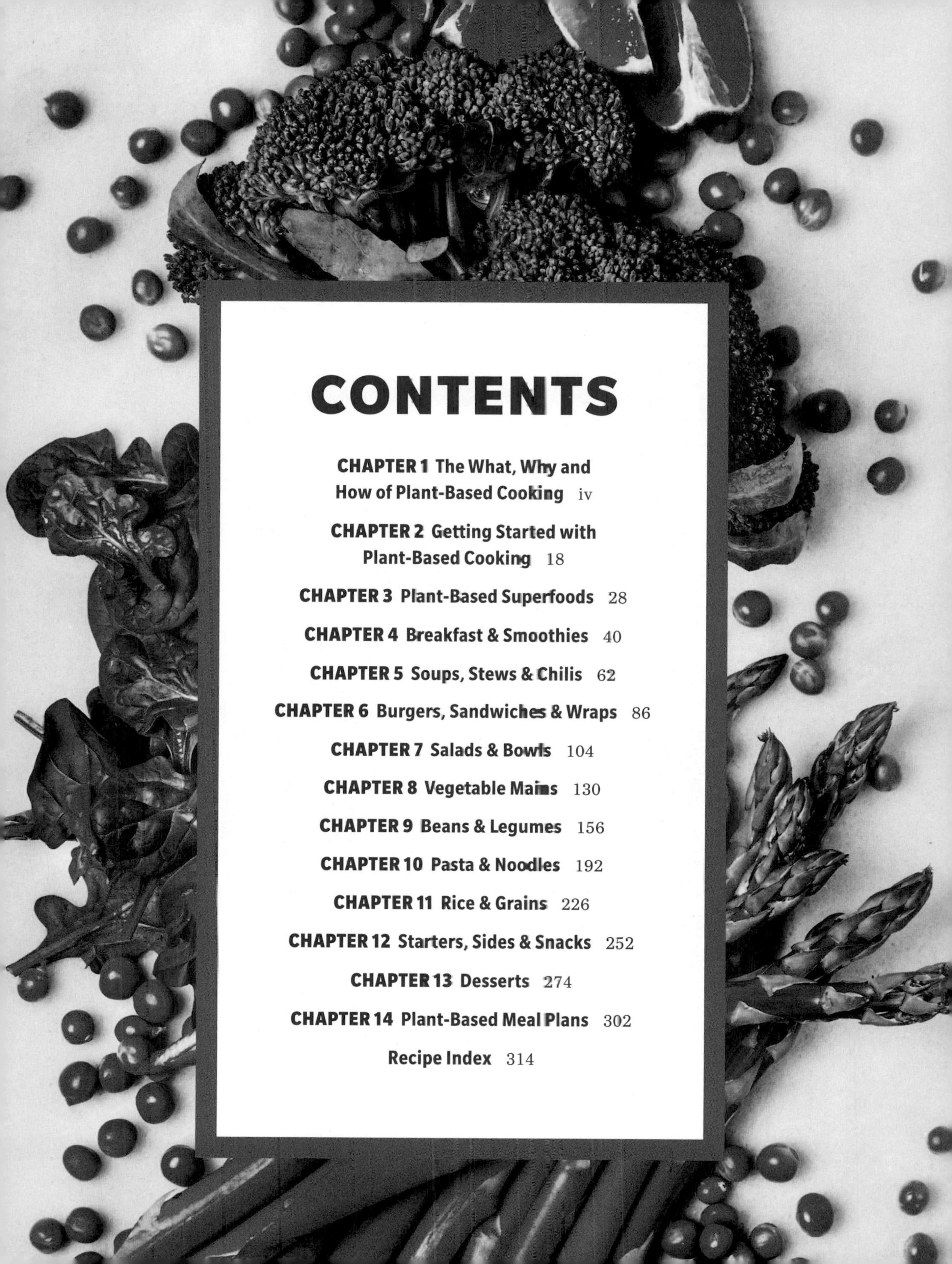

CONTENTS

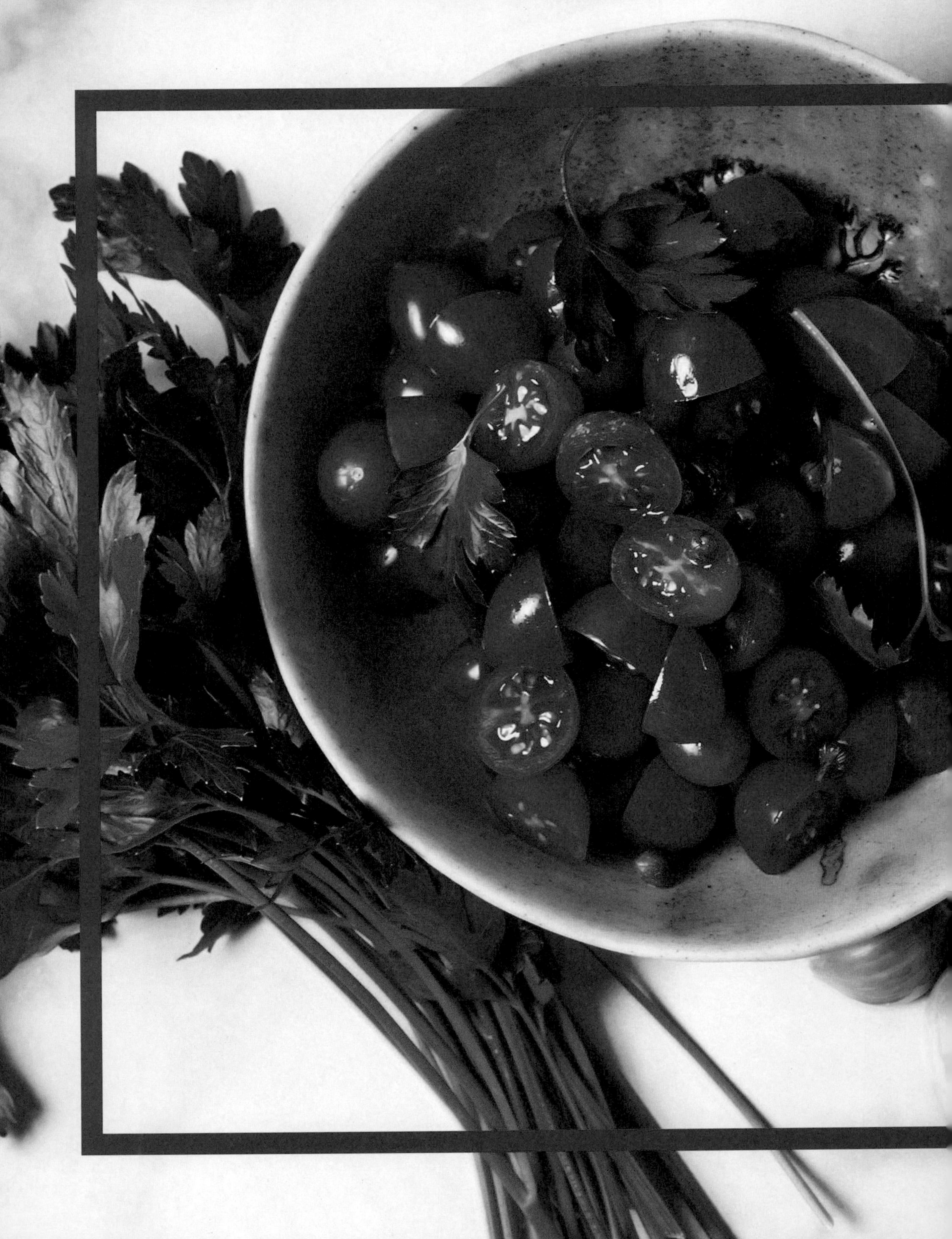

CHAPTER 1

THE WHAT, WHY AND HOW OF PLANT-BASED COOKING

NEWS FLASH! MOM WAS RIGHT. Eating more vegetables is good for you. But it's not just vegetables—fruit, nuts, seeds, beans, grains and pretty much any food that comes from plants are good for you. Now, finally, people are listening to their mothers. They're cutting back on meat, poultry, seafood and other animal foods—or giving them up altogether—as they move toward a plant-based diet of whole grains, legumes, nuts, seeds, fruits and vegetables.

What started as just another food trend continues to grow and appears as though it's here to stay. Approximately 39% of Americans are trying to eat more plant-based foods (according to a 2017 NielsenIQ Homescan survey). Approximately 40% of millennials identify as vegan, compared to 21% each of Generation X and baby boomers. And it turns out that these foods benefit not only our own health, but the health of the environment, our local economies and the animals we use for food.

Of course, there have always been individuals and communities of vegetarians and other people who eat little to no meat or dairy for economic, ethical, religious, health and other reasons. But the numbers are growing as researchers give us more and better reasons why everyone benefits from including more plant foods and fewer animal products in every meal. What they continue to discover is that plant foods

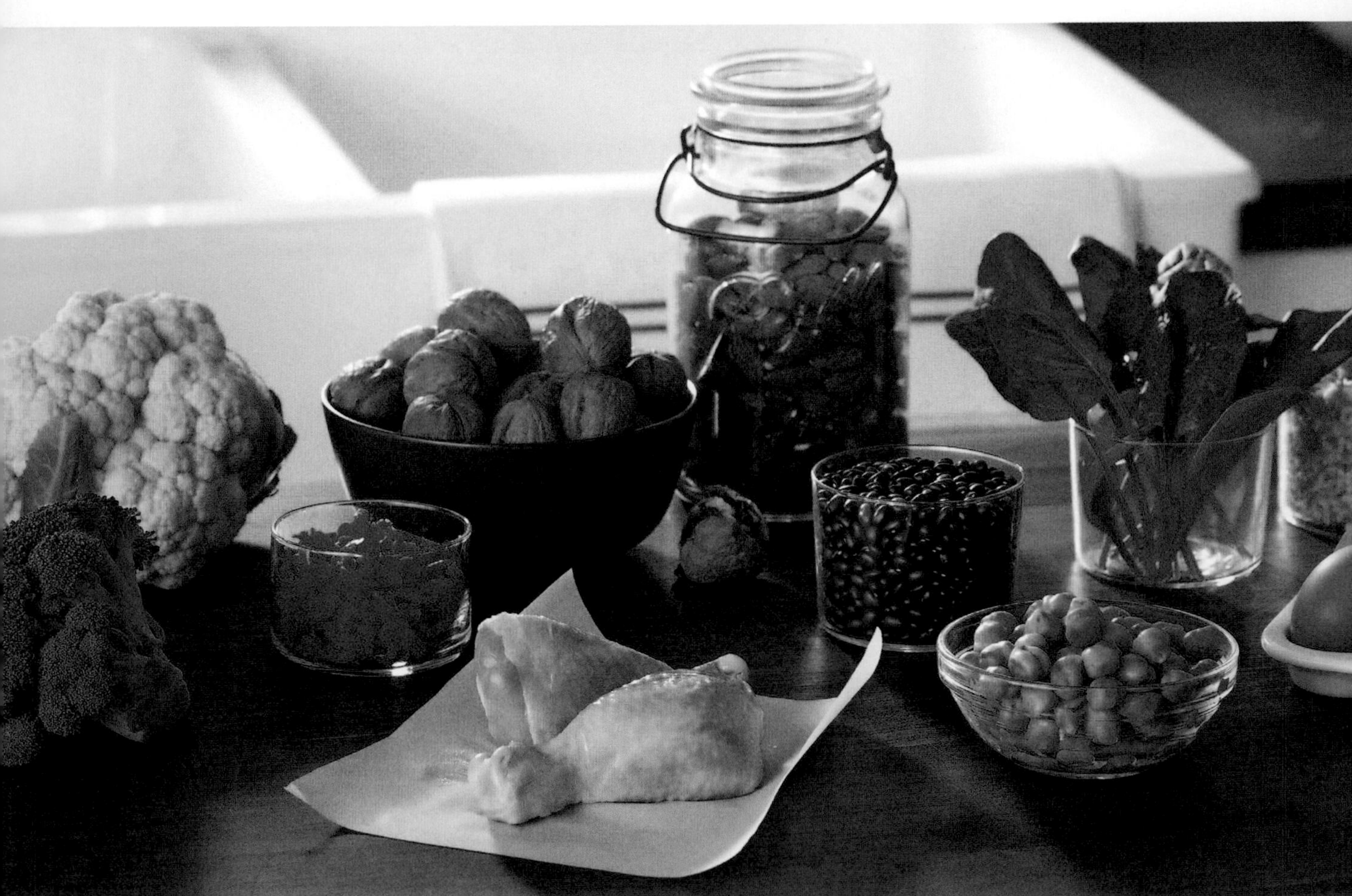

in general are super nutritious and that plant protein, specifically, is healthier and more sustainable than animal protein.

Harvard University researchers, for instance, found that those who consistently follow a healthy plant-based diet may reduce their chances of experiencing a stroke and cardiovascular disease, even if they are genetically at risk. According to the Mayo Clinic, studies comparing the effects of diet on cancer have shown that those who follow a vegan diet have the lowest rates. And a study from the University of Eastern Finland found that those who rely on plant and egg protein, rather than meat protein, have a significantly lower risk of developing type 2 diabetes.

That's why plant-based eating is more than a trend. The popularity of the recent *Reader's Digest* book *Plant-Based Health Basics* was the impetus for this follow-up cookbook. Our editors worked with registered dietitians Susan McQuillan, MS, RD, and Peggy Woodward, RDN, to ensure that the recipes and recommendations in this book reflect the latest science on the health benefits of plant-based foods.

Food manufacturers—big and small—are making it a priority to develop more plant-based foods and ingredients that are better tasting and better for you than ever before. Take a look around any big supermarket and you'll find everything from vegan

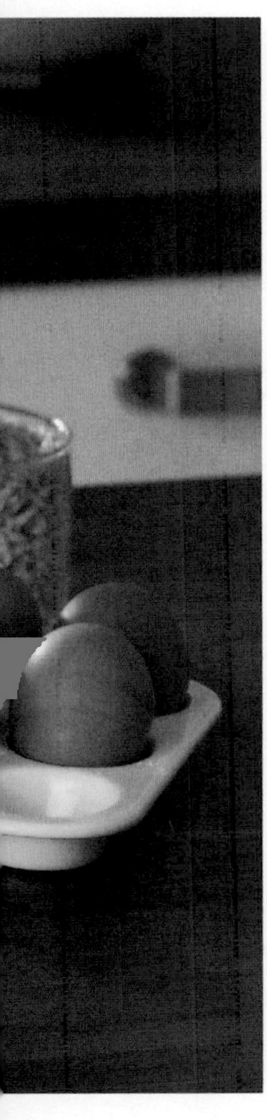

mayonnaise and chicken-free chicken broth, to dairy-free ice cream, plant-based sausage and ground-meat substitutes. Restaurants, including fast-food places such as Burger King and fast-casual chains such as Panera, are likely to have multiple vegetarian and vegan offerings on their menus.

With so many new foods and ingredients on the market, it can be very easy to pick up processed food products that may not be as good for you as they sound. For example, a frozen breaded cutlet can be overloaded with breading and fat—whether it's coating a piece of chicken or a piece of soy protein that resembles chicken.

As with all food products, try to compare different brands of similar foods to make sure you're getting the most nutrition for your money. Keep snack foods and sugary desserts to a minimum. The goal isn't simply to avoid meat and eat any foods sourced from plants, but to eat a varied, well-balanced, whole-food, plant-based diet that is rich in protective nutrients and phytonutrients. Given the wide range of whole foods and ingredients available in markets today, it's not a hard goal to reach.

Because plant-based options are not as readily available in restaurants as in supermarkets—and those that are available may be higher in fat and sodium—cooking at home makes following a plant-based diet not only easier but also less expensive. Another bonus: You control the type, source and amount of the ingredients that go into your meals. Plus, you can customize them to your taste.

Whether you are just now discovering the many benefits of a plant-based diet or you've been incorporating more plant foods into your diet for as long as you can remember, you're sure to find solid information, helpful tips and new recipe ideas in the pages that follow. You'll also find sample meal plans to help you put it all together. Feeding yourself and your family wonderfully delicious and highly nutritious meals and snacks has never been easier.

WHAT IS PLANT-BASED COOKING?

Although a plant-based diet focuses on vegetables, fruits, grains, legumes and other non-meat foods, it doesn't necessarily mean that there's no meat in it at all. In fact, the term plant-based means different things to different people and can take many forms that include or exclude different types of foods. Here are descriptions of common types of plant-based eating plans:

Whole-Food Plant-Based (WFPB), also known as Plant-Forward: Focuses on eating a wide variety of whole-plant foods such as fruits, vegetables, legumes, whole grains, nuts and seeds; may include some meat, poultry, fish, shellfish and eggs, but avoids most processed foods—even those that are plant-based

Vegan: Avoids all animal products, including meat, poultry, fish, shellfish, eggs, cheese and other dairy products; also avoids any products derived from animals, such as honey

Vegetarian: Avoids eating meats, poultry, fish and shellfish, but—depending on the style of vegetarianism—may eat some animal foods and animal-derived products

Lacto-Vegetarian: Avoids all meats, poultry, fish, shellfish and eggs; consumes dairy products

Ovo-Vegetarian: Avoids all meats, poultry, fish, shellfish and dairy products; eats eggs

Lacto-Ovo-Vegetarian: Avoids all meats, poultry and fish; consumes eggs and dairy products

Pescatarian: Avoids all meats and poultry, but eats fish and shellfish; may eat eggs and dairy

Flexitarian: Mostly follows a vegetarian diet, but sometimes eats animal products

No matter which type of plant-based regimen you and your family choose to follow, this book will provide valuable tips for planning and eating the healthiest meals possible.

FOUR REASONS TO GO PLANT-BASED

A plant-forward eating style doesn't just help you, it also helps animals and the environment.

1. REAP HEALTH BENEFITS. Perhaps the most important reason to eat a whole-foods, plant-based diet is that it can help you improve your health and quite possibly extend your life.

Eating more plant foods and less meat lowers your cholesterol and saturated-fat intake while increasing the amount of fiber you get in your diet. It also helps you avoid the potentially cancer-causing substances found in red and processed meat. This, in turn, helps lower your risk of developing serious chronic health conditions—such as heart disease, high blood pressure, type 2 diabetes and some cancers—that can impact your health and longevity.

A plant-based diet can also help you get to and maintain a healthy weight—which, again, can help reduce your risk of developing chronic diseases. Losing weight also helps ease the pain of conditions that affect your bones and joints, such as osteoporosis and arthritis.

Phytonutrients, or phytochemicals—the disease-fighting and immunity-boosting substances exclusively found in all plant foods—are also linked to increased energy, better sleep, improved mood and disease prevention. Phytonutrients act as anti-aging, anti-inflammatory, antimicrobial, antioxidant, anticancer, immunity-boosting and detoxifying agents.

Thousands of these compounds are found in fruits, vegetables, legumes and grains. Each plant food may contain hundreds of phytonutrients that work alone—and together—to protect good health. Kale, for example, has more than 50 phytonutrients, including quercetin, carotenoids and leutin. See the chart on page 14 to find out which nutrients can best help you treat your ailments and which foods are rich in them.

Phytonutrients include prebiotics and probiotics, the "good bacteria" that help maintain a well-balanced gastrointestinal system. A healthy gastrointestinal tract, in turn, protects against the development and progression of inflammation, infectious disease, obesity and chronic conditions—such as type 2 diabetes. The recipes in this book make the best use of foods that are simply packed with phytonutrients.

2. LOWER FOOD COSTS. A whole-food, plant-based diet can be much less expensive than a diet of animal products. Today's supermarkets offer a wide selection of vegetarian and vegan foods. But there are some ways to make plant-based cooking even more affordable.

If you're able to join a community-supported agriculture (CSA) group through local farms, or purchase a membership to a wholesale warehouse that carries store brand foods, you can buy reasonably priced fresh fruits and vegetables as well as frozen and shelf-stable packaged foods that support a plant-based diet.

If you have space for a small garden, grow your own herbs and some of your own vegetables. Basil, thyme, rosemary and cilantro are great ones to grow in pots on the windowsill, balcony or deck.

One of the best things about the staples of a plant-based diet is that the dry foods, such as rice, quinoa, barley and other grains, nuts and seeds, beans, lentils and split peas can be stored for a long time so you can purchase them in bulk—which is cheaper than buying small quantities. The more you cook from scratch, or near-scratch, the less expensive it is to follow a whole-food, plant-based diet.

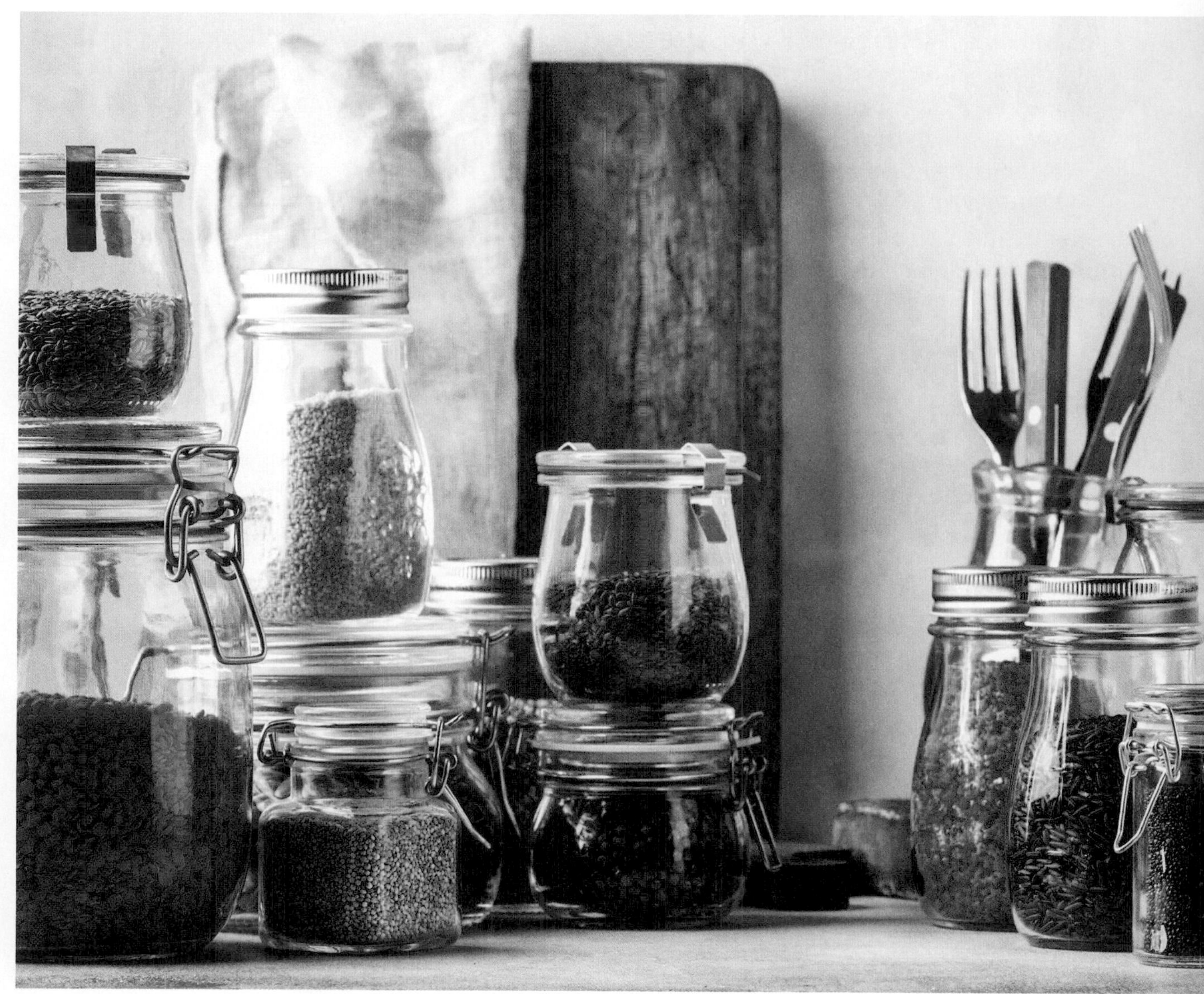

Lastly, a diet that can help keep you out of doctors' offices and hospitals is one that will surely save you some big money in the long run!

3. REDUCE ENVIRONMENTAL CONCERNS. Animal agriculture puts great demands on the environment because of its costly land and water usage and contribution to greenhouse gas emissions. Those, in turn, promote an increase in climate change. Plant-based agriculture, on the other hand, has a less-negative impact on the environment. For example, it takes 1,800 gallons of water to produce a pound of beef as compared to 216 gallons to produce a pound of soybeans. As a result, a plant-based diet is considered a more sustainable practice that promotes environmental as well as human health.

4. SUPPORT ANIMAL RIGHTS. Every year, after a short life in an unnatural and often unsafe environment, billions of chickens, cows, pigs and fish are raised and slaughtered in industrial food factories in the U.S. Often little or no concern is given to their welfare. Animal-rights groups and activists have long tried to persuade the food industry to adopt more ethical practices. It's not hard to figure out that the more people who follow a diet that minimizes or eliminates animal products, the less need there will be to produce those foods in the first place. That could mean less cruelty to agricultural animals, particularly those that are factory-farmed for mass production of food.

DEBUNKING PLANT-BASED EATING MYTHS

You may have some concerns about the cost, convenience, taste, nutritional value or accessibility of the foods that make up plant-based diets. Let's break down these myths and separate fact from fiction:

MYTH 1: Too expensive. Many think that eating a diet based on whole foods is more expensive than eating the standard American diet, which includes a lot of meat. Actually, meat is often the most expensive item on a grocery bill. For example, a 15-ounce can of beans often can be purchased for less than a dollar. Meat prices, on the other hand, can run from about $1.99 to $14.99 or more per pound, and that often includes bones and other inedible components. So, skipping meat is likely to save you a good chunk of money.

While some out-of-season produce may be more expensive, if you plan your menu around fruits and vegetables that are in season, you'll find that they are often relatively inexpensive—not to mention more flavorful. In addition, frozen fruits and vegetables, which are just as healthful, can be a more economical and flavorful choice.

Similarly, while some whole grains—especially trendy ancient grains such as farro or millet—and products made with whole grains can be more expensive than, say, wheat flour or white bread, you can usually find foods made with whole wheat, oat and similar whole grains at a reasonable price. And because whole grains are so rich in fiber, you may find that you need less of a whole-grain product to feel full.

Additionally, to keep costs down, shop in the food section of big-box stores where there is often more brand and price variety and more economy-size packaging. Buy in bulk or large-size packages—but only as much as you'll use in the next six to 12 months. Store grains in airtight containers for six months or freeze for up to a year so they don't become rancid.

Cost-conscious shoppers look for fresh and minimally prepared plant foods such as chopped vegetables, frozen fruits and precooked grains when they're on sale and stock up on these foods for later use. For the sake of meal planning, it helps to look at supermarket ad circulars and clip coupons in advance, when possible.

MYTH 2: Lacks calcium. Calcium is an essential mineral but the belief that it's only present in dairy products is incorrect. Calcium is plentiful in a plant-based diet, especially one that includes a variety of foods. To get the 1,000-1,500 milligrams of calcium most adults need daily for good health, eat a range of leafy green vegetables; cruciferous vegetables such as cabbage, kale, broccoli and bok choy; nuts (especially almonds) and seeds (especially sesame seeds); canned or cooked dried beans; fortified juices and plant-based milks; tofu and tempeh.

MYTH 3: Not enough protein. Some people worry that they won't get enough high-quality protein in a plant-based diet. Not true! Although protein needs vary among individuals, and the actual amount of protein required for healthy living is debatable, many nutrition experts say the average American gets too much protein in their diet.

Most protein in the average person's diet comes from meat and other animal products, but that doesn't mean it has to. All plant foods provide some protein. One way to figure out the minimum amount of protein you need daily is to multiply your weight in pounds by 0.36. Using that formula, a 135-pound woman requires approximately 49 grams of protein each day. From the chart below, it's easy to see how a varied diet of plant-based foods can give you the protein you need.

If you're especially concerned about getting enough protein, look for the recipes

Plant Foods Rich in Protein

SOY PRODUCTS
(per ½ cup)
Edamame 8.5g
Seitan 15.75g
Soy milk 3.5g
Tempeh 15g
Tofu 10g

LEGUMES (per ½ cup)
Black beans 7g
Cannellini beans 7g
Chickpeas 7g
Kidney beans 8g
Lentils 9g
Pinto beans 7.6g

NUTS AND SEEDS
(per 2 tablespoons)
Almonds 3g
Almond butter 7g
Cashews 2.5g
Peanuts 4.7g
Peanut butter 7g
Walnuts 2.5g
Chia seeds 5g
Hemp seeds 6g
Flaxseed 4g
Pumpkin seeds 4.5g
Sesame seeds 3.25g
Sunflower seeds 3g
Tahini 5g

VEGETABLES (per 1 cup)
Asparagus 3g
Artichokes 4g
Avocado 3g
Broccoli 3g
Brussels sprouts 3g
Corn 5g
Kale (cooked) 4g
Mushrooms 2g
Peas 4g
Potatoes (cooked) 3g
Spinach 4g
Sun-dried tomatoes 7.6g
Sweet potatoes (mashed) 3g

GRAINS
(cooked, per ½ cup)
Amaranth 4.7g
Farro 4g
Kamut 4.9g
Millet 3.11g
Oats 5g
Quinoa 4g
Rice, brown 3g
Rice, wild 3.27g
Spelt 5.4g

OTHERS
Nutritional yeast (per 2 tablespoons) 2.5g
Ezekiel bread (2 slices) 8g

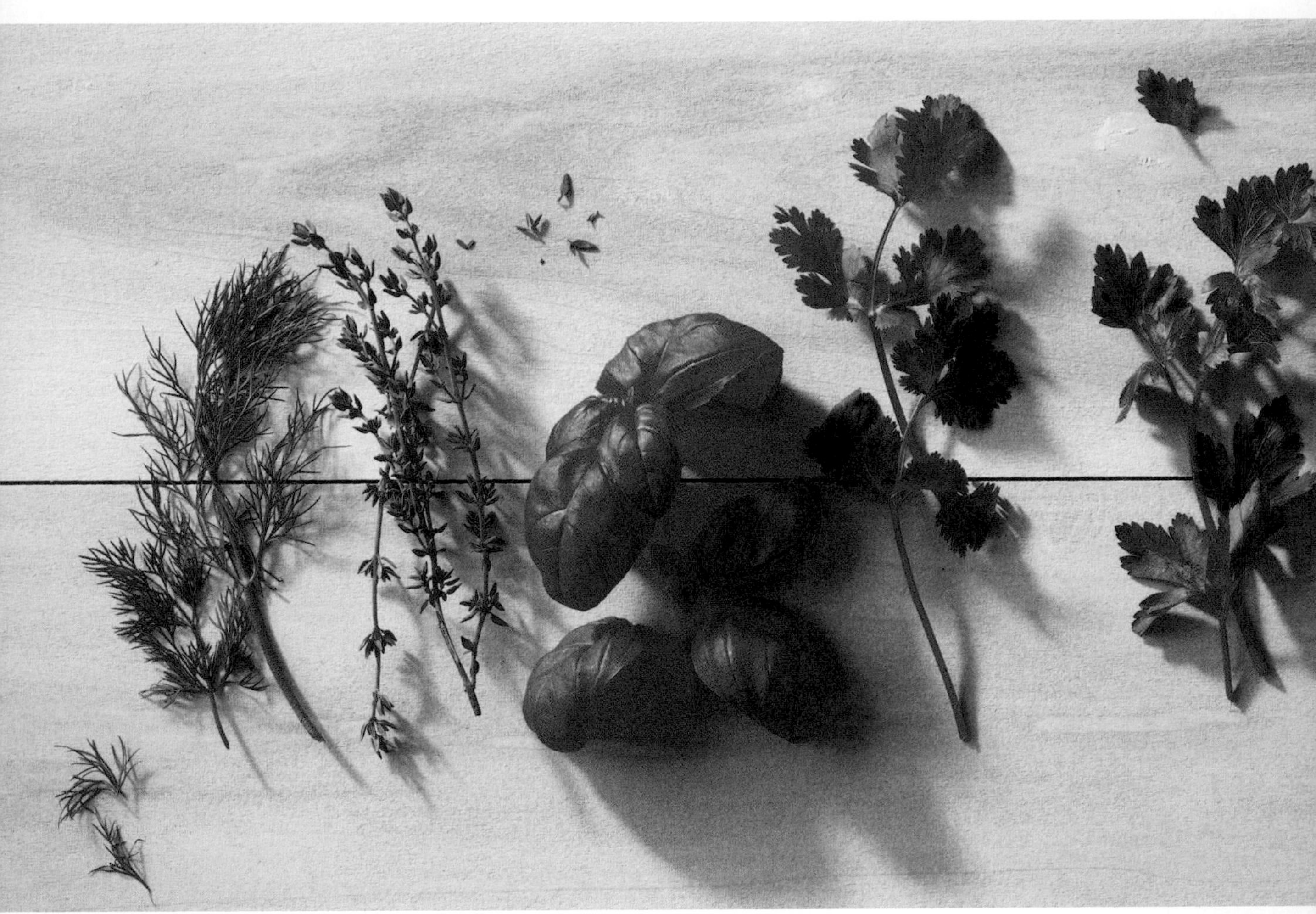

in this book that are marked with the "protein-packed" icon. (See page 39 for more information about our icons.)

MYTH 4: Too much gas. When adopting a plant-based diet, you may consume significantly more fiber than your body is accustomed to digesting at one time. This could cause some intestinal gas, but as your body adapts to this new way of eating, the gas should subside. Go slow when first starting out, adding just one or two high-fiber foods each day.

Raw vegetables are easy to eat and nutritious, but you should also try the steamed or roasted varieties. Cooked vegetables are easier on your digestive tract and won't cause as much gas. Drink plenty of water as you increase the amount of fiber in your diet.

Beans are also high-fiber and can cause flatulence, but certain preparation methods can offset the effects. Thoroughly rinse canned beans with running water. Not only will water rinse off gas-producing substances in the liquid, but it will also send about one-third of the added sodium in the can down the drain. When preparing dried beans, soak them in water with a teaspoon of lemon or lime juice for eight to 24 hours. After the first soaking, drain the liquid and rinse the beans.

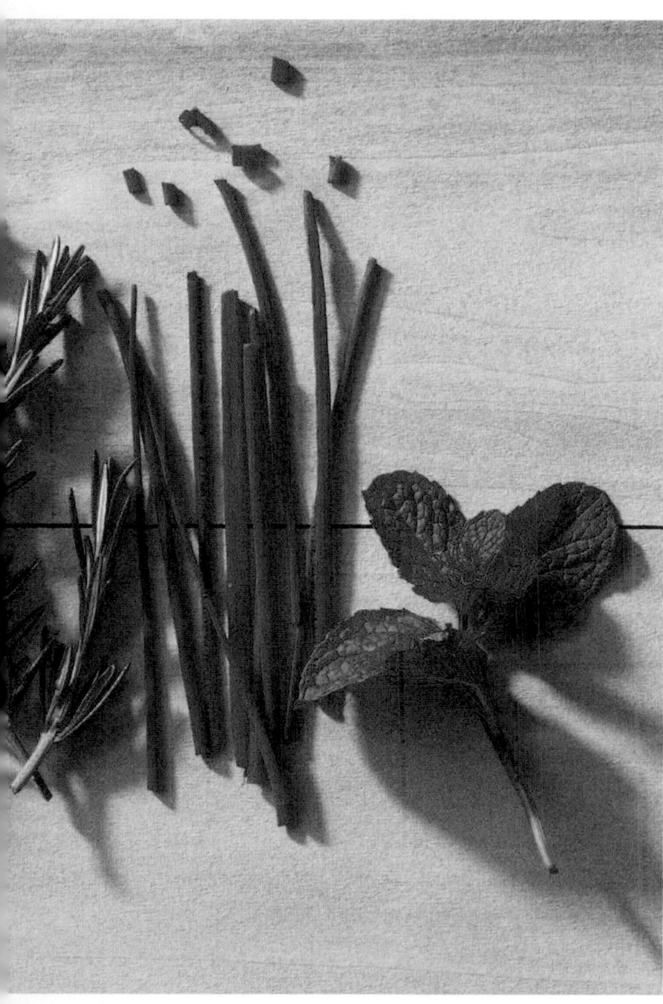

Then cook in a fresh pot of water.

Adding ½ to 1 cup of enzyme-rich pineapple or papaya (fresh, frozen or dried) to meals that include beans can also aid digestion. (The high heat of processing destroys the digestive enzyme in canned fruits.)

Or give ginger a try. Whether in root, powdered or tea form, ginger is known to calm digestive issues. You can also use enzyme-rich supplements, such as Beano, to help prevent the gas and bloating that some people experience.

MYTH 5: Not enough to eat. You never have to worry about going hungry on a whole-food, plant-based diet, because there are so many food options. But be sure to let go of any old dieting philosophies.

You'll be eating plenty of carbohydrates—but they are good, healthy carbs, such as sweet potatoes, brown rice, beans and lentils—and a plethora of vegetables. Don't even think about measuring the volume of your food, especially if your diet consists mostly of low-fat dishes. Instead, just eat until you feel satisfied. You can pile your plate high with fresh, healthful food and the calories will be far less than if you filled a smaller plate with fried or otherwise fatty foods.

This is mindful eating, and the beauty of eating this way is that you don't have to count calories, fat grams or anything else. Instead, you simply eat enough to feel satisfied. You will lose or maintain your weight, and at the same time help yourself deal with other health issues.

Unlike many diet plans, a plant-based diet is not a temporary way to eat until you reach a particular goal. Instead, it's a way of life. Even if you don't follow the plan perfectly, striving to eat whole-food, plant-based meals 80 percent of the time will boost your health and well-being.

MYTH 6: Tasteless. Plant-based dishes are as full of flavor, texture and color as you choose to make them. If you follow the recipes starting on page 40, you'll learn ways to include herbs and spices, condiments and other ingredients that add spectacular flavor. The more you avoid high-sodium, high-fat and sugary processed foods, the more your taste buds will tune into the pure flavors of fruits and vegetables and the earthy goodness of whole grains, legumes, nuts and seeds. You'll start to love and crave wholesome meals and find yourself drooling over a ripe mango or a handful of juicy strawberries!

MYTH 7: Hard-to-find foods. Nothing could be further from the truth. All the recipes in this book are made with ingredients from the supermarket. Seasonal fruits and vegetables are also plentiful at farmers markets, health food stores and even big-box stores. Most whole grains and soy foods also are now readily available in grocery stores. When starting out, take time to go through the aisles of your store to familiarize yourself with different varieties of whole-grain foods on the shelves; soy products in the refrigerated section; and fruits, vegetables and other plant-based foods in the freezer cases.

FOCUS ON WHOLE FOODS

Whether you have been vegan for years or are just starting to add more vegetables to your diet, in order to reap the most benefits from plant-based cooking, you'll want to choose whole foods over processed foods as often as possible. A whole-food, plant-based diet means eating mostly unrefined or minimally refined foods including fruits, vegetables, legumes, nuts, seeds and whole grains. It is centered around foods in their whole, natural state as much as possible—eating a baked potato instead of french fries, whole grain pasta instead of white, and snacks such as hummus and baby carrots instead of onion dip and potato chips.

You may also hear the term "clean eating." It generally focuses on foods that are raised without herbicides, pesticides, additives and preservatives. These choices naturally include many whole foods.

If plant-based eating is new to you, here are the basics to help you get started.

1. EAT VEGETABLES. And lots of them. One easy way to do this is to fill half your plate with vegetables at every meal.

2. FOCUS ON A RAINBOW OF COLORS. Vary the vegetables on your plate throughout the day or week so you are eating all the colors of the rainbow. This ensures you are getting a wide variety of phytonutrients for optimal health.

3. START WITH AN APPETIZER. Why not enjoy a restaurant-style meal at home and serve a first course of vegetable soup or salad? Not only will this increase your veggie intake, it will also take the edge off your appetite so you don't overeat higher-calorie foods.

4. USE WHOLE GRAINS. And avoid refined ones. Opt for brown rice over white, whole-grain breads or tortillas instead of white ones, and whole-wheat flour instead of refined white flour. Experiment with other whole grains you may not have tried, such as the ancient grains amaranth, farro, kamut, millet, quinoa and spelt.

Fiber-rich whole grains are packed with nutrients—such as B vitamins, vitamin E and healthy fats—that are found in the outer bran and germ layers stripped away during the refining process. For example, when these layers are stripped from brown rice and whole wheat to produce white rice and white flour, these nutrients are lost and only the endosperm, or white starchy carbohydrate, remains. Some of these nutrients are added back to refined grain products, such as white flour, through a supplemental enrichment process, but that doesn't include fiber, nor does it encompass all grain products.

5. ADD LEGUMES TO YOUR MEALS. Whether your diet is 100% animal-free or you're just cutting down on meat and dairy, you need to make sure you get enough protein. Legumes—canned or cooked dried beans, split peas and lentils—provide plant protein as well as fiber, both of which help you feel full longer. Eat legumes at least three times per week, ½ to 1 cup cooked per

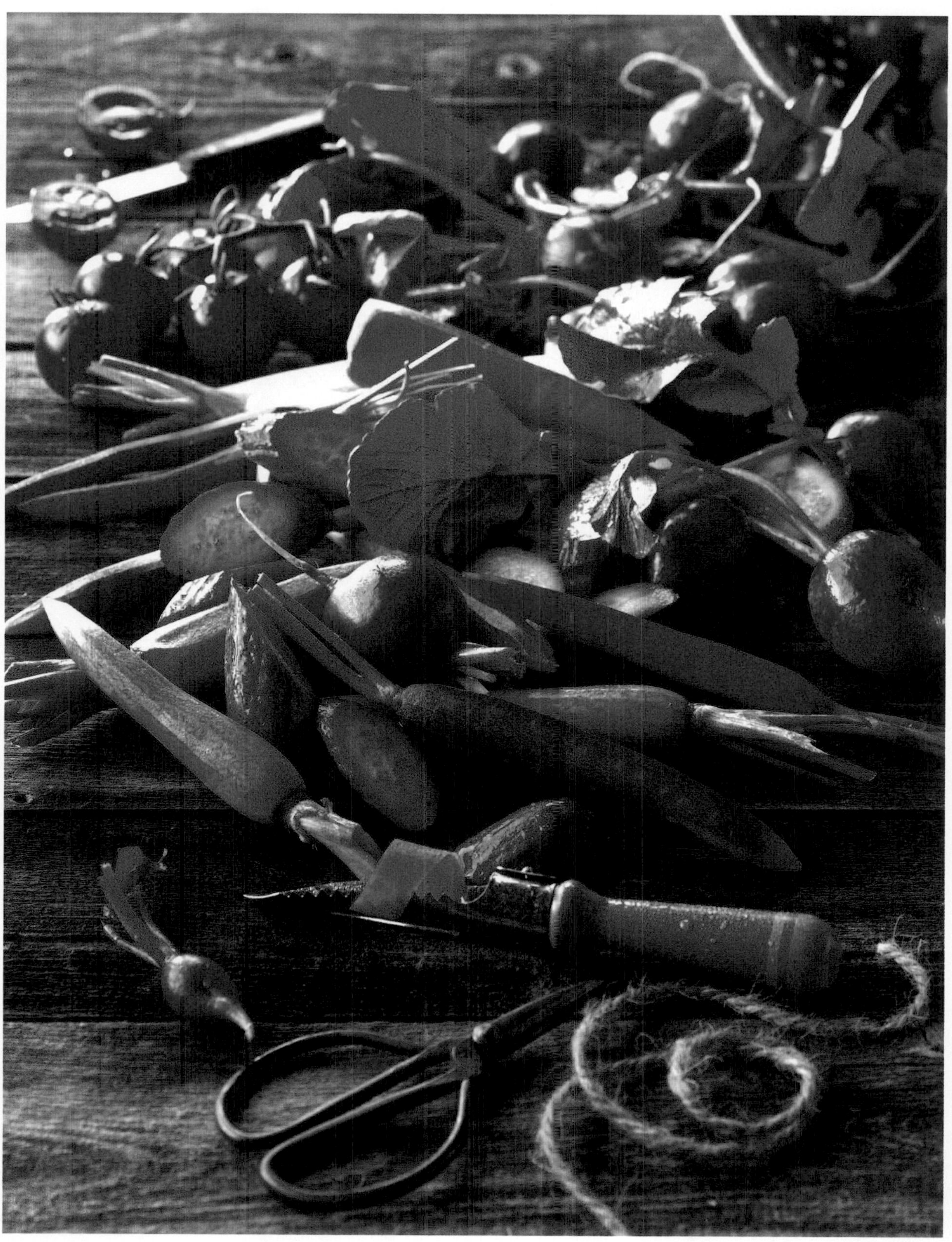

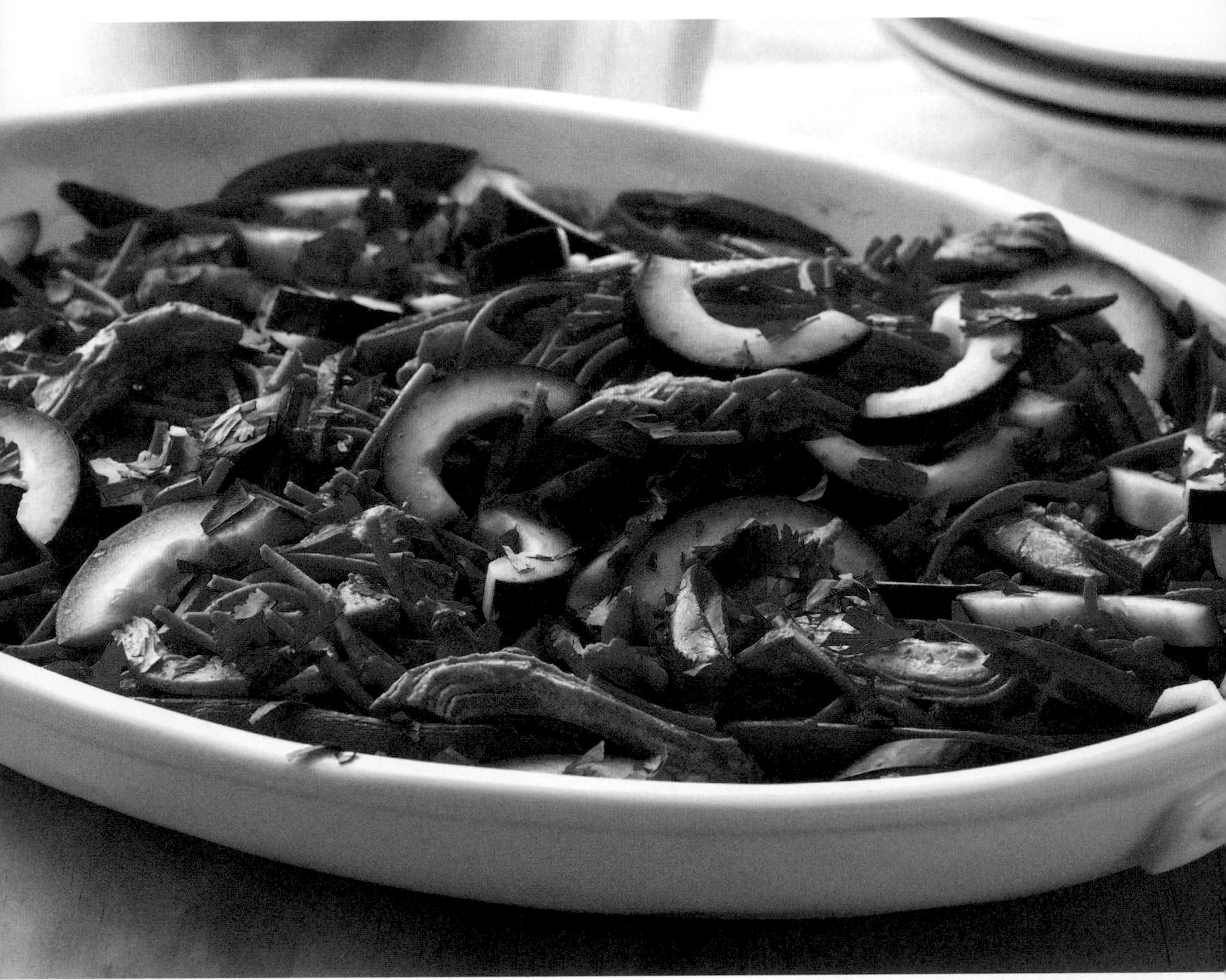

day. If you're using canned beans, reach for low-sodium ones and be sure to rinse them in water before using to remove about one third of the sodium.

6. INCREASE YOUR FIBER INTAKE. Getting enough fiber is key to good health and has been shown to lower LDL cholesterol level, control blood sugar levels, provide fullness after meals to aid weight loss, maintain optimal bowel health and reduce the risk of dying from cancer and heart disease. By choosing whole foods over processed foods of any kind, your diet will naturally be high in fiber. Beans, legumes, avocado, berries, apples, pears and cruciferous vegetables are good sources of fiber.

7. THINK DIFFERENTLY ABOUT MEAT, FISH AND POULTRY. Instead of being at the center of the plate, use small amounts of meat as a condiment or flavoring for your whole grains and vegetables. The world's healthiest cuisines often include just bits of fish, meat,

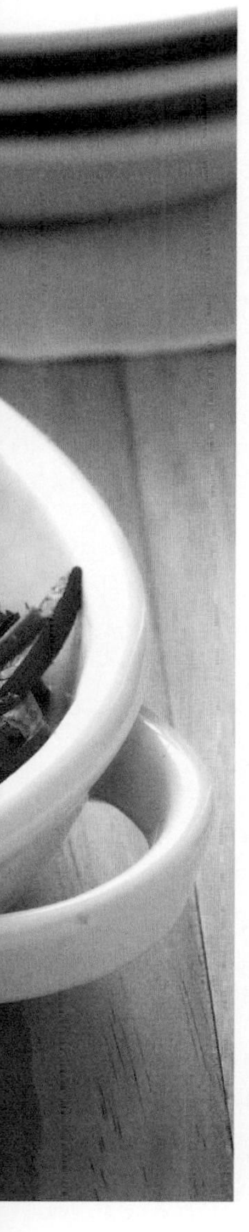

or poultry along with lots of veggies, seasoning the food with great flavor but not adding a lot of cholesterol or saturated fats. Common examples include bean, lentil and split pea soups, curry dishes, stir-fries, chilis with beans, and main-dish salads.

8. TRY MEATLESS MONDAY. This plan encourages vegetarian or vegan meals at least once a week, typically on Monday. Other plans suggest eating animal products only on the weekend or only after 6 p.m., when you have more time to prepare thoughtful meals.

Choose one of these or make your own schedule by preparing meals for one or more days with little or no meat and animal products. This is a great way to gradually move toward a lifetime pattern of eating more plant-based meals.

9. REACH FOR PLANT-BASED MILKS AND CHEESES. Experiment with different plant-based milks such as almond, soy, rice and oat. While some plant-based cheese is high in fat—especially those made from refined oil instead of nuts—adding small portions to your diet will help with the transition off of dairy products. Read labels and opt for nut-based plant-based cheese, which is lower in saturated fat than dairy cheese.

10. FINISH WITH FRUIT. Ending a meal with a sweet treat is always enjoyable but, to keep it healthy, go for sliced raw or poached fruit instead of sugar- and fat-laden desserts. The more you choose fresh, ripe, seasonal fruit as your dessert, the more you will prefer it over other supersweet confections.

11. USE GOOD FATS. In addition to using small amounts of healthy fats such as olive oil for cooking, consider whole-food fats whenever possible.

This means getting your fat from small amounts of chopped or crushed nuts or seeds instead of oil, when possible, or using avocado instead of mayonnaise as the base of a creamy salad dressing or sandwich spread. Sprinkle whole or crushed flaxseed on salads instead of flaxseed oil. Spray a thin coating of olive oil in pots or pans or skip the oil and sauté vegetables in vegetable broth when cooking lower-fat dishes.

Foods that contain an abundance of healthful unsaturated fats often contain other essential nutrients, such as fat-soluble vitamin E. The fats themselves are made up of fatty acids that fight inflammation and can help reduce symptoms of chronic diseases such as diabetes and heart disease, and may also play a role in good mental health.

12. AVOID MOST PROCESSED AND PACKAGED FOODS. There's an abundance of processed vegan, vegetarian or plant-based foods on supermarket shelves these days. However, they don't necessarily promote optimal health as they may contain high fat, salt and refined grains. Keep these in your pantry or freezer for an occasional treat or when you don't have time to cook. Most days, reach instead for recipes prepared with whole foods such as those offered here, starting on page 40.

Your Food Arsenal

Thanks to a vast array of vitamins, minerals, phytonutrients, fibers and healthful carbs, proteins and fats, a whole-food, plant-based diet can help you prevent and treat diseases and disorders of both the body and mind. From treating everyday ailments such as heartburn and mood swings, to reducing the symptoms of life-threatening, chronic conditions, such as high blood pressure and memory loss, plant foods help keep you physically healthy and mentally fit. Find foods in this arsenal to help treat your specific ailment(s).

NUTRIENT	AILMENT	FOODS
allium compounds	cancer, yeast infection	garlic, onion family
anthocyanins	cancer	apples, berries, cherries, red grapes & wine
antioxidants	psoriasis	broccoli, carrots, sweet potatoes, tomatoes
beta-carotene	cancer, eczema, macular degeneration	apricots, Brussels sprouts, carrots, spinach, sweet potatoes, winter squash
bromelain	rheumatoid arthritis	pineapple
calcium	anxiety & stress, high blood pressure, hyperthyroidism, osteoporosis, overweight, perimenopause & menopause, pregnancy, premenstrual syndrome, stroke, tooth & mouth conditions	broccoli, cooking greens, figs, fortified dairy substitutes, kale, sesame seeds, sesame tahini, tofu
carotenoids	immune deficiency	carrots, sweet potatoes, tomatoes
catechins	cancer, tooth & mouth conditions	dark chocolate, green tea, pomegranates
complex carbohydrates	anxiety & stress, diabetes, diarrhea, heartburn, insomnia, memory loss, overweight, premenstrual syndrome, sprains & strains	beans, potatoes, brown rice, winter squash, whole grains
dietary fiber	diabetes, fibrocystic breasts, heartburn, high blood pressure, hypothyroidism, overweight, stroke, varicose veins	apples, asparagus, beans, beets, lentils, pomegranates, whole grains

NUTRIENT	AILMENT	FOODS
essential fatty acids	eczema, fibrocystic breasts, immune deficiency, rosacea	chia seeds, edamame, flaxseed, nuts, seeds, vegetable oils
flavonoids	cancer, high cholesterol, memory loss, rheumatoid arthritis, stroke, varicose veins	apples, berries, broccoli, citrus fruits, onion family
folate	anemia, cancer, depression, heart disease, infertility & impotence, pregnancy	asparagus, beets, black-eyed peas, chicory, lentils, peas, pinto beans, salad greens, spinach
fructooligosaccharides (FOS)	yeast infection	artichokes, onion family
genistein	prostate problems	soy foods
glucosinolates	cancer	broccoli, Brussels sprouts, cabbage
insoluble fiber	constipation, irritable bowel syndrome, kidney stones, tooth & mouth conditions	broccoli, bulgur, cabbage family, flaxseed, peas, salad greens, sweet potatoes
iodine	hypothyroidism	fruits and vegetables, iodized salt, seaweed
iron	anemia, immune deficiency, pregnancy	amaranth, beans, cashews, lentils, quinoa, tofu
isoflavones	memory loss, osteoporosis	lentils, soy foods
lycopene	cancer, high cholesterol, infertility & impotence, macular degeneration, prostate problems	apricots, pink & red grapefruit, guava, tomatoes, watermelon
lysine	cold sores	fenugreek seeds, spirulina, soybeans, tofu
lutein & zeaxanthin	cataracts, macular degeneration	collard greens, corn, kale, kiwifruit, peas, peppers, spinach, sweet potatoes
magnesium	allergies & asthma, anxiety & stress, chronic fatigue syndrome, diabetes, high blood pressure, kidney stones, migraine, premenstrual syndrome	amaranth, avocados, quinoa, sunflower seeds, wheat germ, winter squash

NUTRIENT	AILMENT	FOODS
monounsaturated fat	cancer, heart disease, high cholesterol, memory loss	avocados, olives/olive oil, peanuts/peanut oil, walnuts
omega-3 fatty acid	bronchitis, depression, heart disease, high blood pressure, osteoarthritis, perimenopause & menopause, psoriasis, rheumatoid arthritis, stroke	chia seeds, edamame, flaxseed, seaweed, soy foods, walnuts
pectin	diarrhea	applesauce, bananas
phenolic acids	cancer	apples, berries, green tea, pomegranates, turmeric
phytoestrogens	cancer, perimenopause & menopause	flaxseed, legumes, pomegranates, soy foods
potassium	high blood pressure, kidney stones, stroke	avocados, bananas, potatoes, quinoa
probiotics	immune deficiency, irritable bowel syndrome, urinary tract infection, yeast infection	fermented foods, kimchi, kombucha, tempeh
protein	sprains & strains	amaranth, legumes, quinoa, soy foods
quercetin	allergies & asthma, cataracts, colds & flu	apples, berries, cherries, plums & prunes, red onion
resveratrol	stroke	peanuts, red grapes, red wine
riboflavin	migraine	broccoli, mushrooms, quinoa
selenium	allergies & asthma, cancer, infertility & impotence, macular degeneration, prostate problems	barley, Brazil nuts, fortified cereals, mushrooms, whole grains, whole-wheat bread, seeds
shogaols & gingerols	rheumatoid arthritis	ginger
soluble fiber	constipation, heart disease, high cholesterol, irritable bowel syndrome	apricots, beans, carrots, figs, flaxseed, oats, plums & prunes
soy protein	heart disease, high cholesterol	soy foods

NUTRIENT	AILMENT	FOODS
sulforaphane	cancer	broccoli, cabbage family, cooking greens
sulfur compounds	high cholesterol	garlic, onions
tannins	kidney stones, urinary tract infection, varicose veins	blueberries, cranberries
tryptophan	anxiety & stress, chronic fatigue syndrome, depression, insomnia	bananas, peas, spirulina, turnips, wheat germ
vitamin B6	anxiety & stress, depression, premenstrual syndrome	acorn squash, avocados, bananas, peas, potatoes
vitamin B12	anemia, depression	fortified cereals, nutritional yeast
vitamin C	allergies & asthma, anemia, bronchitis, cataracts, cold sores, colds & flu, diabetes, high blood pressure, hyperthyroidism, immune deficiency, infertility & impotence, macular degeneration, osteoarthritis, osteoporosis, rheumatoid arthritis, rosacea, sinusitis sprains & strains, stroke, tooth & mouth conditions, urinary tract infection, varicose veins	bell peppers, berries, broccoli, citrus fruit, kiwifruit, melons, pineapple, strawberries
vitamin D	osteoarthritis, osteoporosis, perimenopause & menopause	fortified milk substitutes, mushrooms
vitamin E	cancer, cataracts, eczema, hyperthyroidism, immune deficiency, infertility & impotence, macular degeneration, memory loss, osteoarthritis, prostate problems, rheumatoid arthritis	avocados, broccoli, nuts, olive oil, peanut butter, seeds, whole grains
vitamin K	osteoporosis	kale, spinach
zinc	chronic fatigue syndrome, colds & flu, eczema, immune deficiency, infertility & impotence, macular degeneration, sinusitis	almonds, beans, cashews, fortified cereal, pumpkin seeds, whole grains

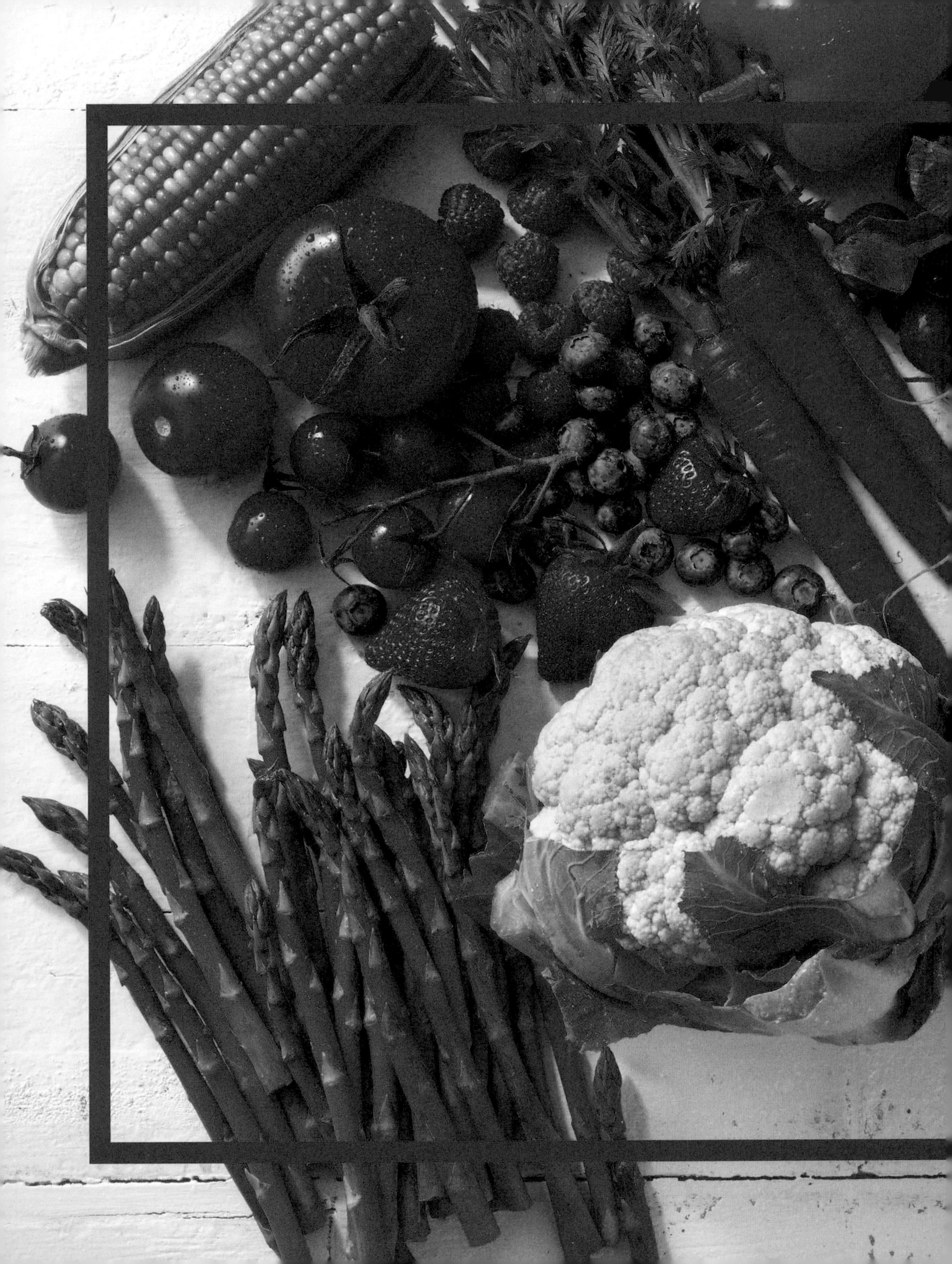

CHAPTER 2

GETTING STARTED WITH PLANT-BASED EATING

NOW THAT YOU KNOW WHAT TO EAT on your plant-based diet—and why—the information in this chapter will help you learn how to cook your plant-based meals. Here you'll find guidelines to help you plan nutritious meals, advice on how to shop for plant-based foods, tips and tricks for feeding your family (even if they don't want to jump on the plant-based wagon with you right now) and much more.

When you embark on a whole-food, plant-based diet, start where you are. You don't need to completely clean out your kitchen and discard everything. Instead, just focus on eating more plants. Perhaps start by adding a salad to lunch or dinner. This might be a green salad loaded with a variety of vegetables, a whole grain salad such as the Feta Bulgur Bowl (page 122) or a corn and bean salad such as the Colorful Taco Salad (page 110). Dishes such as these will have you putting more plants on the plate and no one will miss their old favorites.

MEAL PLANNING FOR OPTIMAL HEALTH

A healthful, balanced, plant-based meal looks like any other well-balanced meal, but with a limited amount of meat—or none at all. Recommendations vary somewhat, but generally

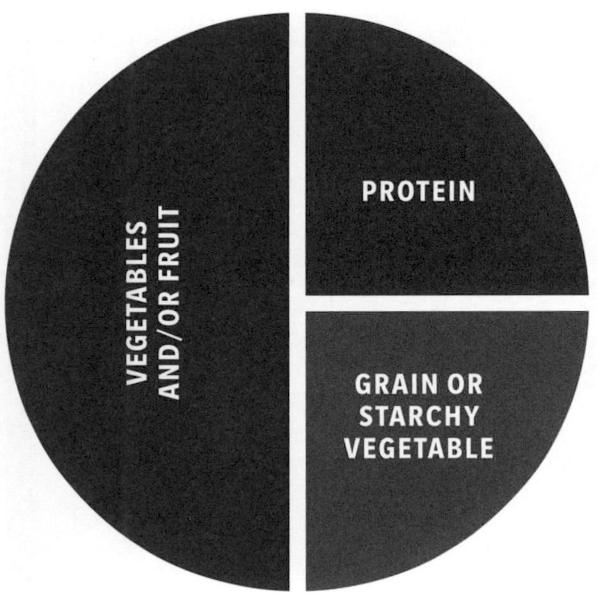

an overall balanced diet should contain approximately 50-60% carbohydrates, 12-20% protein and 20-35% fat.

In order to meet that overall goal, it helps to break down each meal (and even snacks) the same way whenever possible. You can use the nutritional information for each recipe to help you do this. (If you have diabetes, look for recipes with diabetic exchanges; only those with low enough amounts of sodium, saturated fat and carbohydrates have them.)

Besides knowing how much protein, fat and carbs to include in your diet, it's perhaps just as important to mix up the specific foods you eat within each of those categories. For instance, sometimes your fat can come from an avocado, sometimes from nuts or seeds and occasionally from olive oil or other vegetable oils. Your carbs can come from tomatoes, green beans, rice, kale, sweet potatoes, quinoa, whole grain bread or any other grains or vegetables. You may get your protein from beans, lentil soup or baked tofu. Just keep switching it up and you'll get all the vitamins, minerals and phytonutrients you need from eating a wide variety of foods.

To keep it simple and avoid having to do math at every meal, nutrition experts recommend filling half your plate with vegetables (and/or fruit) and dividing the other half of the plate evenly between a protein and a grain or starchy vegetable, such as a sweet potato. Some of these foods will provide a little healthy fat as well.

Of course, not all meals are served on a flat plate. Combination foods such as soups, stews and casserole-type dishes might seem like a challenge, but once you understand the portion sizes involved in planning a healthful, plant-based diet, you can simply eyeball your foods and ingredients and you'll know how much of each to add to any dish.

For instance, you may just add extra fresh veggies (sauteed in olive oil) and some brown rice to a bowl of prepared lentil soup. You'll still have a good balance of carbohydrates (from the veggies and rice), protein (from the lentils) and a little healthy fat (from the olive oil).

How about a breakfast of seeded whole-grain toast spread with almond butter and topped with sliced bananas and blueberries, with a glass of fortified soy milk? Your carbohydrates come from the fruit and the bread, protein from the almond butter and soy milk, plus a little healthy fat from the almond butter as well.

Don't let meal planning overwhelm you as you begin this journey. Many of the meals will be similar to the ones you've been eating. Oatmeal or dry cereal topped with fruit, plant-based milk and perhaps some chopped nuts is still a great way to start the day. For heartier morning options, scramble up some plant-based eggs or tofu with onion, bell pepper and garlic for a delicious, savory meal.

For lunch or dinner, you may fill half your plate with stir-fried mixed vegetables, and the other half with equal portions of steamed rice and seasoned cubed tofu. Or you may choose to have bean tacos—filling whole-grain tortillas with shredded cabbage or sautéed mixed vegetables and topping with ripe avocado and tomato salsa. Sandwiches with nut butter and sliced apple or banana are ready in minutes. Or turn a favorite tuna or chicken salad recipe into a plant-based lunch by folding coarsely mashed drained chickpeas into the dressing instead of meat.

If you eat lunch at takeout places, Tex-Mex restaurants offer vegetable burritos or tacos, Chinese restaurants feature stir-fried vegetables and brown rice, and most burger places are now featuring a veggie patty or meat alternative burger (pass on the fries). Diners with salads or a salad bar can be the best choices.

Need more ideas? With more than 150 recipes in this book, you'll be off to a good

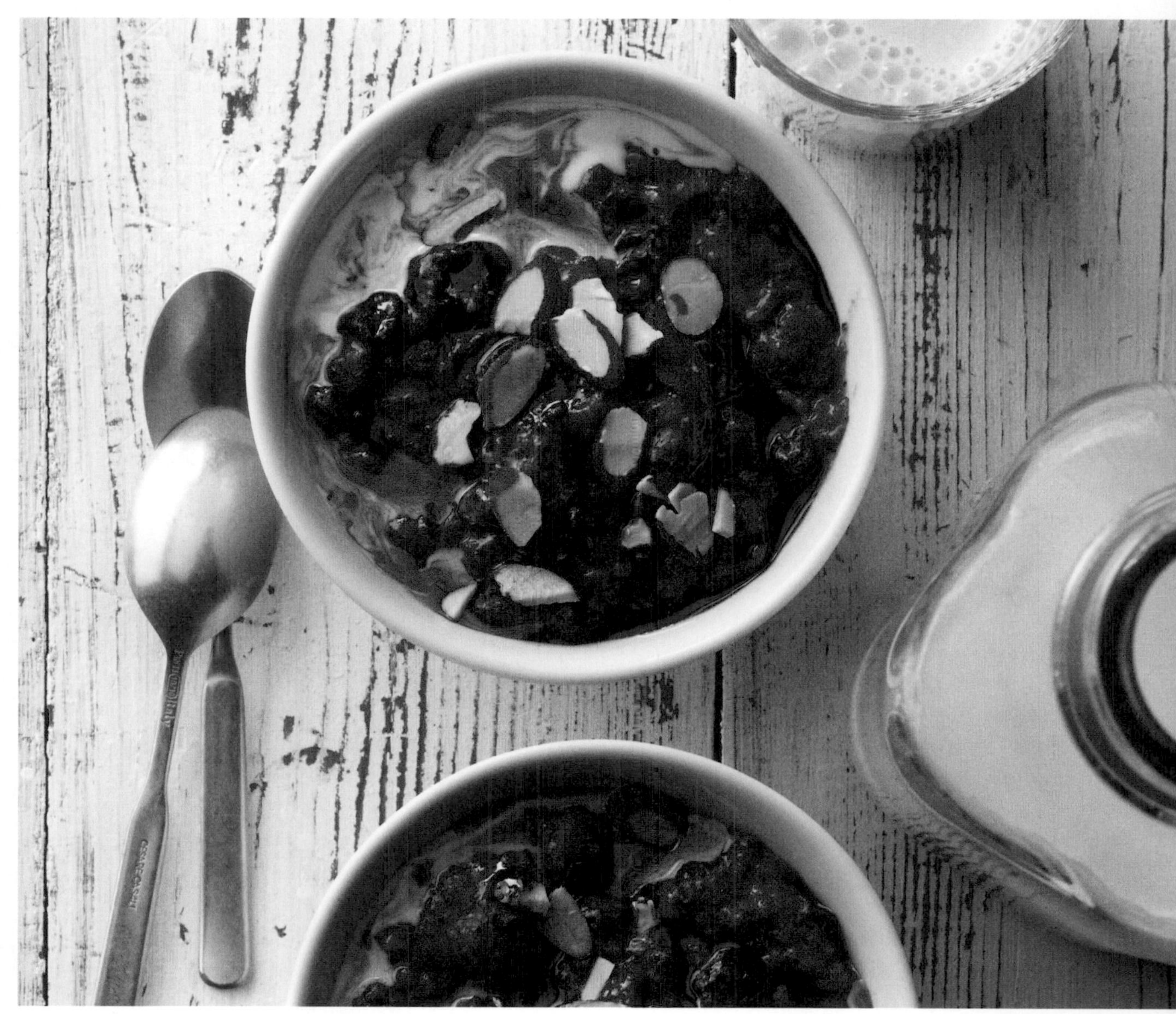

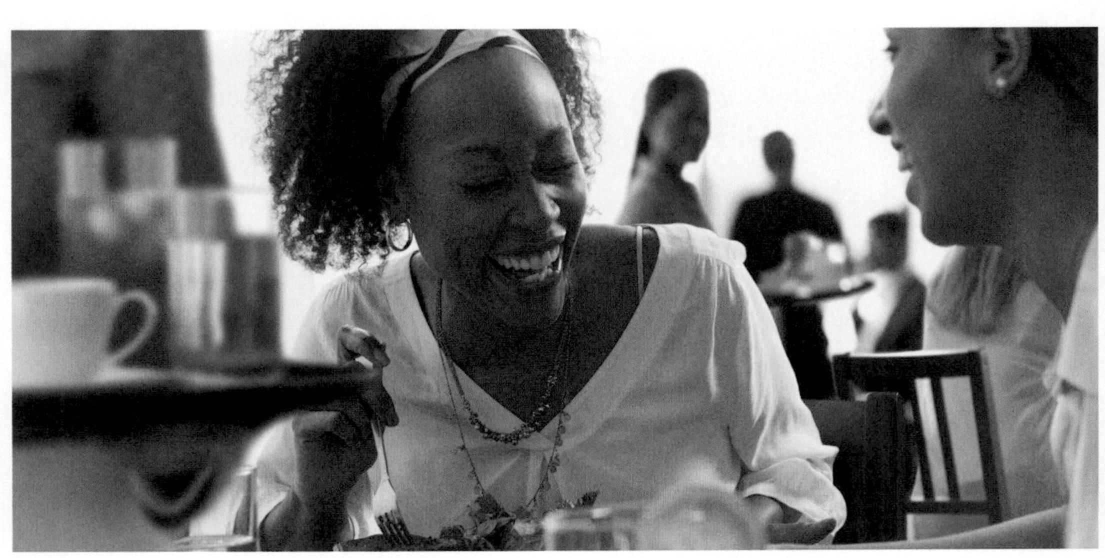

Special Occasions

It's easy to manage your diet when cooking your own meals, but more challenging when eating away from home. Whether you're going out for a simple meal, heading to a friend's dinner party or holiday gatherings, these tips will help you stick to your plant-based ways.

RESTAURANT DINING. Go to the restaurant's website and view the menu before you head out. If you can't find any meat-free dishes (or if you can't tell what's in each dish), plan to ask the waiter if something can be prepared without the animal ingredients—for example, by leaving off the butter or cheese. If you are looking for a plant-based eatery, go to happycow.net for listings in your area.

HOLIDAY AND BIRTHDAY PARTIES. This is easiest when you are the host and can make simple unnoticeable changes to the recipes such as using plant-based butter and vegetable broth for the stuffing. Be sure to also include some additional new plant-based dishes on the menu. If you are attending a gathering away from home, check with the host to see what's on the menu. Ask if they can make some simple substitutes such as topping the steamed veggies with plant-based butter that you will bring along. Offer to bring a dish or two that you will enjoy and be able to share at the table. Finally, pick your battles! Would it be OK to eat a bit of the traditional dishes just once a year?

OTHER GATHERINGS. Whether you're attending a dinner party, church potluck or picnic, if you plan ahead, you can stay plant-based. If you're going to someone's home, let your hosts know you've made this switch in your diet and ask if there are ways they can help you stay on track. Offering to bring a dish or two allows you to quietly introduce new foods to friends and also ensures there will be enough for you to eat. But, always focus more on connecting with people than on the food.

start. Still want to prepare your family's favorite meals? Just eat half of the meat you normally would, filling your plate with more vegetables instead.

And don't feel that you need to spend hours in the kitchen to cook plant-based. Popular Buddha bowls can come together in minutes, especially if you use precut or precooked items. Line individual bowls or plates with mixed greens, top with a pile of beans, steamed or raw chopped vegetables, grains and tofu or hummus. Drizzle with vinaigrette and enjoy!

Finally, when you think ahead about the meals you plan to eat during the week, you can prepare some or all the ingredients ahead of time. Making a large pot of soup or stew and chilling or freezing portions for later in the week makes mealtime a breeze. Washing and cutting salad vegetables or steaming vegetables ahead of time helps the meals to come together quickly.

Preparing ahead of time may start with collecting recipes you can easily make in bulk on the weekends and serve again during the week. We've indicated make-ahead dishes in this book with a special icon.

MAKING IT WORK FOR THE WHOLE FAMILY

If your family members are not sure they want to join you on this journey—or if they are adamant that they don't—here's how to prepare food in ways that won't have you cooking two meals each night and will help prevent others from derailing your progress.

1. COOK THE MEAT SEPARATELY. Prepare the meats separately from the veggies and grains and then just add the meat to their plates. If you're preparing a stew or other recipe with everything mixed together, remove a portion of the dish for yourself before stirring the meat into the remaining portion to be served to your family.

2. MAKE MEALS IN WHICH THEY WON'T MISS THE MEAT. Try preparing dishes with so many other ingredients that they don't miss the meat. Lentils, tofu and mushrooms make a great substitute for meat in chilis, pasta sauces, burritos or tacos.

3. MAKE SOUPS WITHOUT MEAT. Pea, lentil or vegetables soups don't need added meat. Try adding a few drops of liquid smoke or smoked paprika so the lack of ham flavor will go unnoticed.

4. ASK FOR THEIR COOPERATION. See if your family will go meat-free for at least one day a week. This would give you the opportunity to feature many meatless recipes (see Vegetable Mains on page 130) that can become new family favorites. Let them know how important this is to you and how their involvement will help you achieve your goals.

If you don't want to give up your family favorites, try preparing them without the usual meat or dairy. Follow the recipe as written but use more vegetables to pump up the dish. Here are some simple ingredient changes to convert your meat and dairy favorites to plant-based meals:

Cheese. Substitute plant-based cheese, such as cashew cheese, and add a few tablespoons of nutritional yeast.

Milk and creams. Use plant-based milks. Soy and oat milk are the thickest and creamiest when substituting for whole milk, half-and-half or cream. Look for dairy-free sour cream and yogurt. You can even find plant-based whipping cream. But when you're ready to delve deeper into plant-based cooking, try making our homemade plant-based whipped cream (page 31).

Butter. Oils are healthier than butter but when you need that buttery flavor, plant-based butters are readily available.

Eggs. Flaxseed and chia seeds make a great egg substitute for baking (see page 34). Or look for JUST Egg products that cook up very similarly to eggs.

Broth. Use vegetable or mushroom broth in place of beef or chicken broth.

Ground beef. Start by switching to plant-based meats such as Beyond Beef®. Or cook minced mushrooms or eggplant browned with onion and garlic before adding to dishes for a meaty texture and flavor.

Shredded pork. Jackfruit, an Asian fruit, is readily available in markets in canned or packaged form. Start with a version that's seasoned and ready to eat before working with the plain variety.

Sausage. Look for both breakfast and Italian-style in the refrigerated or frozen food sections.

Mayonnaise. There are several brands of plant-based or vegan mayo on shelves next to traditional mayonnaise.

Salad dressings. Look for dressings labeled vegan or even paleo, which may be free of dairy ingredients.

Making the switch to plant-based foods should be a slow and steady experience, not a race to the finish line. Take your time and try to focus each day on adding plants to meals. Over time it will be a habit and you'll find yourself (and hopefully your family) eating fewer animal and more plant-based meals.

SETTING UP YOUR PLANT-BASED PANTRY

As you switch from the meat-centered standard American diet to one that is plant-based, you may be adding some new ingredients to your pantry and fridge while still using much of what you already have on hand. Discovering some of these new food items—mostly seasoning ingredients—are part of what makes plant-based cooking and eating both tasty and exciting.

To fill your pantry, start shopping for the following ingredients or condiments often used in plant-based recipes. These are your staples. Don't feel the need to purchase them all at once; just pick up one or two a week to help get you on your way. They are listed in order of importance so you can start with those that are used most.

- **Ground flaxseed** (see page 34 to make egg substitute)
- **Nutritional yeast**
- **Balsamic and other flavored vinegars**
- **Low-sodium soy sauce or Bragg's Amino Acids** (a gluten-free, soy-based alternative)
- **Low-sodium vegetable or mushroom broth**
- **Nut and seed butters such as almond, cashew or tahini**
- **Herbs and spices**
- **Mustard—Dijon and yellow if desired**
- **Liquid smoke**
- **Miso** (adds umami flavor to dishes)
- **Plant-based butter**

Besides these ingredients, the most exciting part of adapting a plant-based diet is that it is packed with superfoods that are simply bursting with nutrients. So not only will you be adding fun new ingredients to your meals, you will be adding some of the most delicious healthful ones. Learn more about them in the following chapter.

SHOPPING FOR SUCCESS

A healthy, plant-forward diet starts with making smart, selective choices in the supermarket. Here's how to do that:

- **Shop the perimeter of the store** for fresh foods, such as fruits and vegetables; non-dairy milk, cheese and

Plant-Based 'Meats'

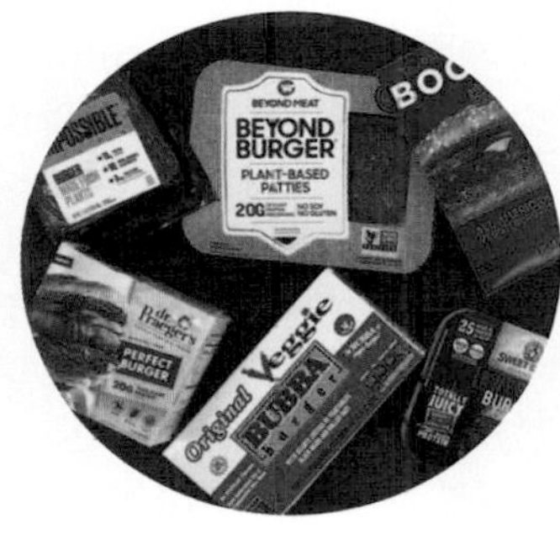

AS MORE AND MORE people have become aware of the downsides of eating an animal product-based diet, and have started eating more plant foods, the food industry has taken note. While veggie burgers have been around for decades, they have never resembled meat. Instead they have typically been a mix of mashed beans and minced vegetables.

Today, there are new players in the field, and plant-based burgers (or ground "meat") have been created to mimic beef. They even "bleed" on the burger roll as meat does.

These mixtures combine vegetable protein such as soy, bean, pea, rice or potato; fats from oils such as coconut, sunflower or cocoa butter; salt and other seasonings; flavor and other enhancers (beets are used to add the pink drippings); and food starches to help bind.

The most common brands of these products are Beyond Meat® and Impossible™ but new brands continue to hit shelves as the demand for these products continues to grow.

In addition to burgers, there are plant-based sausages (both breakfast and Italian-style), beef-like crumbles and ground "pork." There are also "chickenless nuggets and patties," "meatless meats" and "fishless seafood."

Nutritionally speaking, however, not all meat, poultry and seafood alternatives are created equal. Many, such as plant-based "deli slices" and hot dogs, are high in sodium and not necessarily any better for your health than processed and deli meats. Others, such as breaded and fried vegan shrimp and crab, can be loaded with starchy fillers, such as tapioca starch and powdered rice.

Though they are plant-based, these are still processed convenience foods and should be treated as such. They may not align with your diet goals and ought to be used sparingly.

Compare similar products and look for the options with a limited number of ingredients that also provide at least 10 to 15g protein per serving and are comparatively low in sodium, fats and filler carbs.

It may be easier to keep track of sodium, fat or carbs throughout the day rather than to track the grams per serving of every individual food. The adult daily recommendations are:

- **sodium:** no more than 2,400 milligrams per day.
- **fat:** no more than 30% of total calories (for a 1,500-calorie diet, that's about 50 grams of fat; for a 2,000- calorie diet, about 67 grams; and for a 2,500-calorie diet, about 83 grams of fat daily)
- **carbohydrates:** approximately 130 grams per day

If you choose, you could divide up the daily numbers and allocate a certain amount to each meal and snack.

yogurt alternatives; and some meat substitutes that can be found in the regular refrigerated meat cases.

- **Check your shopping cart while you're in the produce section** and be sure you've chosen a variety of different colored fruits and vegetables. You might want to try a new fruit or vegetable every week.
- **To make cooking easier, look for prewashed, pre-cut vegetables** including cooking greens, slaw mixes, carrot sticks and broccoli or cauliflower florets. If your store doesn't carry packaged pre-cut veggies, use the salad bar to provide these. They could be a bit more expensive but may be worth it to get more nutritious vegetables into your meals quickly. Don't overlook frozen vegetables—they are bursting with nutrients and ready in minutes. You can throw these into the water with whole grain pasta during the last few minutes of cooking to bulk up your plant quotient.

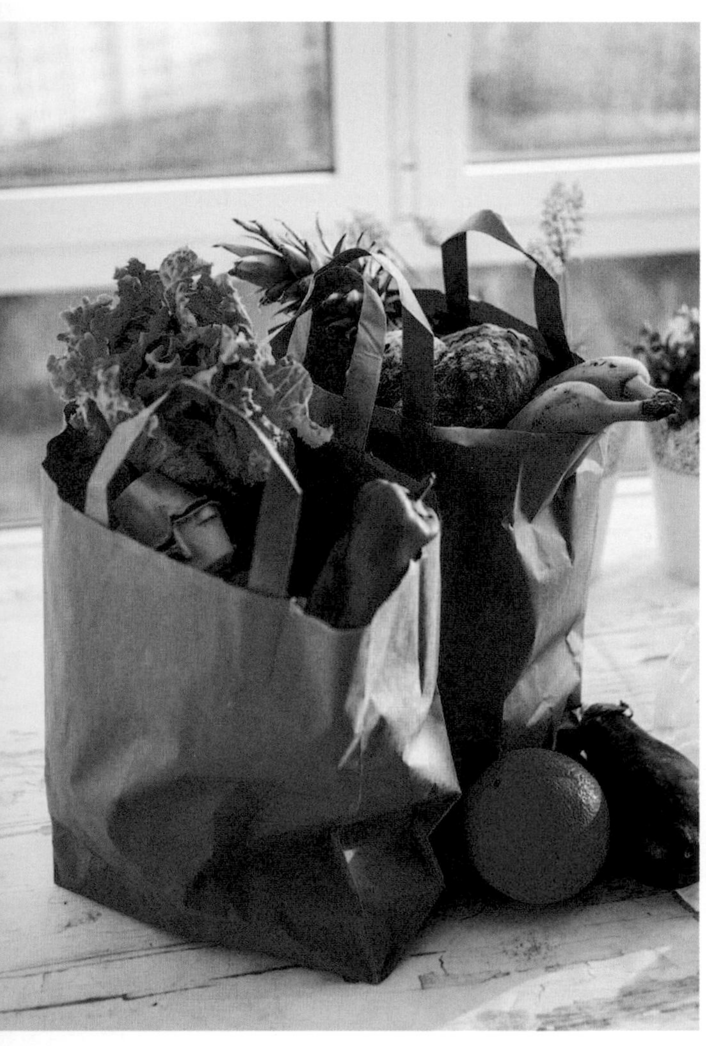

- **Choose cereals, breads and grain products such as pastas that are 100% whole-grain and provide at least 4 grams of fiber per serving, if possible.** Reach for a pouch or bowl of precooked brown rice or quinoa for last minute meals. You can toss them with drained canned beans and salsa, serve with a premade salad and you've got dinner in minutes.
- **Resist the temptation to buy complete frozen meals** and instead focus on frozen individual items, such as cut-up fruits and vegetables, as well as some meat alternatives and whole-grain foods (which, again, should provide 4 grams fiber or more per serving).
- **Select canned, bottled, "pouched" and dried foods with no added salt, fat or sugar whenever possible.** Compare similar products and choose those that are made with the fewest ingredients, making them closer to a whole food. Carefully chosen and conveniently packaged fruits and vegetables, tomato products, soups, broths, nut butters and beans can all be healthful additions to your pantry stock and very helpful when you can't cook completely from scratch.

Fresh, Frozen, Canned or Dried?

When it comes to the healthiest, tastiest, most economical and flavorful form of plant-based foods, whole and fresh are generally best. But when fresh fruits or vegetables are unavailable or out of season, frozen, canned, bottled, dried or otherwise-commercially packaged food is your best bet. Here are the top choices of each category:

FRESH: The "fresh is best" motto goes for most foods and ingredients that are actually available in fresh form, but for some, fresh is not only best, it's practically essential for true flavor and/or best texture.

Best bets for fresh food:

- Avocados
- Salad greens, including spinach and kale, that are intended to be eaten raw
- Most tender-leaf herbs, including basil and cilantro
- Fruits and vegetables in-season
- Ginger and seasoning vegetables such as onions, celery and garlic

FROZEN: Vegetables and fruits that are commercially frozen are generally picked during their peak growing season, so they can be tastier and contain more nutrients than fresh fruits and vegetables that are off-season, or shipped from a great distance.

Best bets for frozen food:

- Sweet corn
- Green peas
- Spinach, kale and other leafy greens that are intended to be cooked or blended
- Berries
- Mango
- Pineapple
- Precooked rice
- Strongly flavored herbs such as rosemary, sage and thyme

CANNED OR BOTTLED: Canned or jarred tomatoes and tomato products, such as puree and paste, beat out-of-season or commercially grown supermarket tomatoes for both flavor and nutrition. And as long as you avoid added salt or sugar, canned beans, fruits and vegetables are convenient to have on hand.

Best bets for canned foods:

- Legumes such as black beans, kidney beans and garbanzo beans (no salt added)
- Tomatoes and tomato products (including tomato sauce)
- Corn kernels (off the cob with no salt added)
- Chiles, such as chipotle and diced green
- Applesauce (no added sugar)
- Pear halves (no added sugar)
- Pumpkin

DRIED, DEHYDRATED OR FREEZE-DRIED: Dried food is especially helpful to keep for emergencies or while traveling or on a hike.

Best bets for dried foods:

- Legumes such as beans, lentils or split peas
- Grains, including barley and rices
- Mushrooms (especially for making soups, stews and broths)
- Whole chiles, such as ancho, habanero and New Mexico red
- Fruits such as dried plums/prunes, apricots, dates, figs, raisins and cranberries
- Most herbs, spices and seasoning mixes

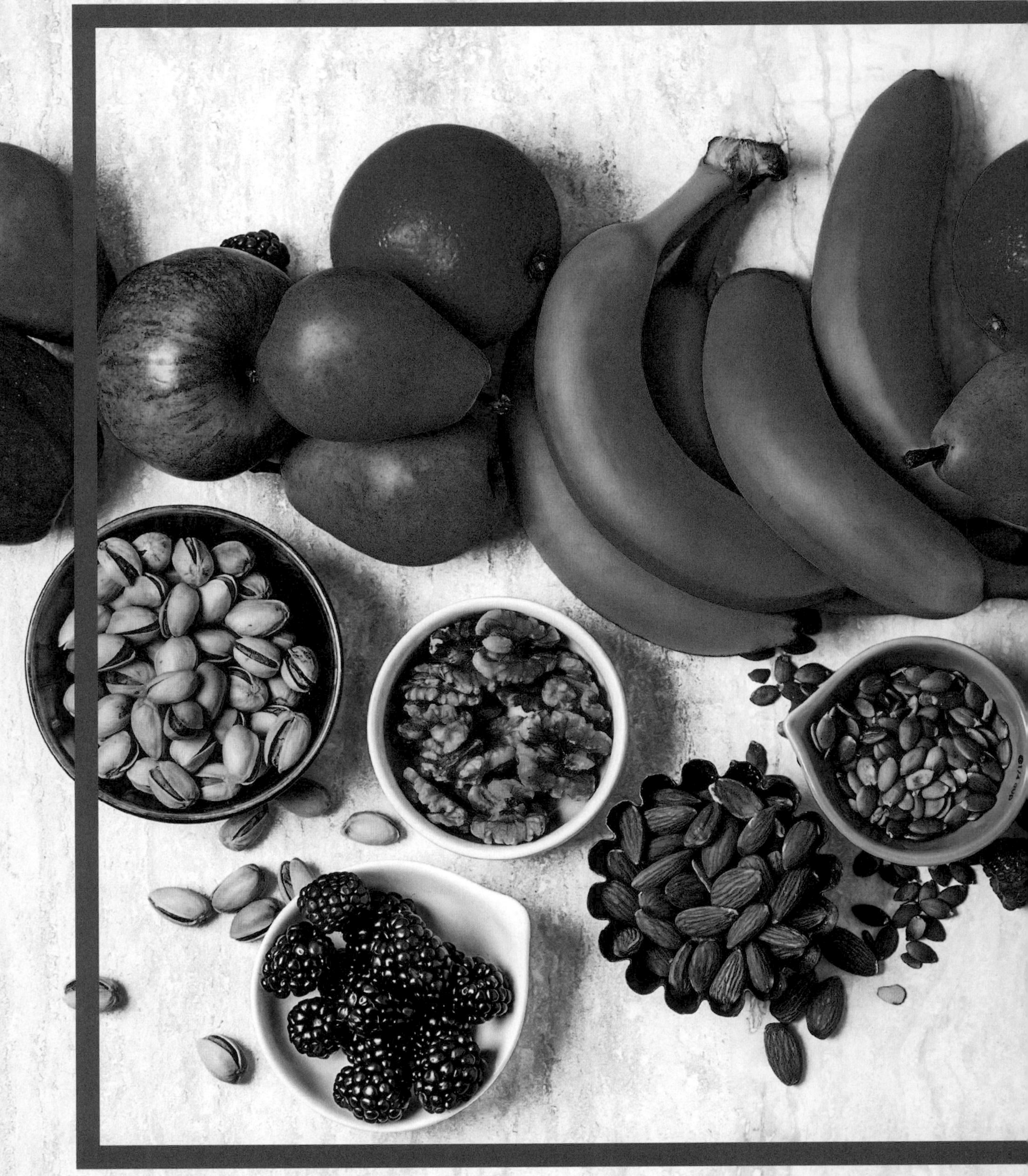

CHAPTER 3

PLANT-BASED SUPERFOODS

BECAUSE THEY ARE RICH IN NUTRIENTS, phytonutrients and other healthful substances, these superfoods are key to the healthiest whole-food, plant-based kitchen you could design. You'll see many familiar foods on this list, but you may not know just how healthful they really are. In order for a plant-based diet to be good for you, it's important to stay focused on whole foods and avoid using too many commercially prepared, processed, plant-based meals and ingredients. Stocking your kitchen with a rotating supply of these superfoods will make homemade meal prep quicker and easier.

APPLES

Apples are packed with beneficial substances, including pectin, vitamin C and numerous phytonutrients that may help prevent heart disease and certain cancers, and also alleviate symptoms of allergies and asthma.

MAXIMIZE THE BENEFITS For vitamin C and glutathione, eat apples uncooked, as these nutrients are diminished by heat. For pectin, cook the apples to release it. For insoluble fiber and anthocyanins, which are found in the apple skin, use unpeeled apples (choose organic if you are concerned about pesticides).

PUMP UP YOUR RECIPES Add chopped apples to tossed salads or steamed vegetables. Stir shredded apple into dips and spreads. Throw an apple or two into cream soups or sauces before cooking. They will add a slight sweetness, especially to winter squash or tomato-based soups and sauces.

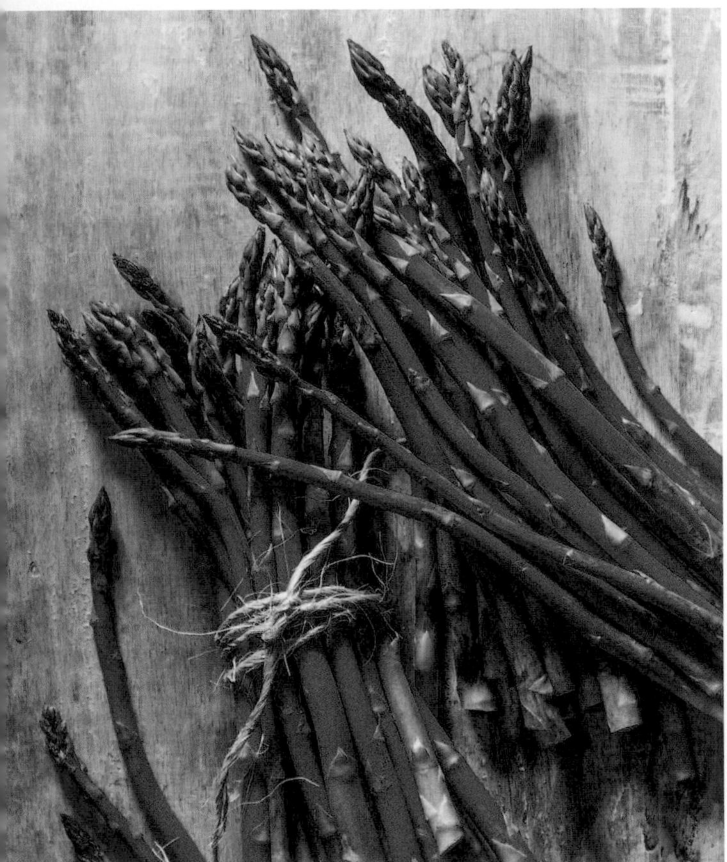

ASPARAGUS

Asparagus is delicious, low in fat and low in sodium. A nutrient-dense superfood, asparagus may help prevent heart disease, cancer and certain birth defects.

MAXIMIZE THE BENEFITS To reap the full health benefits from this nutritional powerhouse, steam or microwave asparagus. When you're trimming the tough ends from asparagus stalks, save them and cook them in water until very tender. Use this B-vitamin-enriched water to boost the nutrition of an asparagus (or other) soup or pasta sauce.

PUMP UP YOUR RECIPES Add steamed asparagus to salads, sandwiches, or grain dishes. Roast with red pepper and onion in a splash of olive oil for a delicious side to whole grains, roasted potatoes or pasta.

AVOCADOS

Avocados are a terrific way to add beneficial monounsaturated fats to your diet. These fats help to lower LDL ("bad") cholesterol levels and the risk for heart disease.

PUMP UP YOUR RECIPES Mash avocado with a lemon or lime juice and a pinch of an herb and salt. Substitute this mixture for mayonnaise or dairy-based salad dressings. Add avocado to smoothies along with spinach or kale, banana and a handful of berries.

BANANAS

Bananas may help relieve anxiety, and ward off heart disease, stroke and certain gastrointestinal woes.

MAXIMIZE THE BENEFITS Cooking partially destroys vitamin B6, so to improve mood, it's best to eat bananas raw. If you want extra pectin, cook the bananas.

PUMP UP YOUR RECIPES While they're perfect to eat as is, bananas can also be added to a fruit salad, mashed and stirred into pancake batter, or frozen and pureed with 1 tablespoon each cocoa powder and maple syrup for "nice cream."

BEANS

Beans and legumes may help reduce LDL cholesterol levels, stabilize blood sugar and control weight. They may prevent certain types of birth defects and cancer.

PUMP UP YOUR RECIPES Probably one of the most versatile ingredients in a plant-based kitchen, beans can be stirred into a vegetable sauté, tossed in a pasta dish or sprinkled on a salad. But they have more uses than just that. Mash chickpeas or other beans to make homemade hummus, which can be used as a dip, as a spread on sandwiches or whisked with vinegar and mustard for a creamy salad dressing. Puree white beans in the food processor and stir into soups or stews to add creaminess. Or use them in place of sour cream as the base of a sauce or salad dressing.

Save the liquid from canned beans, which is called aquafaba. You can beat this viscous liquid until lightly foamy and use it as a substitute for eggs in baked goods (3 tablespoons equals 1 large egg, 2 tablespoons per egg white), whip it like egg whites until fluffy to make meringue, or sweeten and whip for a whipped cream-like dessert topping. You can also use aquafaba in place of eggs as the base of a plant-based mayonnaise.

BEETS

Beets provide fiber, folate, potassium and such phytonutrients as anthocyanins and saponins. Beet greens are also bursting with phytochemicals and are delicious steamed or sautéed with garlic and onions, added to salads or tossed into smoothies.

MAXIMIZE THE BENEFITS To preserve the anthocyanin in beets, it's best to roast, bake, or microwave whole beets in their skins. If you cook peeled or chopped beets in water, some of the anthocyanins and water-soluble B vitamin, folate, will leach into the cooking water. Canned beets are a convenient way to get these nutrients in your diet.

PUMP UP YOUR RECIPES A simple way to prepare beets is to wrap them in foil and bake until fork tender at 350° for about an hour. Let cool, then rinse under cold water while peeling off the skin if you wish. Cut up the beets to serve immediately, tossed in a touch of honey and cardamom. Or store in the refrigerator for up to five days and toss into salads or reheat for a quick side.

BERRIES

Berries are tiny powerhouses of nutrition, bursting with healthy compounds, including folate, fiber and phytonutrients, which may help improve memory in people with mild cognitive impairment and reduce the risk for developing heart disease and type 2 diabetes.

MAXIMIZE THE BENEFITS Cooking does not seem to destroy the antioxidant ellagic acid in berries. However, it will destroy some of their folate and vitamin C, so you'll get the most benefit from eating them raw.

PUMP UP YOUR RECIPES Aside from eating them as is, you can stir berries into muffins, smoothies or cooked cereal. Toss with a touch of good-quality balsamic vinegar and serve over arugula or mixed greens.

BROCCOLI

Broccoli has a high level of phytonutrients, including beta-carotene, folate, lutein, potassium and a good amount of calcium.

MAXIMIZE THE BENEFITS Boiling broccoli can diminish its glucosinolates, folate and vitamin C content. Steam, microwave, or stir-fry it instead. Don't ignore frozen broccoli—it may contain 35% more beta-carotene by weight than fresh broccoli.

PUMP UP YOUR RECIPES Add broccoli to pasta dishes by tossing the florets into the pasta water for the last 4 minutes of cooking. Drain with the pasta and toss with sauce. Peel stems and cut into thick sticks for dipping into roasted garlic hummus. Scatter steamed florets atop a pizza, open-faced sandwich or mashed potatoes.

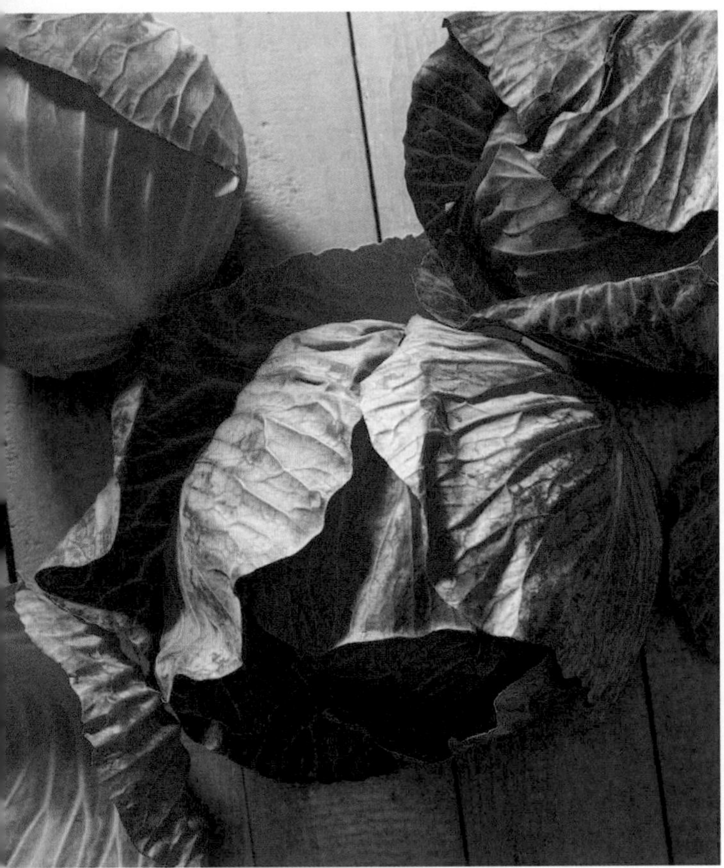

CABBAGES

Cabbages are nutritional kings, as are their relatives, bok choy, kale and Brussels sprouts. Nutrient-rich and loaded with protective compounds, these members of the cabbage family may all help to fight off cancer and heart disease.

MAXIMIZE THE BENEFITS To retain the most vitamin C, raw or very lightly cooked cabbage is best. Vitamin C is lost to high heat and can leach out into cooking water that is then discarded. Overall, it's best to steam, microwave or stir-fry to get the most nutrients from cabbage (and most other vegetables as well). Light cooking not only retains some nutrients, it also helps release more of others, such as beta-carotene, making them more available to your body.

PUMP UP YOUR RECIPES Sauté shredded cabbage, sliced celery, red bell pepper and onion, then stir in broth and dill to make soup. Toss shredded red cabbage, carrot and onion in Thai peanut sauce for an Asian-inspired salad. Top tacos with shredded Napa cabbage instead of lettuce.

CARROTS

Carrots may help to protect against heart disease, certain types of cancer, skin disorders, eye conditions, constipation and high cholesterol.

MAXIMIZE THE BENEFITS Cooking carrots, especially with a little bit of fat (preferably monounsaturated fat, such as olive oil), makes beta-carotene more available for absorption by the body.

PUMP UP YOUR RECIPES Serve shredded carrots, tossed with lemon and garlic, on cucumber slices over a bed of dark leafy greens. Add sliced carrots when preparing mashed or roasted potatoes. For a bit of sweetness, stir shredded carrots into soups and sauces before cooking.

CELERY

Celery may help lower blood pressure and reduce the risk for certain types of cancer.

MAXIMIZE THE BENEFITS If possible, include the celery leaves when cooking. They contain high concentrations of nutrients, such as potassium and vitamin C.

PUMP UP YOUR RECIPES Cut ribs into pieces and fill with reduced-fat refried beans and a drizzle of salsa. Or fill with hummus and sprinkle with flaxseed. Sauté chunks of celery, carrot and red onion with sage. Shave stalks into ribbons with a vegetable peeler and toss with thin strips of colorful bell peppers and greens tossed with vinaigrette.

CITRUS FRUITS

Citrus fruits have an abundance of vitamin C, potassium, pectin and phytonutrients, which may benefit numerous conditions, including allergies, asthma, cancer, cataracts, heart disease, stroke and the common cold.

MAXIMIZE THE BENEFITS Don't spend too much time removing the pith (the spongy white layer between the zest and pulp), because a good amount of the fiber and phytonutrients, particularly the flavonoids, are found in both the pulp and the pith. Freshly squeezed citrus juice also has more nutrients than frozen or bottled juices. If you're reducing your salt intake, squeeze lemon or lime over your vegetables or grain dishes instead. The acid hits the same area on the tongue as salt, so it boosts flavor without the added sodium.

PUMP UP YOUR RECIPES Make a simple salad of grapefruit sections, avocado slices, a drizzle of olive oil, salt and pepper. Serve over shredded romaine leaves. Simmer dates and orange wedges in orange juice to make a compote, then sprinkle walnuts on top. Sauté tangerine sections and drizzle with brown sugar and cinnamon. Combine blood oranges, red onion and spinach leaves in salad.

COOKING GREENS

Cooking greens—kale, Swiss chard, and collard, beet, turnip and mustard greens—are packed with vitamins, minerals, fiber and an array of phytonutrients that may reduce heart disease risk, eye diseases and certain cancers.

MAXIMIZE THE BENEFITS To enhance the bioavailability of beta-carotene in cooking greens, cook them with a small amount of olive oil. If you cook greens in water, which can diminish folate levels, use the cooking water in the recipe or add it to a smoothie.

PUMP UP YOUR RECIPES Add some raw slivered curly kale to salads. Make kale chips by tossing kale pieces in a small amount of oil and sprinkling with garlic and onion powder. Bake at 275° for 20 to 30 minutes or until crisp. Braise chopped mustard greens with plenty of chopped garlic. Layer chopped cooked chard in lasagna.

CORN

Corn may help to fight type 2 diabetes, heart disease, certain cancers, macular degeneration and obesity. The phytonutrients lutein and zeaxanthin, which are abundant in corn, are associated with better test scores on cognition, memory and executive function in adults age 50 and older.

MAXIMIZE THE BENEFITS To preserve the water-soluble B vitamins in corn (folate and thiamin), it's best to steam rather than boil corn. If this isn't practical, then be sure to cook for no longer than 10 minutes in boiling water to minimize nutrient loss. Or cook in the microwave.

PUMP UP YOUR RECIPES Add corn kernels and salsa to guacamole to extend the avocado. Make a corn salsa with chopped red onion and orange bell pepper, chopped green chiles, olive oil, lime juice and ground cumin. Cook corn kernels, celery, diced red potatoes and thyme in vegetable broth until veggies are tender. Mash half the mixture and return to the pot for tasty corn chowder.

FLAXSEED

Flaxseed is rich in fiber and omega-3 fatty acids. Adding flaxseed to your diet may help to ward off heart disease and diabetes.

MAXIMIZING THE BENEFITS To get the most out of flaxseed, they must be ground, or they simply pass through the body, and you don't reap their health benefits. In addition, don't heat flaxseed oil—this will destroy its beneficial alpha-linolenic (omega-3 fatty acid) content as well as make the oil taste bitter and unpleasant.

PUMP UP YOUR RECIPES Sprinkle ground flaxseed on salads or stir-fries. Stir 2 tablespoons ground flaxseed into the batter of any baked goods for added fiber. Make a vegan egg substitute for baking by combining 1 tablespoon of ground flaxseed with 3 tablespoons water and let stand for 5 minutes to thicken. Substitute flaxseed oil for olive oil in salad dressings.

GARLIC

Garlic has been shown to reduce blood pressure in people with high blood pressure by as much as 7% to 8%. In addition, garlic seems to reduce atherosclerosis, the hardening of arteries brought on by age. It has also been shown to reduce the risk of heart disease and ward off infections and some cancers.

MAXIMIZE THE BENEFITS After chopping or crushing garlic, let it stand for 10 minutes before cooking. This allows allicin and its potent derivatives to be activated. If you're concerned about garlic breath, eating parsley might help to reduce these unpleasant odors, possibly because of its chlorophyll.

PUMP UP YOUR RECIPES Drop peeled cloves in with any simmering vegetable that will be pureed for soup. Add minced garlic to rice or other grain dishes before cooking. Replace the butter in mashed potatoes or pasta dishes with tender roasted garlic. Tightly wrap a bulb of garlic in foil and bake in a 400° oven for 45 minutes or until the cloves are tender. Let cool slightly and squeeze onto baked potatoes or toast, or into a sauce. Chill for later use.

GRAPES

Grapes contain phytonutrients that may help to reduce the risk for heart disease, cancer, diabetes and strokes. In addition to grapes, red wine, grape juice and raisins are also rich in disease-fighting phytonutrients.

MAXIMIZE THE BENEFITS To reap the full benefits of grapes, it is best to select red or purple varieties, which contain the highest concentrations of healthful compounds.

PUMP UP YOUR RECIPES Make a grape salad by tossing halved grapes, minced celery, sour cream (dairy or non-dairy) and lemon juice. Top with chopped nuts. Add halved grapes to a Caesar salad. Halve or chop grapes or raisins and toss into cooked whole grains with chopped nuts for a quick pilaf.

LENTILS

Lentils are low-fat, protein-rich legumes that offer substantial phytonutrient power, folate and an impressive amount of fiber, more than a quarter of which is the heart-healthy soluble type. They also contain decent amounts of iron and calcium.

MAXIMIZE THE BENEFITS Eat foods high in vitamin C along with lentils to enhance iron absorption. To prevent B vitamins from leaching out into water that may ultimately be discarded, cook lentils in just enough water to cover them by 1 inch. Soluble fiber in lentils is made available as they cook and the fiber dissolves (this also softens the lentils).

PUMP UP YOUR RECIPES Toss cooked, cooled lentils with peeled orange slices, chopped fennel, minced garlic and red wine vinaigrette for a hearty salad. Substitute cooked lentils for ground meat in chili or tomato-based meat sauce recipes. Add protein and fiber to pilafs by substituting lentils for some of the rice.

MUSHROOMS

Mushrooms contain abundant disease-fighting compounds that may help manage cancer, heart disease, high blood pressure, high cholesterol and viral infections.

MAXIMIZE THE BENEFITS Since the B vitamins in mushrooms leach into water when heated, if you soak dried mushrooms to reconstitute them, try to use the soaking water in the recipe—it's packed with flavor. Since some people may react to the allergens and other substances in raw mushrooms, it's best to eat them cooked.

PUMP UP YOUR RECIPES Quickly sauté and add to grain dishes, soups and stews, or use them to top a pizza. Make soup with sautéed mushrooms, broth, diced tomatoes, garlic and rosemary. Sauté sliced mushrooms with onion, garlic and herbs for a flavorful topping to baked potatoes.

NUTS

Nuts are energy-packed and protein-rich and may also lower the risk for cancer and cardiovascular disease. Studies show that nuts protect against heart disease by improving blood levels of fat, reducing inflammation and contributing unsaturated fats and plant sterols.

MAXIMIZE THE BENEFITS Refrigerate or freeze nuts to prevent their oils from going rancid. To enhance the flavor of nuts, toast them in the oven for 5 to 10 minutes, or until fragrant.

PUMP UP YOUR RECIPES Sprinkle chopped walnuts or peanuts over oatmeal, salads or stir-fries. Thicken sauces or salad dressings by whisking in a tablespoon of peanut or almond butter. Drizzle melted dark chocolate (70% or higher) over hazelnuts and let stand to set. Roll small balls of peanut butter in oats for a family-friendly snack.

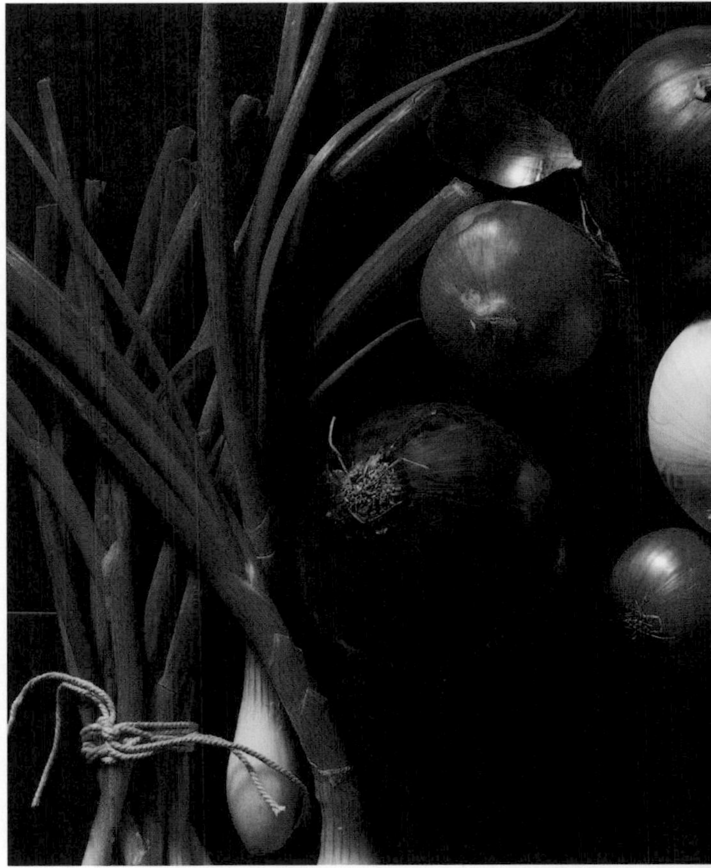

ONIONS

Onions and all members of the onion family—onions, chives, leeks, scallions and shallots—are noted for their powerful phytonutrients and fiber, which may protect against cancer, cardiovascular disease, neurodegenerative disorders, constipation, hypertension, allergic conditions and atherosclerosis.

MAXIMIZE THE BENEFITS High-heat cooking significantly reduces the benefits of diallyl sulfides, an important group of phytonutrients in the onion and garlic family. Fresh, raw onion has the most health benefits, and mincing (or even chewing) the onion helps to release the phytonutrient power.

PUMP UP YOUR RECIPES Grill thick slices of onion to place on sandwiches or veggie burgers. Brush scallions with olive oil and grill until charred. Sprinkle with lime juice and salt and eat in warm tortillas. Cut red onions into wedges and drizzle with olive oil, minced herb and salt. Roast in a 350° oven for 45 to 60 minutes or until tender and browned. Place sliced or minced raw onion in a small container and top with red wine or rice vinegar. Allow to stand for at least 1 hour or up to 3 days in the fridge. This will mellow the flavor slightly for adding raw onion to salads or sandwiches.

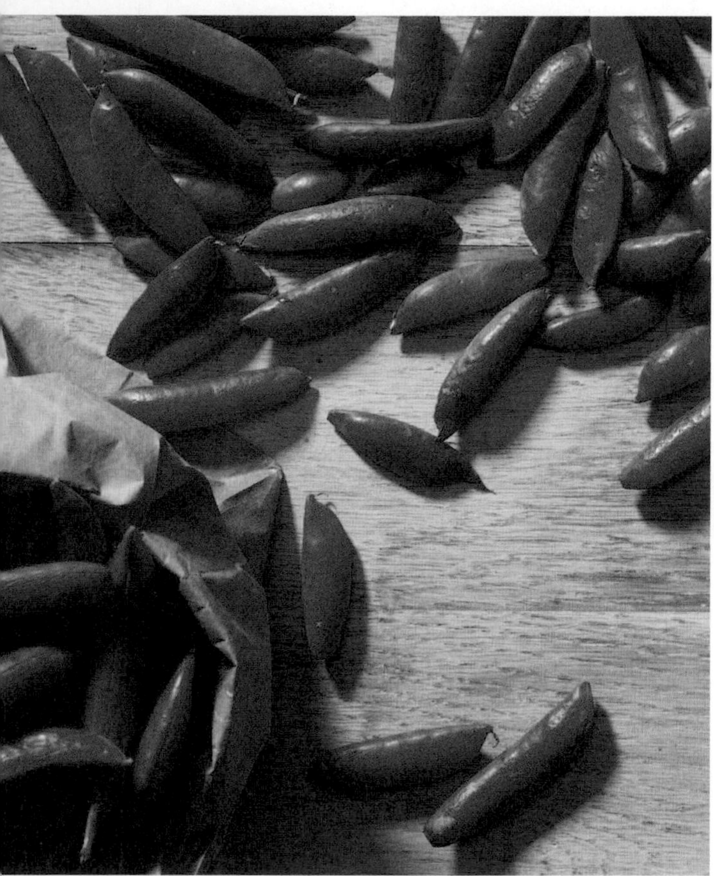

PEAS

Peas are a good source of plant-based protein and iron, making them an excellent food for plant-based diets. Peas may help reduce the risk for developing certain cancers, depression, high cholesterol and macular degeneration.

MAXIMIZE THE BENEFITS Heat-sensitive vitamin C and water-soluble B vitamins (folate and B6) are best preserved if you quickly steam or microwave peas instead of boiling or cooking them for long periods of time.

PUMP UP YOUR RECIPES Puree with mint and a pinch of salt until smooth. Spread on bread, top baked potatoes, or toss with hot pasta. Toss into grain dishes with sliced roasted red peppers. Blend cooked peas with avocado and lemon juice in food processor for creamy cold soup.

PEPPERS

Peppers, including sweet bell peppers and spicy chili peppers, add color and zest to your favorite dishes, while offering protection against heart disease, vision loss and nasal congestion. Red bell peppers are richer in vitamin C and supply more than ten times the beta-carotene of green peppers. But all peppers are rich in both nutrients.

MAXIMIZE THE BENEFITS For vitamin C, eat uncooked peppers, since this vitamin is easily destroyed by heat. To maximize the bioavailability of beta-carotene and also preserve other nutrients, cook peppers until they are crisp-tender and eat with a little monounsaturated fat, such as olive oil, to aid absorption.

PUMP UP YOUR RECIPES Stuff poblanos for grilling with rice pilaf, corn, tomatoes and queso fresco. Puree roasted red peppers, almonds, olive oil and sherry vinegar for a dip. Top a veggie pizza with banana peppers. Slice strips of red pepper and serve as a snack with a dip such as hummus or guacamole.

POTATOES

Potatoes may increase the production of memory-enhancing brain chemicals.

MAXIMIZE THE BENEFITS For the most nutrients, eat potatoes with their skin, and bake, microwave or steam. If peeling, remove the thinnest layer possible. If boiling, leave the skin on and try to reuse the cooking water, where many of the B vitamins wind up after cooking. Avoid frying or adding lots of butter or other fats when you prepare potatoes.

PUMP UP YOUR RECIPES Cut into chunks and toss with olive oil and herbs. Roast at 400° for 40 minutes, turning once, or until crisp. Make healthy potato chips by placing thinly sliced potatoes on parchment paper in the microwave. Cook for 2 to 3 minutes or until lightly browned and crisp. Combine steamed quartered potatoes with chopped scallion and celery, toss with apple cider vinegar and mustard dressing.

QUINOA

Quinoa, pronounced KEEN-wah, is a gluten-free, protein-packed, nutrient-dense seed that is prepared like a grain. Quinoa has been shown to protect against cancer and heart disease, help regulate blood sugar and high blood pressure and help fight obesity.

MAXIMIZE THE BENEFITS A source of iron and B vitamins, quinoa should be cooked in the amount of water as directed in recipes to prevent nutrient loss.

PUMP UP YOUR RECIPES Add some cooked quinoa to a corn relish. Use quinoa flour in place of half of the all-purpose flour in muffin recipes. You will need the all-purpose flour for the muffins to raise properly. Cook quinoa with raisins and cinnamon for breakfast. Change up rice or barley dishes by using quinoa instead.

RICE

Rice is an important source of complex carbohydrates, fiber and essential nutrients. Free of gluten, rice is a natural choice for people with celiac disease or wheat gluten allergies. Choose brown rice, because it has more vitamins and minerals than plain milled white rice, which has been stripped of many of its nutrients. Brown rice is also high in insoluble fiber and oryzanol, an oil with cholesterol lowering properties.

MAXIMIZE THE BENEFITS Unless package directions say otherwise, when cooking rice, do not rinse it before (or after), because that washes away essential nutrients. To retain B vitamins, avoid cooking with excess water.

PUMP UP YOUR RECIPES Toss with black beans and salsa for a quick Tex-Mex dish. Combine with pesto for a bright green alternative to pasta—stir in roasted red pepper strips and green peas for a hearty main dish. Toss with Italian vinaigrette and chopped greens and stuff into tomatoes.

SEEDS

Pumpkin, sesame and sunflower seeds are rich in heart-healthy fats, possess plenty of phytonutrients that may protect against cancer, cardiovascular disease, cataracts, chronic fatigue syndrome and macular degeneration.

MAXIMIZE THE BENEFITS To preserve their essential fats and nutrients (and to prevent them from going rancid), refrigerate or freeze seeds in airtight containers.

PUMP UP YOUR RECIPES Sprinkle pumpkin or sunflower seeds on muffins before baking. Sprinkle pumpkin seeds over soups or salads in place of croutons. Top Asian-style dishes with sesame seeds. Add seeds to cereals or yogurt bowls.

SOY FOODS

Soy foods include tofu, edamame, dried soybeans, soy milk, miso and tempeh, which contribute high-quality plant protein, soluble fiber and a wealth of phytonutrients to the diet. Soy foods help lower cholesterol and may help manage blood sugar.

MAXIMIZE THE BENEFITS To preserve phytoestrogen content, minimize cooking time for tofu and miso by adding them late in the cooking process.

PUMP UP YOUR RECIPES Look for dried edamame to sprinkle on salads or eat as a snack. Replace the beans in salads with cooked edamame or replace half the avocado in guacamole with edamame. Slice tofu into slabs and marinate overnight in mixture of soy sauce, rice vinegar and ginger, turning to coat. Grill or air-fry to cook. Process drained tofu with salt, lemon juice and nutritional yeast for a ricotta cheese substitute.

SPINACH

Spinach helps protect against cancer, high cholesterol and vision loss. Vitamin K, found in dark greens such as spinach, is necessary for proper blood clotting and may play a role in preserving bone health. Consult with your doctor before consuming if you are on blood-thinning medications.

MAXIMIZE THE BENEFITS Serve spinach either raw or cooked, but avoid overcooking. To preserve water-soluble B vitamins, steam or stir-fry spinach. Cooking helps to convert the protein, lutein and beta-carotene in spinach into more well-absorbed forms. To enhance carotenoid absorption, eat spinach along with heart-healthy fat.

PUMP UP YOUR RECIPES Chop and stir into soups and stews at the end of cooking. Substitute spinach for the basil in your favorite pesto recipe. Throw handfuls of baby spinach into smoothies or salads. Sauté garlic in olive oil and cook spinach until wilted; toss into pasta or grain dishes or fill baked sweet or white potatoes with the mixture.

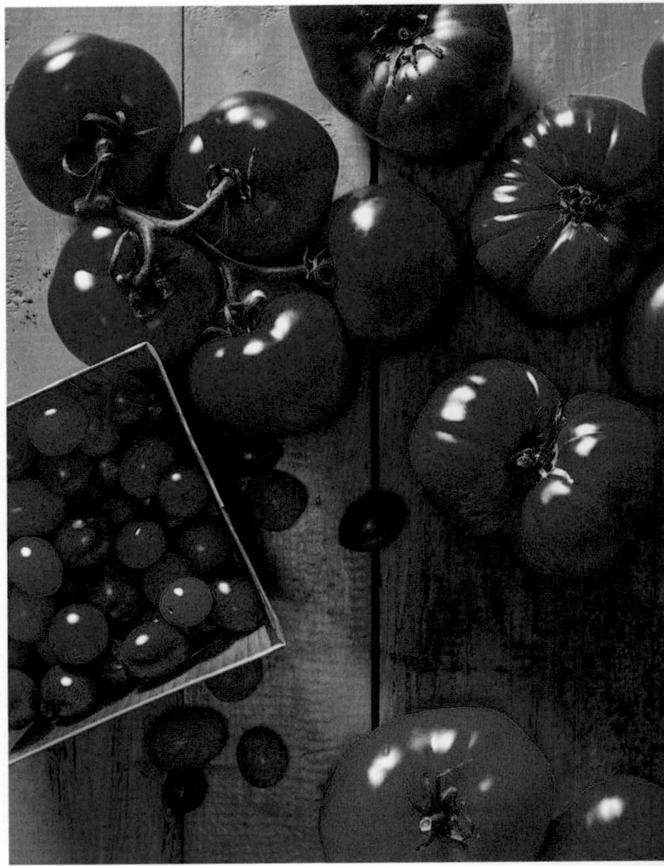

TOMATOES

Tomatoes and tomato products are full of phytonutrients such as lycopene that protect against cancer, clogged arteries and skin conditions. Lycopene-rich foods such as tomatoes and tomato paste may reduce the risk of developing prostate cancer.

MAXIMIZE THE BENEFITS Lycopene is best absorbed from concentrated forms of tomatoes, such as ketchup and tomato paste, juice, sauce and soup. The more concentrated the tomato source, the more concentrated the lycopene. Heat and oil enhance absorption of lycopene and beta-carotene, though some vitamin C is lost.

PUMP UP YOUR RECIPES Stir tomato paste into lentil soup, stew recipes or grain dishes. Add tomato paste to veggie burgers or lentil loaf. Sauté halved grape tomatoes in olive oil with minced garlic and basil for a quick pasta sauce. Make a veggie-rich pasta sauce by sautéing onion, garlic, carrots and celery until tender. Add canned tomatoes and simmer with Italian seasoning until very tender. Process until smooth.

WHOLE GRAINS

Whole grains include the nutritious germ and bran layers of the grain and are packed with phytonutrients and both soluble and insoluble fiber. Consuming whole grains, such as barley, buckwheat, bulgur, oats, rye and wheat, is linked to a lower risk for cancer, cardiovascular disease and diabetes. Ancient grains, such as amaranth, farro, kamut, spelt and teff, are high in protein and rich in fiber, B vitamins and phytonutrients.

MAXIMIZE THE BENEFITS Cook these grains in a minimal amount of water and only until tender as indicated on package cooking directions; overcooking or cooking in too much water will diminish the nutrient and phytonutrient content of the grain and dilute the flavor.

PUMP UP YOUR RECIPES Stir quick-cooking barley into soups instead of orzo. In a food processor, pulse oats until coarsely ground and use in place of bread crumbs or some of the flour in recipes. Cook buckwheat noodles (soba) in broth with shredded vegetables and miso for a rich ramen soup. Mix wheat germ into pizza dough or quick breads, or sprinkle over breakfast cereal. Stir crushed wheat bran flakes into veggie burgers to provide more texture and add fiber.

PUTTING THE SUPERFOODS TO WORK

Now that you know the healthiest foods to eat and best ways to prepare them, the following section will provide delicious recipes for these ingredients. Some you may be familiar with, such as the Bean and Bulgur Chili on page 82, only this recipe replaces much of the meat with vegetables. Other recipes, such as Spicy Orange Quinoa on page 231, will teach you how to prepare these superfoods for the first time. Each recipe has been tested to ensure it will work for you.

For ease when preparing a meal, look for the icons highlighting the features of each recipe:

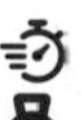 meals ready in 30 minutes or less
recipe bursting with protein
recipe that can be prepared ahead and served last minute
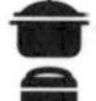 recipe made in a slow-cooker
recipe made in a pressure-cooker

Following the recipe section are suggested meal plans to show how these dishes fit into anyone's lifestyle. Created by registered dietitian Peggy Woodward, these meal plans give you a starting point to show you how to mix and match the recipes in the book if you are short on time, on a budget, looking for diabetes-friendly meals, or watching your salt, sugar or fat intake.

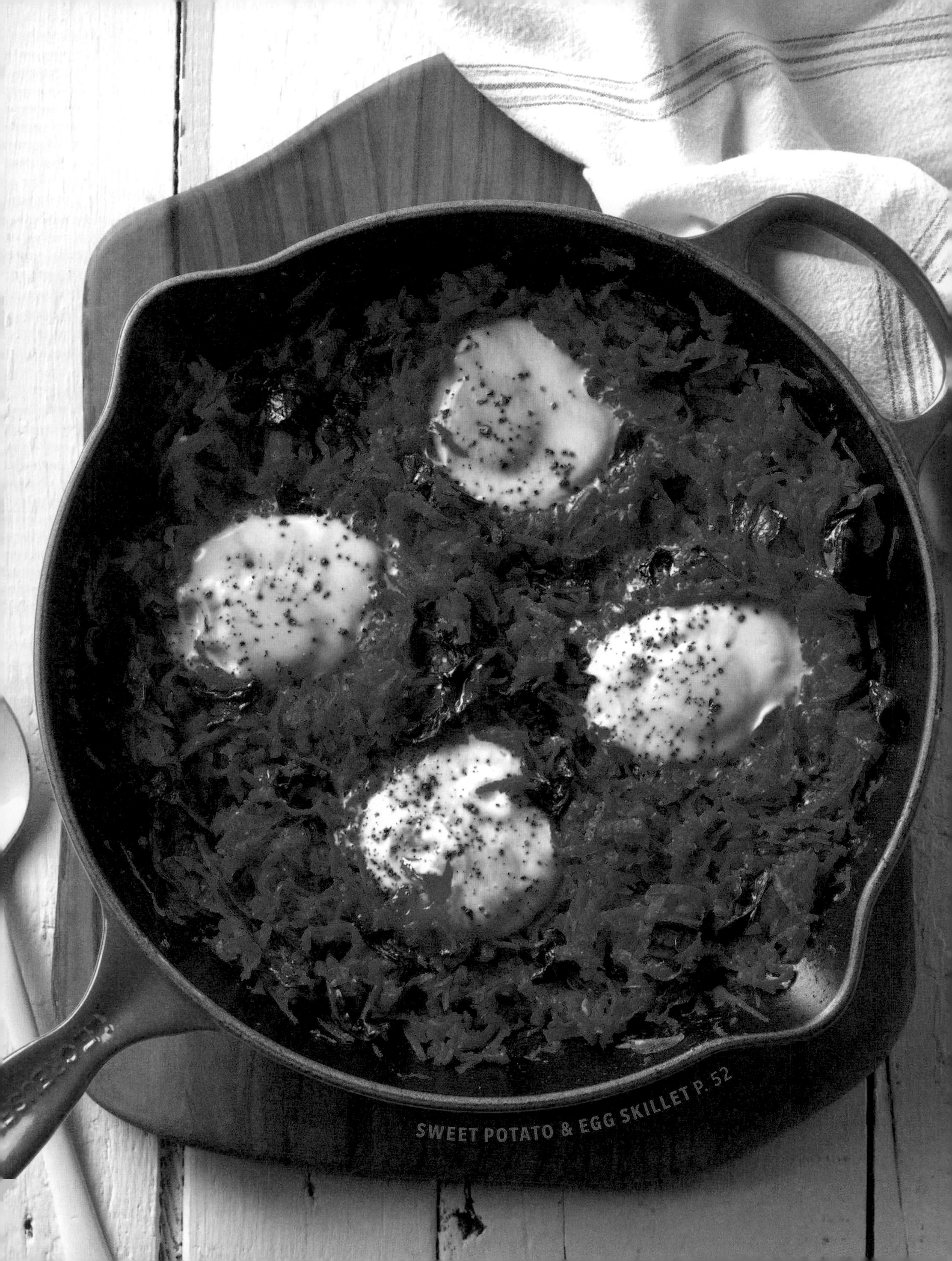

SWEET POTATO & EGG SKILLET P. 52

CHAPTER 4

BREAKFAST & SMOOTHIES

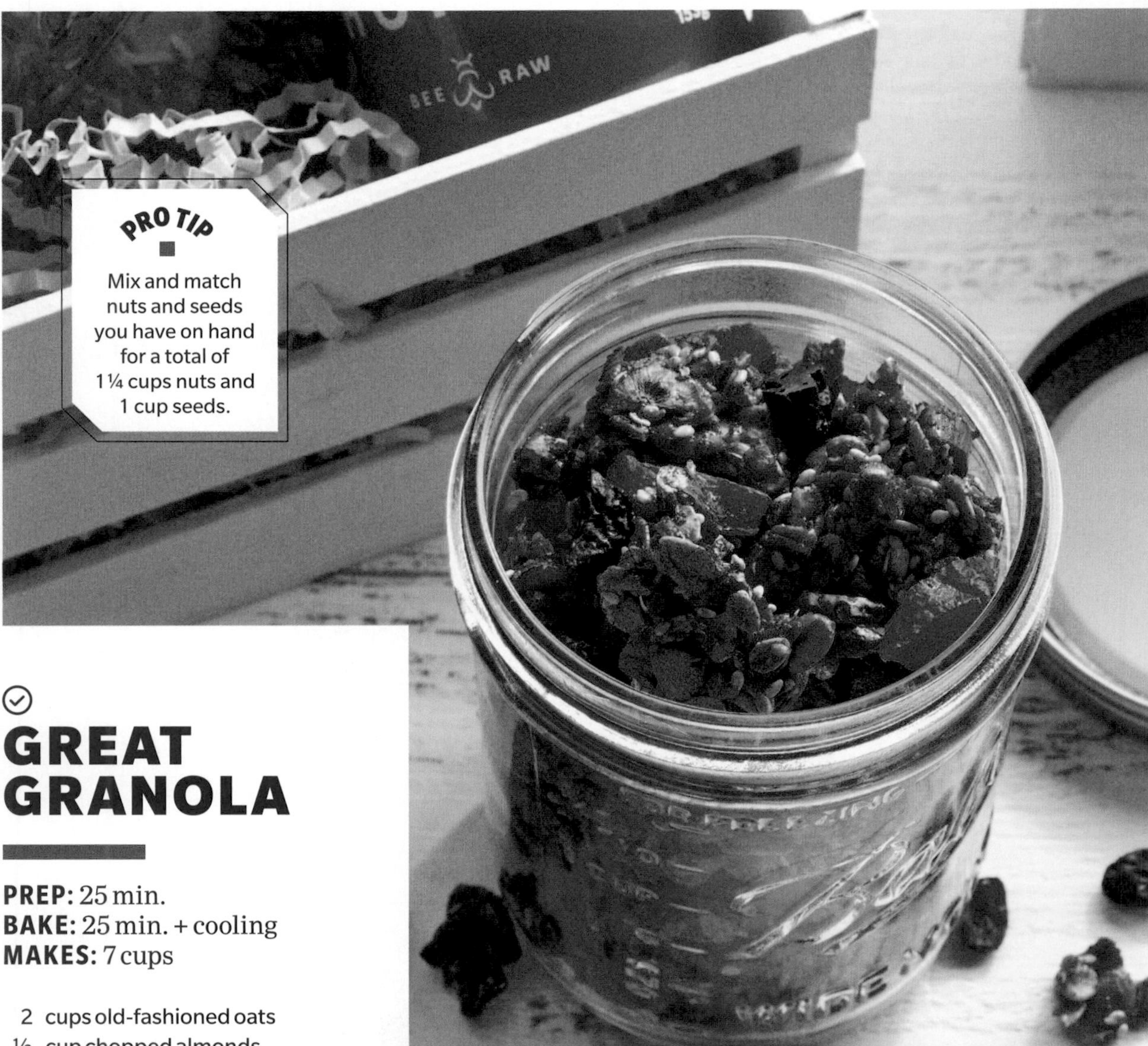

PRO TIP

Mix and match nuts and seeds you have on hand for a total of 1¼ cups nuts and 1 cup seeds.

GREAT GRANOLA

PREP: 25 min.
BAKE: 25 min. + cooling
MAKES: 7 cups

- 2 cups old-fashioned oats
- ½ cup chopped almonds
- ½ cup salted pumpkin seeds or pepitas
- ½ cup chopped walnuts
- ¼ cup chopped pecans
- ¼ cup sesame seeds
- ¼ cup sunflower kernels
- ⅓ cup agave nectar
- ¼ cup packed brown sugar
- ¼ cup maple syrup
- 2 Tbsp. toasted wheat germ
- 2 Tbsp. canola oil
- 1 tsp. ground cinnamon
- 1 tsp. vanilla extract
- 7 oz. mixed dried fruit (about 1⅓ cups)

1 In a large bowl, combine the first 7 ingredients; set aside.

2 In a small saucepan, combine the agave, brown sugar, syrup, wheat germ, oil and cinnamon. Cook and stir over medium heat until smooth, 4-5 minutes. Remove from the heat; stir in the vanilla. Pour over the oat mixture and toss to coat.

3 Transfer mixture to a greased 15x10x1-in. baking pan. Bake at 350° until golden brown, stirring occasionally, 22-27 minutes. Cool completely on a wire rack. Stir in dried fruit. Store the granola in an airtight container.

½ CUP *290 cal., 14g fat (2g sat. fat), 0 chol., 49mg sod., 38g carb. (25g sugars, 4g fiber), 6g pro.*

OVERNIGHT FLAX OATMEAL

PREP: 10 min.
COOK: 7 hours
MAKES: 4 servings

- 3 cups water
- 1 cup old-fashioned oats
- 1 cup raisins
- ½ cup dried cranberries
- ½ cup ground flaxseed
- ½ cup 2% milk or milk alternative
- 1 tsp. vanilla extract
- 1 tsp. molasses
- Sliced almonds, optional

In a 3-qt. slow cooker, combine all ingredients. Cover and cook on low for 7-8 hours or until liquid is absorbed and oatmeal is tender. If desired, top with sliced almonds and, if desired, additional milk and molasses.

1 CUP *322 cal., 9g fat (1g sat. fat), 2mg chol., 28mg sod., 63g carb. (34g sugars, 8g fiber), 9g pro.*

PRO TIP

If you're trying to cut refined sugar from your diet, skip the (sweetened) dried cranberries and use 1½ cups total raisins instead.

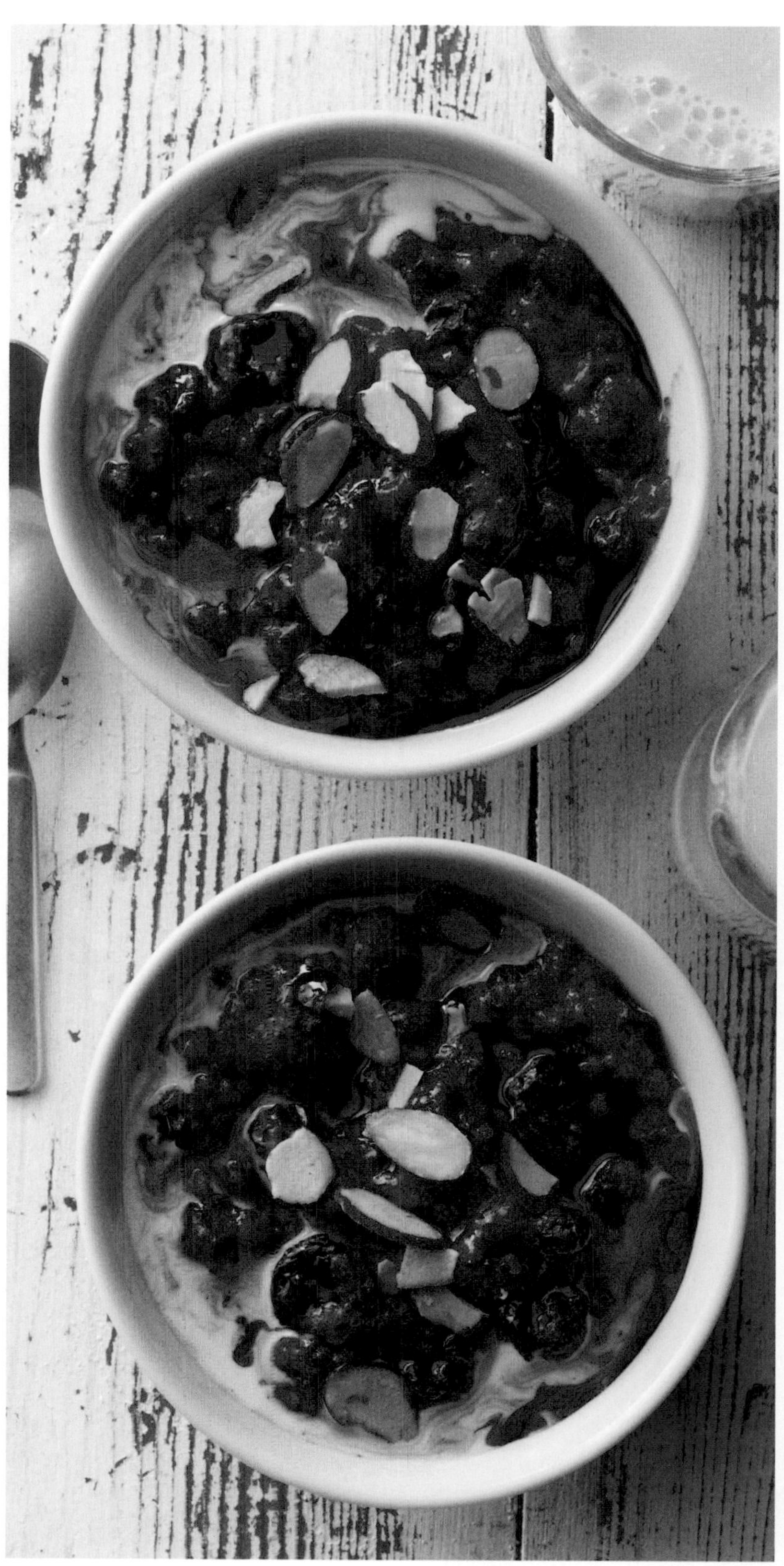

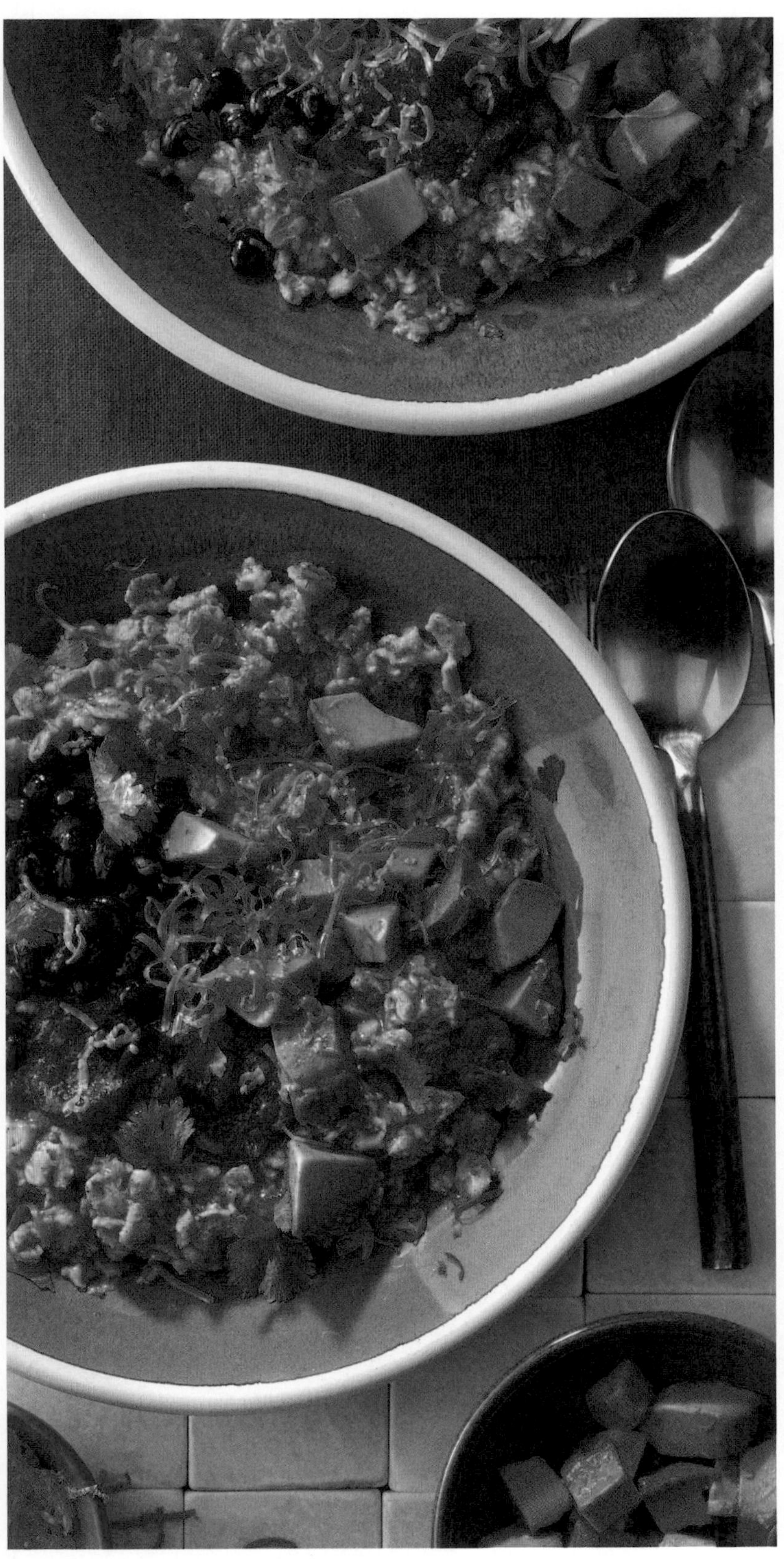

TEX-MEX GRAIN BOWLS

TAKES: 20 min.
MAKES: 4 servings

- 4 cups water
- 2 Tbsp. reduced-sodium taco seasoning
- 2 cups old-fashioned oats or multigrain hot cereal
- 1 cup black beans, rinsed, drained and warmed
- 1 cup salsa
- ½ cup finely shredded cheddar or vegan cheddar-style cheese
- 1 medium ripe avocado, peeled and cubed
- Optional toppings: Pitted ripe olives, sour cream and chopped cilantro

In a large saucepan, bring water and taco seasoning to a boil. Stir in the oats; cook for 5 minutes over medium heat, stirring occasionally. Remove from heat. Divide oatmeal among 4 bowls. Top with beans, salsa, cheese, avocado and toppings as desired. Serve immediately.

1 BOWL *345 cal., 13g fat (4g sat. fat), 14mg chol., 702mg sod., 46g carb. (5g sugars, 9g fiber), 12g pro.*

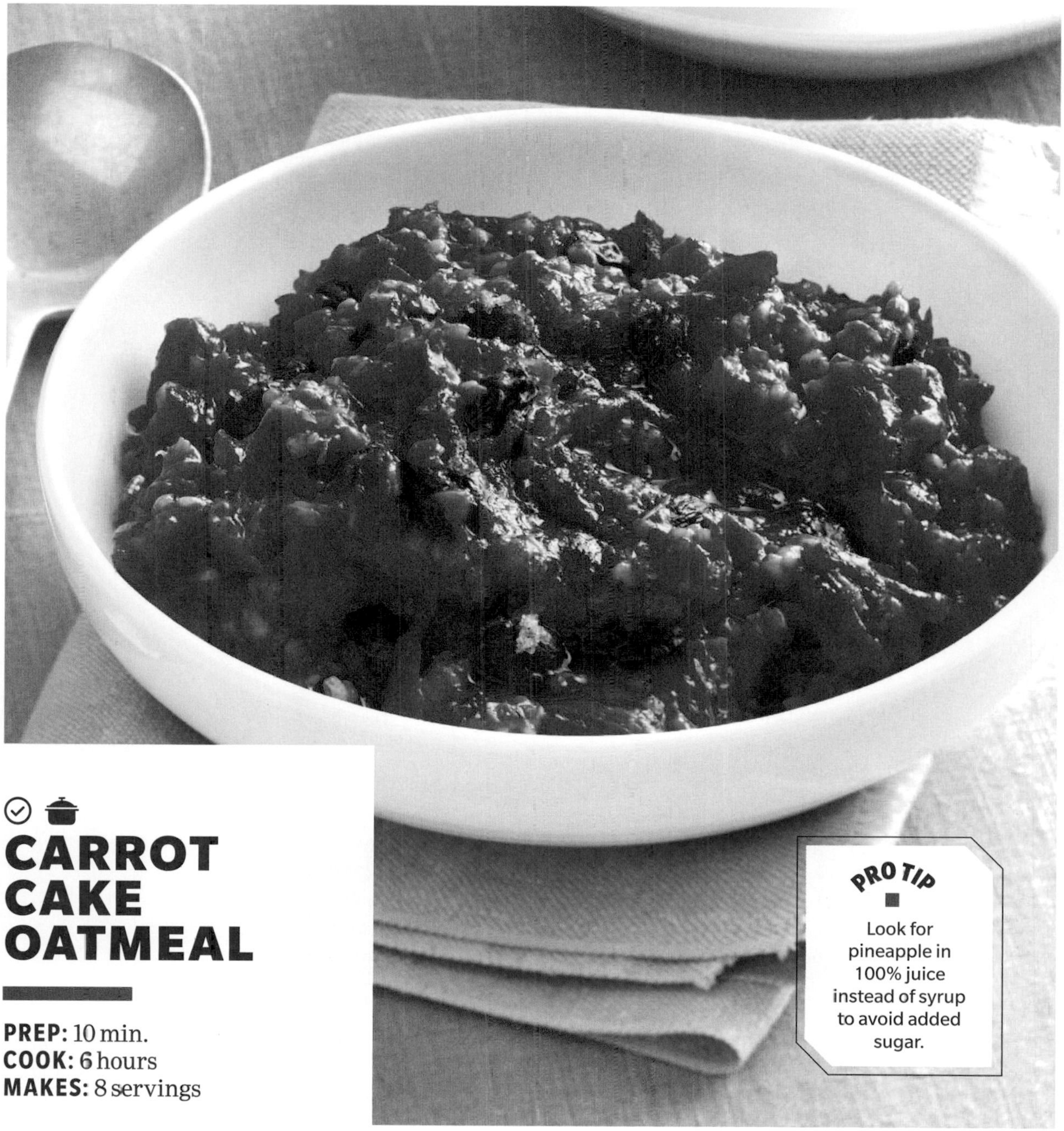

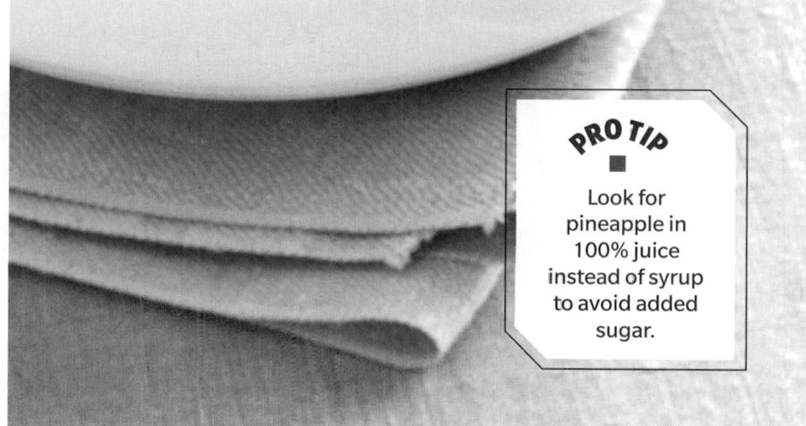

CARROT CAKE OATMEAL

PREP: 10 min.
COOK: 6 hours
MAKES: 8 servings

PRO TIP

Look for pineapple in 100% juice instead of syrup to avoid added sugar.

- 4½ cups water
- 1 can (20 oz.) crushed pineapple, undrained
- 2 cups shredded carrots
- 1 cup steel-cut oats
- 1 cup raisins
- 2 tsp. ground cinnamon
- 1 tsp. pumpkin pie spice
- Brown sugar, optional

In a 4-qt. slow cooker coated with cooking spray, combine the first 7 ingredients. Cover and cook on low for 6-8 hours or until oats are tender and liquid is absorbed. Sprinkle oatmeal with brown sugar if desired.

1 CUP *197 cal., 2g fat (0 sat. fat), 0 chol., 23mg sod., 46g carb. (26g sugars, 4g fiber), 4g pro.*

ROASTED VEGETABLE STRATA

PREP: 55 min. + chilling **BAKE:** 40 min. **MAKES:** 8 servings

- 3 large zucchini, halved lengthwise and cut into ¾-in. slices
- 1 each medium red, yellow and orange peppers, cut into 1-in. pieces
- 2 Tbsp. olive oil
- 1 tsp. dried oregano
- ½ tsp. salt
- ½ tsp. pepper
- ½ tsp. dried basil
- 1 medium tomato, chopped
- 1 loaf (1 lb.) unsliced crusty Italian bread
- ½ cup shredded sharp cheddar or vegan sharp cheddar-style cheese
- ½ cup shredded Asiago or vegan Asiago-style cheese
- 6 large eggs
- 2 cups fat-free milk or milk alternative

1 Preheat oven to 400°. Toss the zucchini and peppers with oil and seasonings; transfer to a 15x10x1-in. pan. Roast until tender, 25-30 minutes, stirring once. Stir in tomato; cool slightly.

2 Trim ends from the bread; cut bread into 1-in. slices. In a greased 13x9-in. baking dish, layer half of each of the following: bread, roasted vegetables and cheeses. Repeat layers. Whisk together eggs and milk; pour evenly over top. Refrigerate, covered, 6 hours or overnight.

3 Preheat oven to 375°. Remove casserole from refrigerator while oven heats. Bake, uncovered, 40-50 minutes or until golden brown. Let stand 5-10 minutes before cutting.

TO FREEZE Cover and freeze unbaked casserole. To use, partially thaw in refrigerator overnight. Remove from the refrigerator 30 minutes before baking. Preheat oven to 375°. Bake casserole as directed, increasing time as necessary to heat through and for a thermometer inserted in center to read 165°.

1 PIECE *349 cal., 14g fat (5g sat. fat), 154mg chol., 642mg sod., 40g carb. (9g sugars, 4g fiber), 17g pro.* ***Diabetic exchanges:*** *2 starch, 1 vegetable, 1 medium-fat meat, 1 fat*

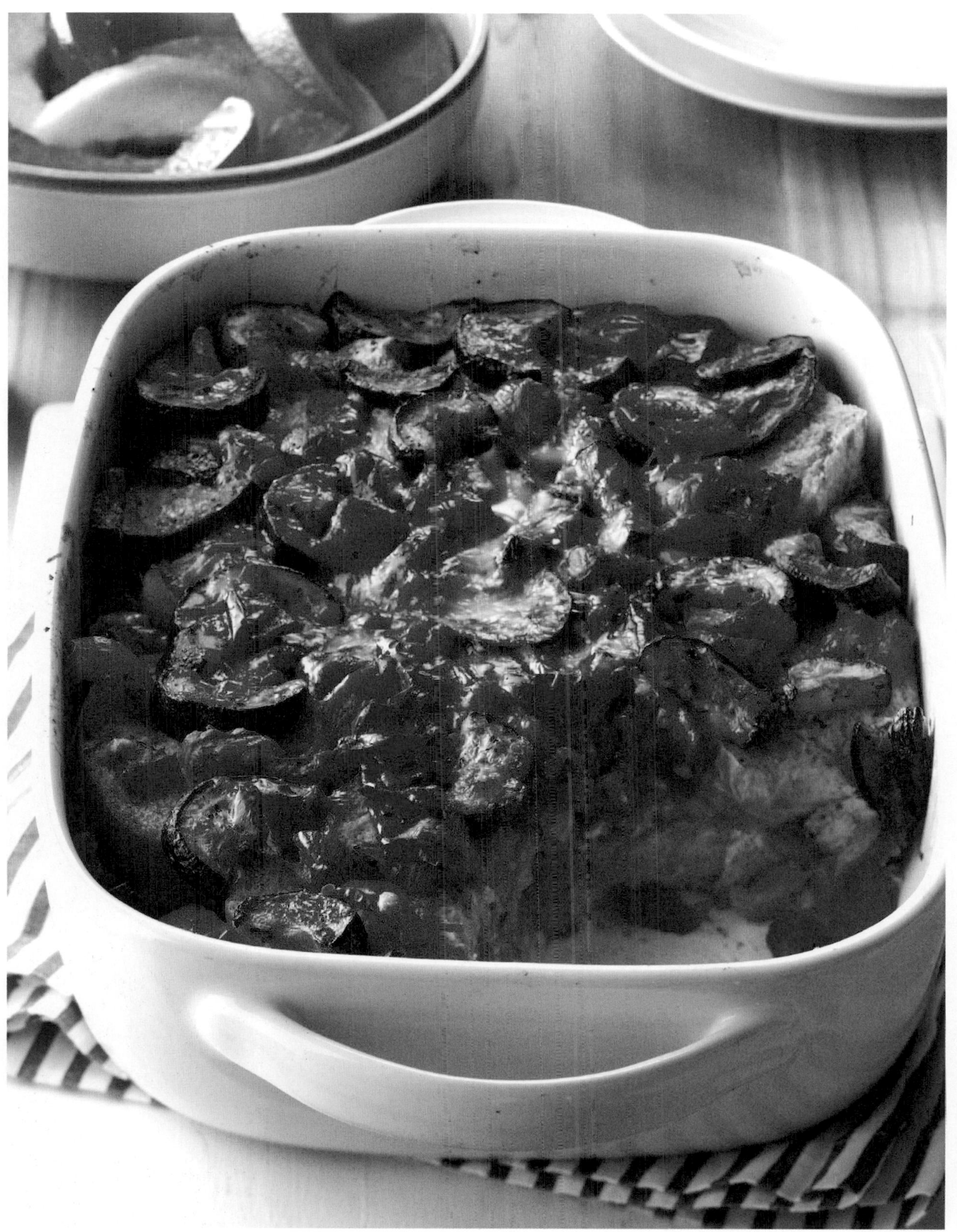

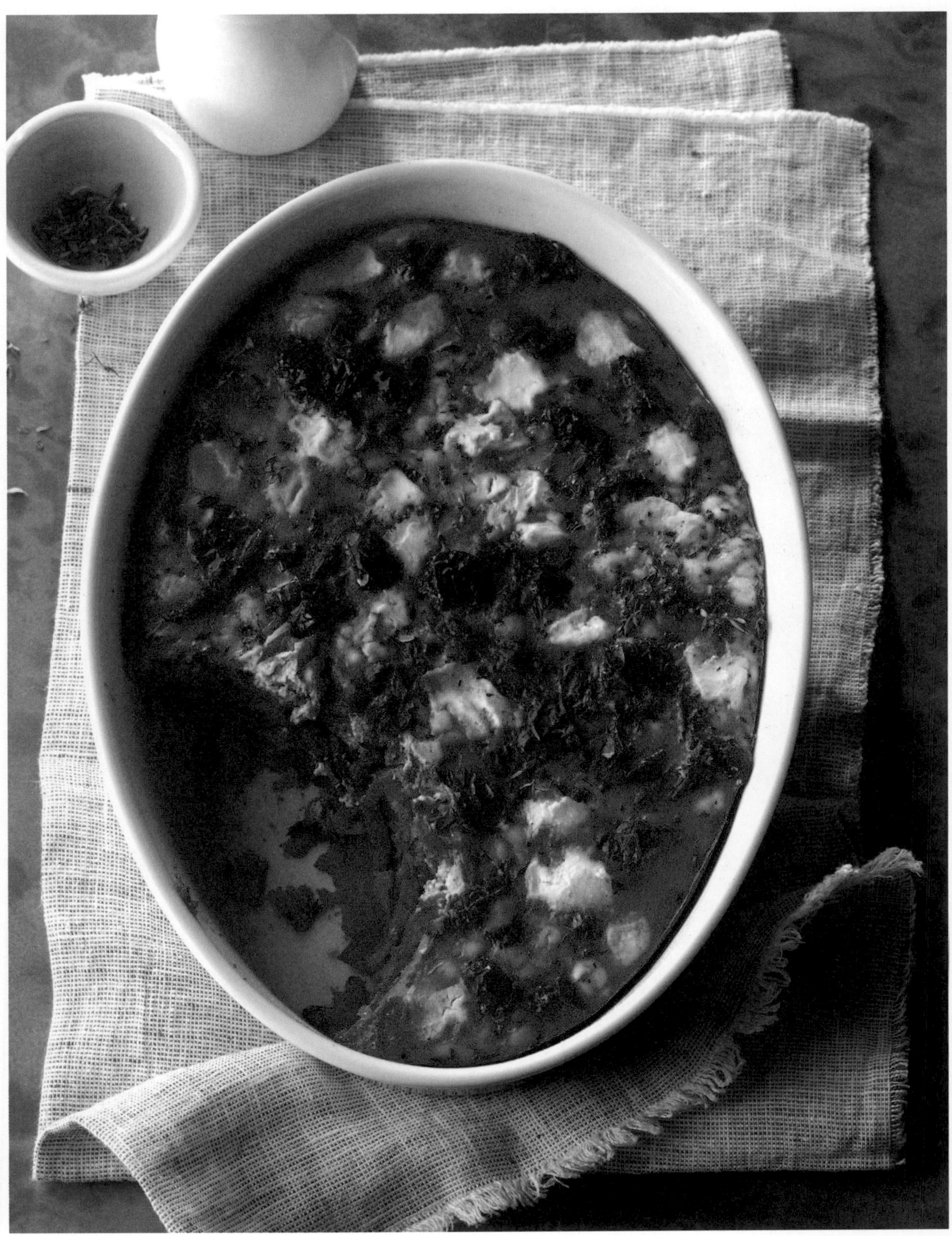

SLOW-COOKER FRITTATA PROVENCAL

PREP: 30 min. **COOK:** 3 hours **MAKES:** 6 servings

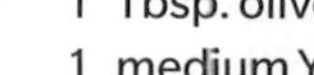
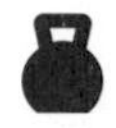
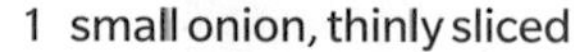

- ½ cup water
- 1 Tbsp. olive oil
- 1 medium Yukon Gold potato, peeled and sliced
- 1 small onion, thinly sliced
- ½ tsp. smoked paprika
- 12 large eggs
- 1 tsp. minced fresh thyme or ¼ tsp. dried thyme
- 1 tsp. hot pepper sauce
- ½ tsp. salt
- ¼ tsp. pepper
- 1 log (4 oz.) fresh goat cheese or vegan goat-style cheese, coarsely crumbled, divided
- ½ cup chopped soft sun-dried tomatoes (not packed in oil)

1 Layer two 24-in. pieces of aluminum foil; starting with a long side, fold up foil to create a 1-in.-wide strip. Shape strip into a coil to make a rack for bottom of a 6-qt. oval slow cooker. Add water to slow cooker; set foil rack in water.

2 In a large skillet, heat oil over medium-high heat. Add potato and onion; cook and stir for 5-7 minutes or until potato is lightly browned. Stir in paprika. Transfer to a greased 1½-qt. baking dish (dish must fit in slow cooker).

3 In a large bowl, whisk eggs, thyme, pepper sauce, salt and pepper; stir in 2 oz. cheese. Pour over potato mixture. Top with tomatoes and remaining goat cheese. Place dish on foil rack.

4 Cook, covered, on low for 3-4 hours or until eggs are set and a knife inserted in center comes out clean.

1 WEDGE *245 cal., 14g fat (5g sat. fat), 385mg chol., 338mg sod., 12g carb. (4g sugars, 2g fiber), 15g pro.* ***Diabetic exchanges:*** *2 medium-fat meat, 1 starch, ½ fat*

SOUTHWEST HASH WITH ADOBO-LIME CREMA

PREP: 20 min. **BAKE:** 25 min. **MAKES:** 4 servings

- 3 medium sweet potatoes (about 1½ lbs.), cubed
- 1 medium onion, chopped
- 1 medium sweet red pepper, chopped
- 1 Tbsp. canola oil
- 1 tsp. garlic powder
- 1 tsp. smoked paprika
- ¾ tsp. ground chipotle pepper
- ½ tsp. salt
- ¼ tsp. pepper
- ⅔ cup canned black beans, rinsed and drained
- 4 large eggs
- ½ cup reduced-fat dairy or vegan sour cream
- 2 Tbsp. lime juice
- 2 tsp. adobo sauce
- ½ medium ripe avocado, peeled and sliced, optional
- 2 Tbsp. minced fresh cilantro

1 Preheat oven to 400°. Place sweet potatoes, onion and red pepper in a 15x10x1-in. baking pan coated with cooking spray. Drizzle with oil; sprinkle with seasonings. Toss to coat. Roast 25-30 minutes or until the potatoes are tender, adding black beans during the last 10 minutes of cooking time.

2 Place 2-3 in. of water in a large saucepan or skillet with high sides. Bring to a boil; adjust heat to maintain a gentle simmer. Break cold eggs, 1 at a time, into a small bowl; holding bowl close to surface of water, slip each egg into water.

3 Cook, uncovered, 3-5 minutes or until whites are completely set and yolks begin to thicken but are not hard. Using a slotted spoon, lift eggs out of water.

4 In a small bowl, mix sour cream, lime juice and adobo sauce. Divide the sweet potato mixture among 4 bowls; top each with an egg, sour cream mixture and, if desired, avocado. Sprinkle with cilantro.

1 SERVING *304 cal., 12g fat (3g sat. fat), 222mg chol., 520mg sod., 37g carb. (15g sugars, 6g fiber), 13g pro.* ***Diabetic exchanges:*** *2 starch, 1½ fat, 1 medium-fat meat*

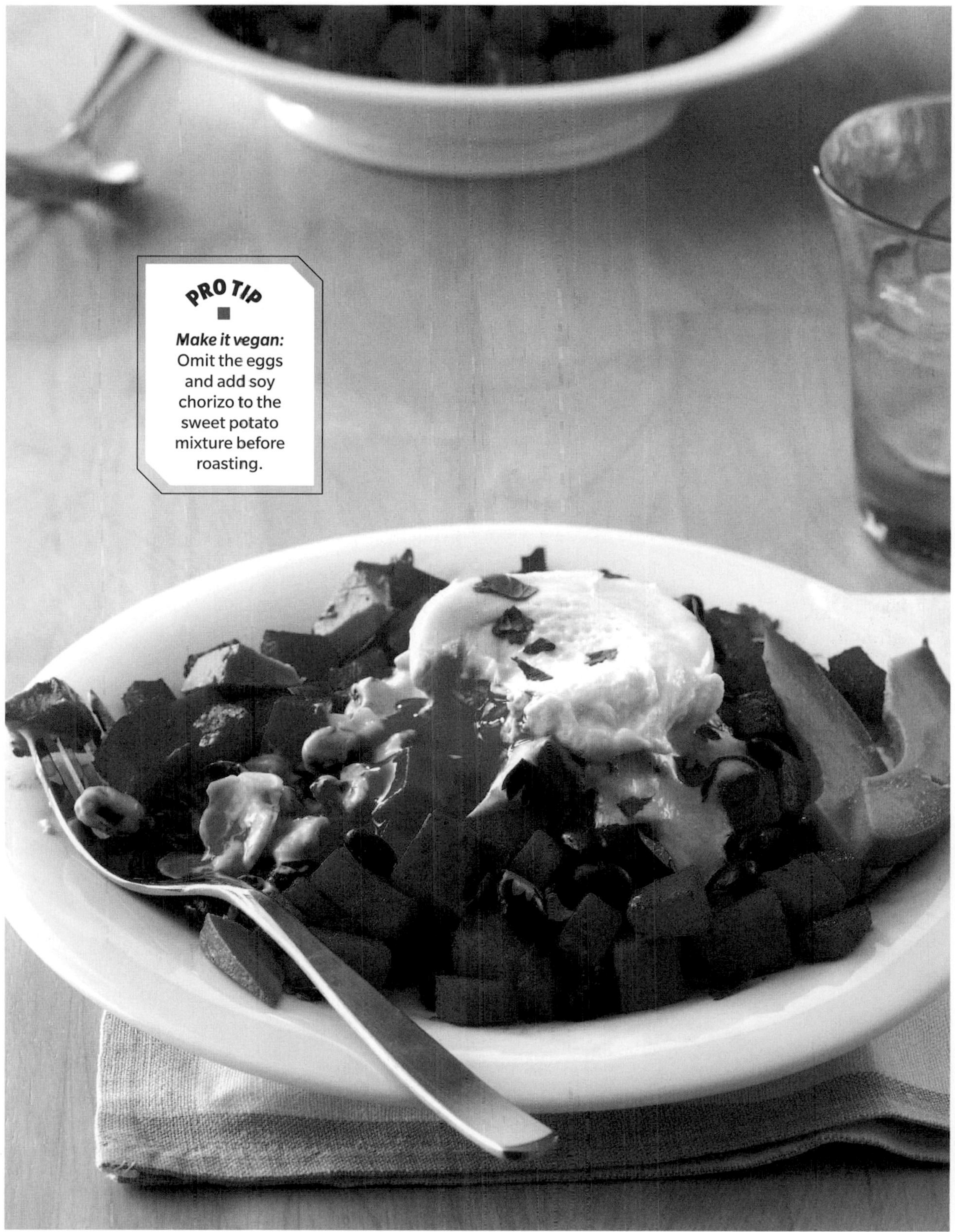

PRO TIP

Make it vegan: Omit the eggs and add soy chorizo to the sweet potato mixture before roasting.

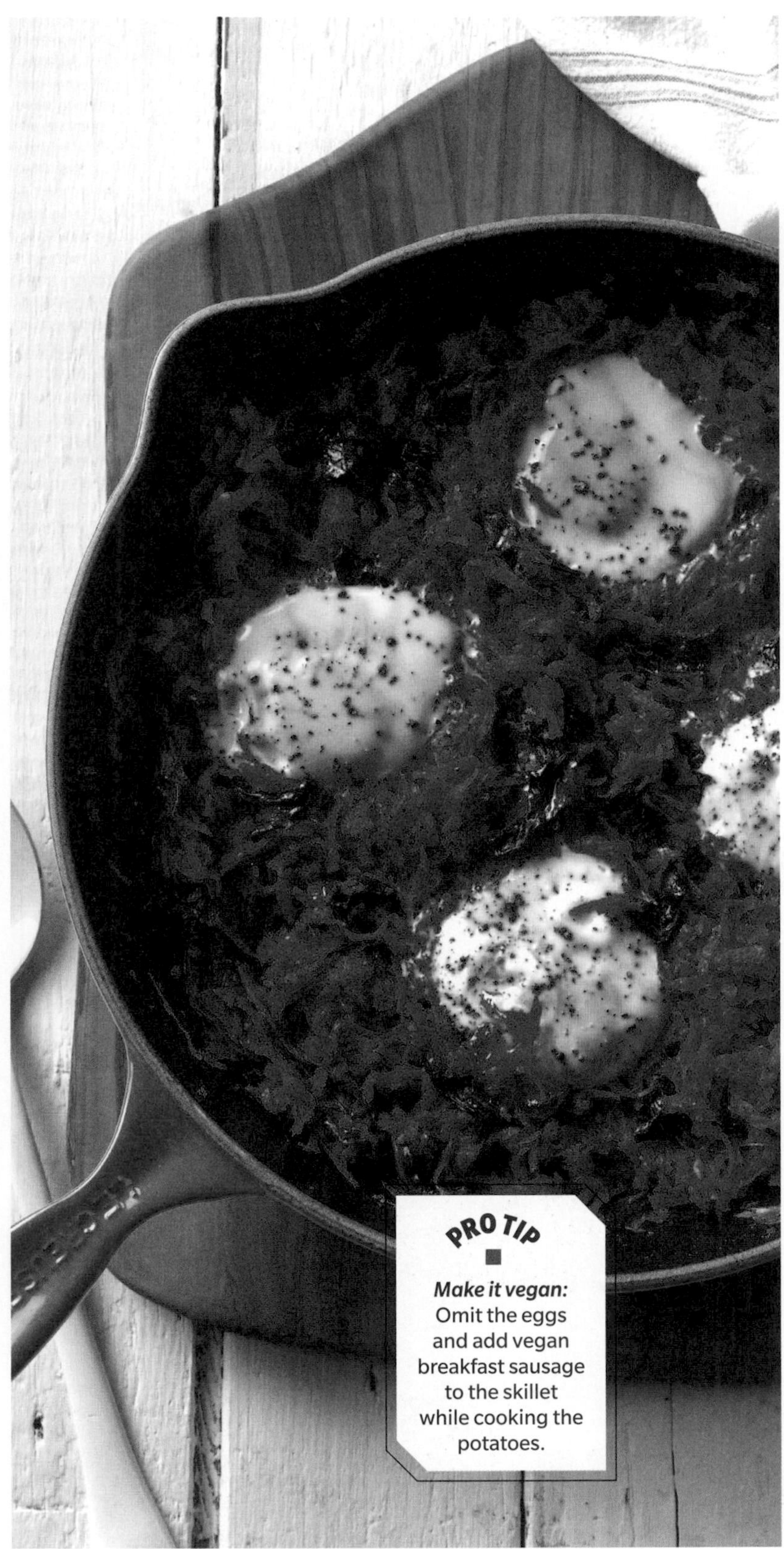

PRO TIP

Make it vegan: Omit the eggs and add vegan breakfast sausage to the skillet while cooking the potatoes.

SWEET POTATO & EGG SKILLET

TAKES: 25 min.
MAKES: 4 servings

- 2 Tbsp. butter or canola oil
- 2 medium sweet potatoes, peeled and shredded (about 4 cups)
- 1 garlic clove, minced
- ½ tsp. salt, divided
- ⅛ tsp. dried thyme
- 2 cups fresh baby spinach
- 4 large eggs
- ⅛ tsp. coarsely ground pepper

1 In a large cast-iron or other heavy skillet, heat butter over low heat. Add sweet potatoes, garlic, ¼ tsp. salt and thyme; cook, covered, until potatoes are almost tender, 4-5 minutes, stirring occasionally. Stir in spinach 2-3 minutes or just until wilted.

2 With the back of a spoon, make 4 wells in potato mixture. Break an egg into each well. Sprinkle eggs with pepper and remaining salt. Cook, covered, on medium-low 5-7 minutes or until egg whites are completely set and yolks begin to thicken but are not hard.

1 SERVING *224 cal., 11g fat (5g sat. fat), 201mg chol., 433mg sod., 24g carb. (10g sugars, 3g fiber), 8g pro.* ***Diabetic exchanges:*** *1½ starch, 1½ fat, 1 medium-fat meat*

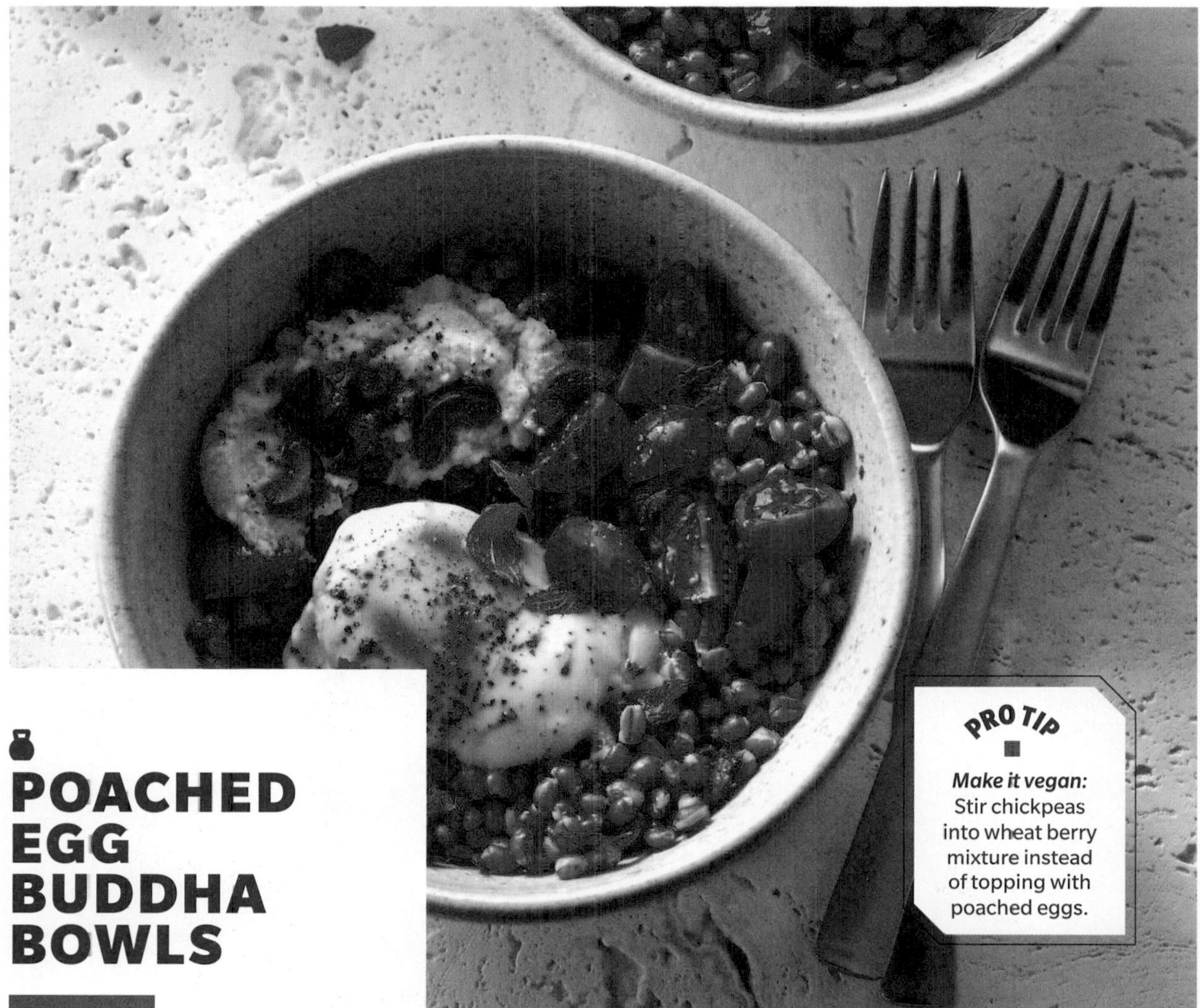

PRO TIP

Make it vegan: Stir chickpeas into wheat berry mixture instead of topping with poached eggs.

POACHED EGG BUDDHA BOWLS

PREP: 10 min.
COOK: 65 min.
MAKES: 2 servings

- ¾ cup wheat berries
- 2 Tbsp. olive oil
- 2 Tbsp. lemon juice
- 1 Tbsp. thinly sliced fresh mint leaves
- ¼ tsp. salt
- ⅛ tsp. freshly ground pepper
- ½ cup quartered cherry tomatoes
- ½ cup reduced-fat ricotta or vegan ricotta-style cheese
- 2 Tbsp. sliced Greek olives
- 2 large eggs

1 Place wheat berries and 2½ cups water in a large saucepan; bring to a boil. Reduce heat; simmer, covered, until tender, about 1 hour. Drain; transfer to a bowl. Cool slightly.

2 Stir in oil, lemon juice, mint, salt and pepper; divide between 2 bowls. Top with the tomatoes, ricotta cheese and olives.

3 To poach each egg, place ½ cup water in a small microwave-safe bowl or glass measuring cup. Break egg into water. Microwave, covered, on high for 1 minute. Microwave in 10-second intervals until white is set and yolk begins to thicken; let stand 1 minute.

4 Using a slotted spoon, transfer egg to 1 of the bowls. Repeat. If desired, drizzle with additional olive oil and sprinkle with more pepper.

1 BOWL *526 cal., 24g fat (5g sat. fat), 201mg chol., 563mg sod., 58g carb. (5g sugars, 10g fiber), 21g pro.*

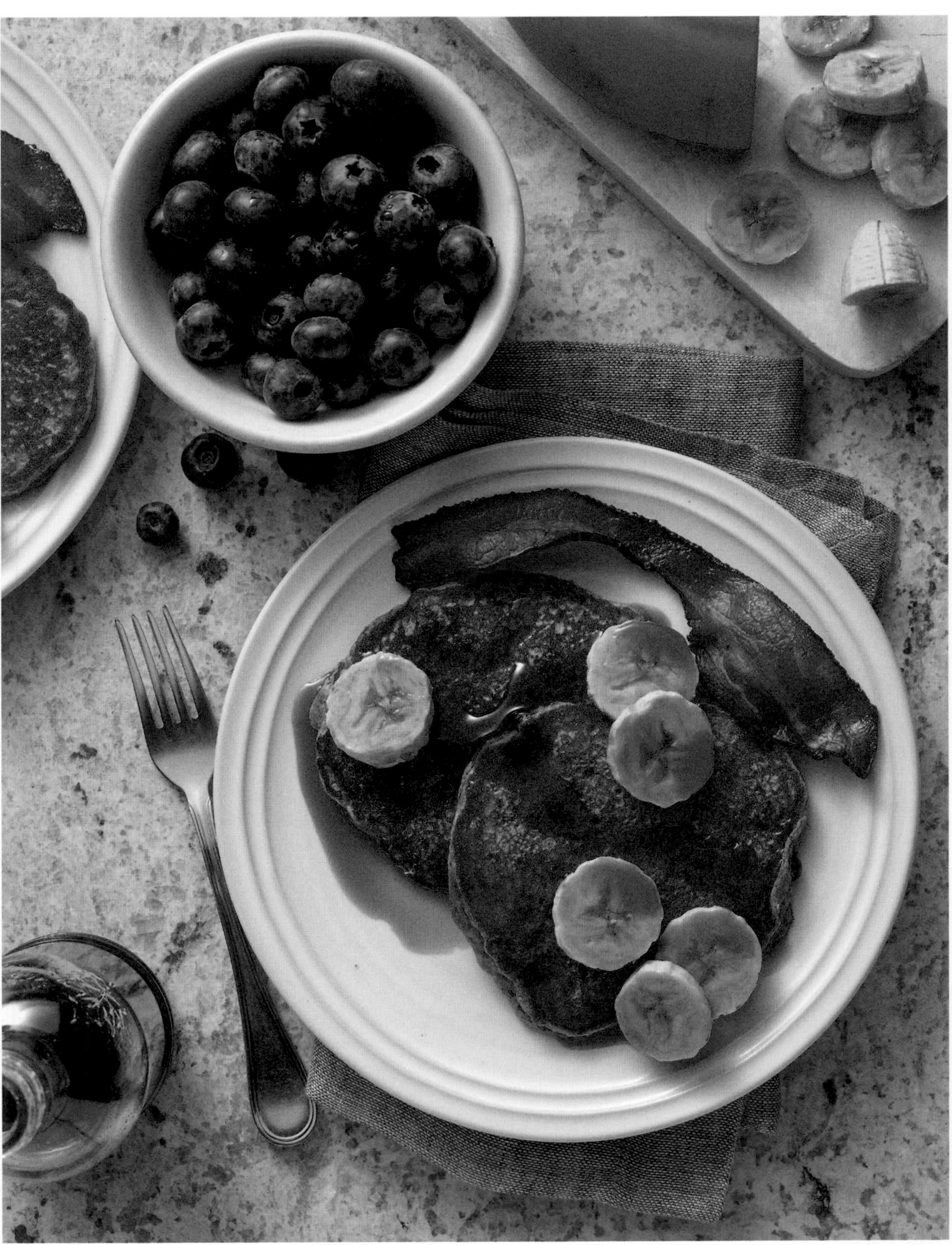

BANANA BLUEBERRY PANCAKES

PREP: 15 min. **COOK:** 5 min./batch **MAKES:** 14 pancakes

- 1 cup whole wheat flour
- ½ cup all-purpose flour
- 2 Tbsp. sugar
- 2 tsp. baking powder
- ½ tsp. salt
- 1 large egg, room temperature, lightly beaten, or vegan egg substitute
- 1¼ cups fat-free milk or milk alternative
- 3 medium ripe bananas, mashed
- 1 tsp. vanilla extract
- 1½ cups fresh or frozen blueberries
- Optional: Maple syrup and sliced bananas

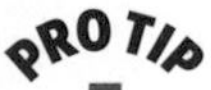

To make a vegan egg substitute, combine 1 Tbsp. ground flaxseed with 3 Tbsp. water; let stand 5 minutes to thicken.

1 In a large bowl, combine the flours, sugar, baking powder and salt. In a second bowl, combine egg, milk, bananas and vanilla; stir into the dry ingredients just until moistened.

2 Pour batter by ¼ cupfuls onto a hot griddle coated with cooking spray; sprinkle with blueberries. (If using frozen blueberries, do not thaw.) Turn when bubbles form on top; cook until second side is golden brown. If desired, serve pancakes with syrup and sliced bananas.

TO FREEZE Freeze cooled pancakes between layers of waxed paper in a resealable freezer container. To use, place the pancakes on an ungreased baking sheet, cover with foil, and reheat in a preheated 375° oven for 6-10 minutes. Or, place a stack of 3 pancakes on a microwave-safe plate and microwave on high 1¼-1½ minutes or until heated through.

2 PANCAKES *195 cal., 2g fat (0 sat. fat), 31mg chol., 317mg sod., 41g carb. (19g sugars, 4g fiber), 6g pro.* ***Diabetic exchanges:*** *1½ starch, 1 fruit*

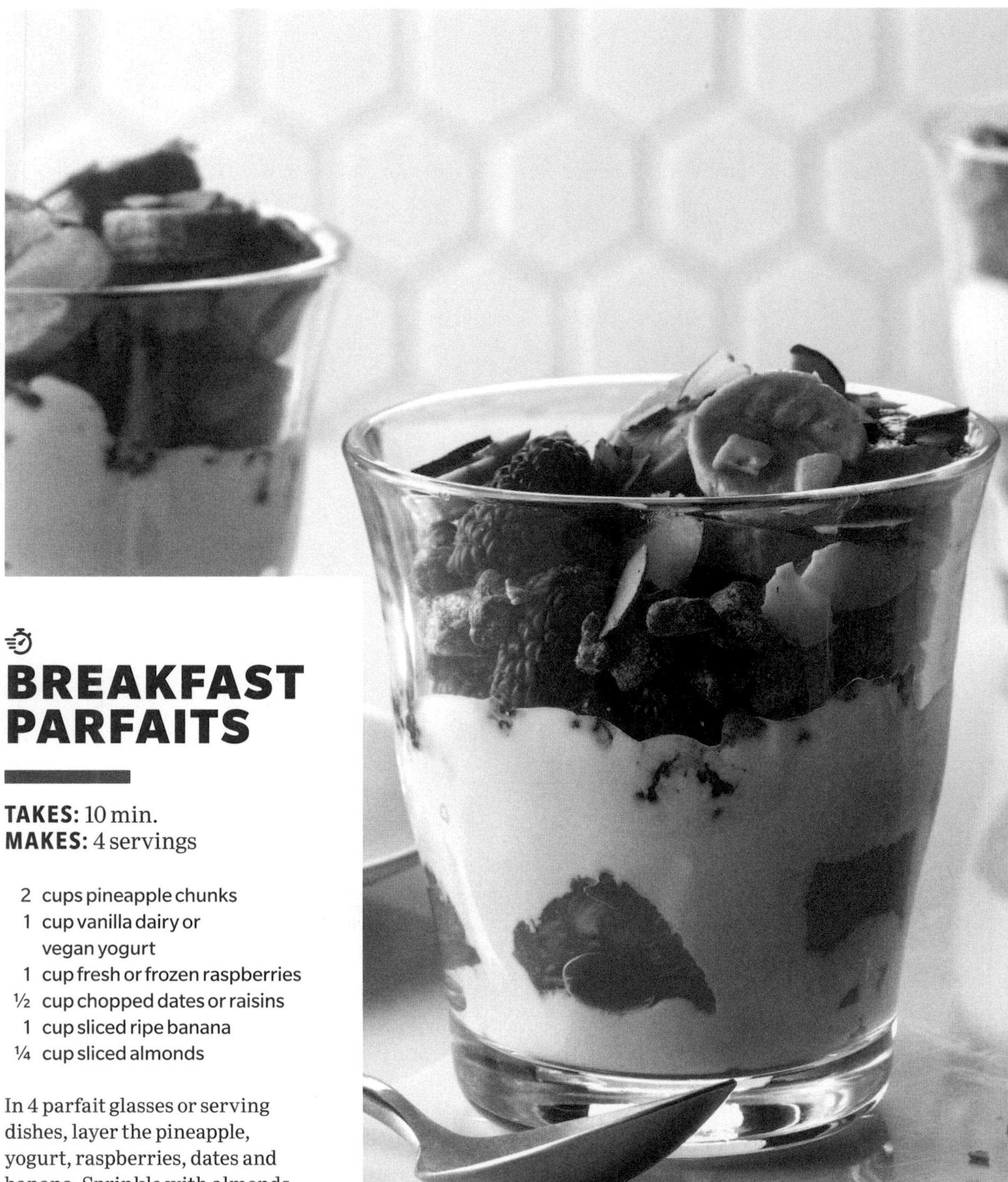

BREAKFAST PARFAITS

TAKES: 10 min.
MAKES: 4 servings

- 2 cups pineapple chunks
- 1 cup vanilla dairy or vegan yogurt
- 1 cup fresh or frozen raspberries
- ½ cup chopped dates or raisins
- 1 cup sliced ripe banana
- ¼ cup sliced almonds

In 4 parfait glasses or serving dishes, layer the pineapple, yogurt, raspberries, dates and banana. Sprinkle with almonds. Serve immediately.

1 PARFAIT *277 cal., 4g fat (1g sat. fat), 3mg chol., 52mg sod., 60g carb. (48g sugars, 6g fiber), 5g pro.*

TROPICAL SMOOTHIE BOWLS

TAKES: 10 min.
MAKES: 2 servings

- 2 Tbsp. frozen orange juice concentrate, thawed
- ¾ cup peeled fresh or frozen mango chunks, thawed
- ¾ cup (½ lb.) fresh or frozen pineapple cubes
- ¼ cup quick-cooking oats
- ¼ cup vanilla soy or whey protein powder
- 2 Tbsp. ground flaxseed
- ¼ tsp. ground cinnamon
- ¼ tsp. ground nutmeg
- 1 cup cold water
- Optional toppings: Granola, chopped mango and pineapple

Place orange juice concentrate in a blender. Add fruit, oats, protein powder, flax, seasonings and water. Cover and process until smooth. If desired, add optional toppings. Serve immediately.

1¼ CUPS *239 cal., 5g fat (1g sat. fat), 5mg chol., 70mg sod., 43g carb. (28g sugars, 6g fiber), 10g pro.*

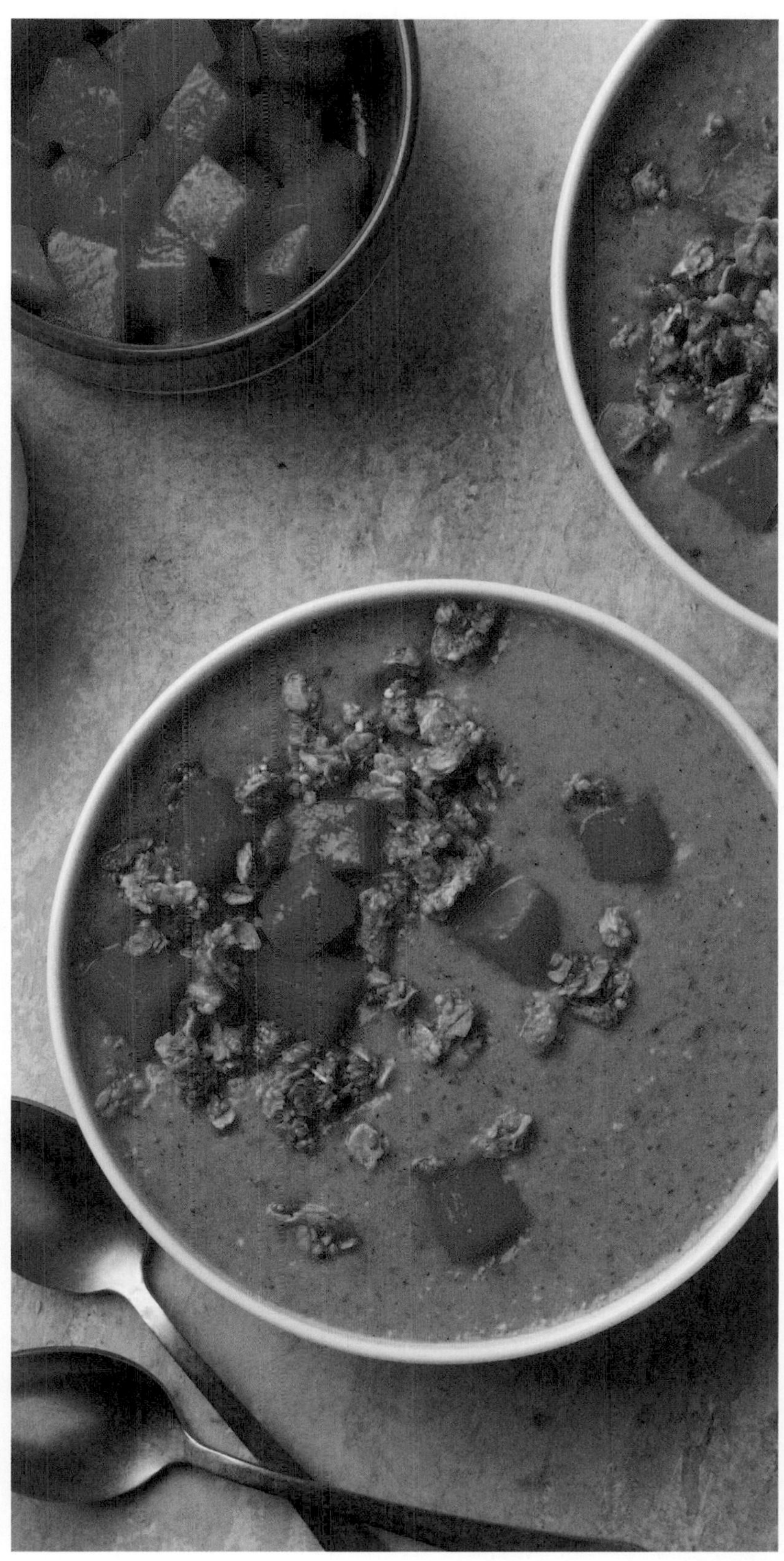

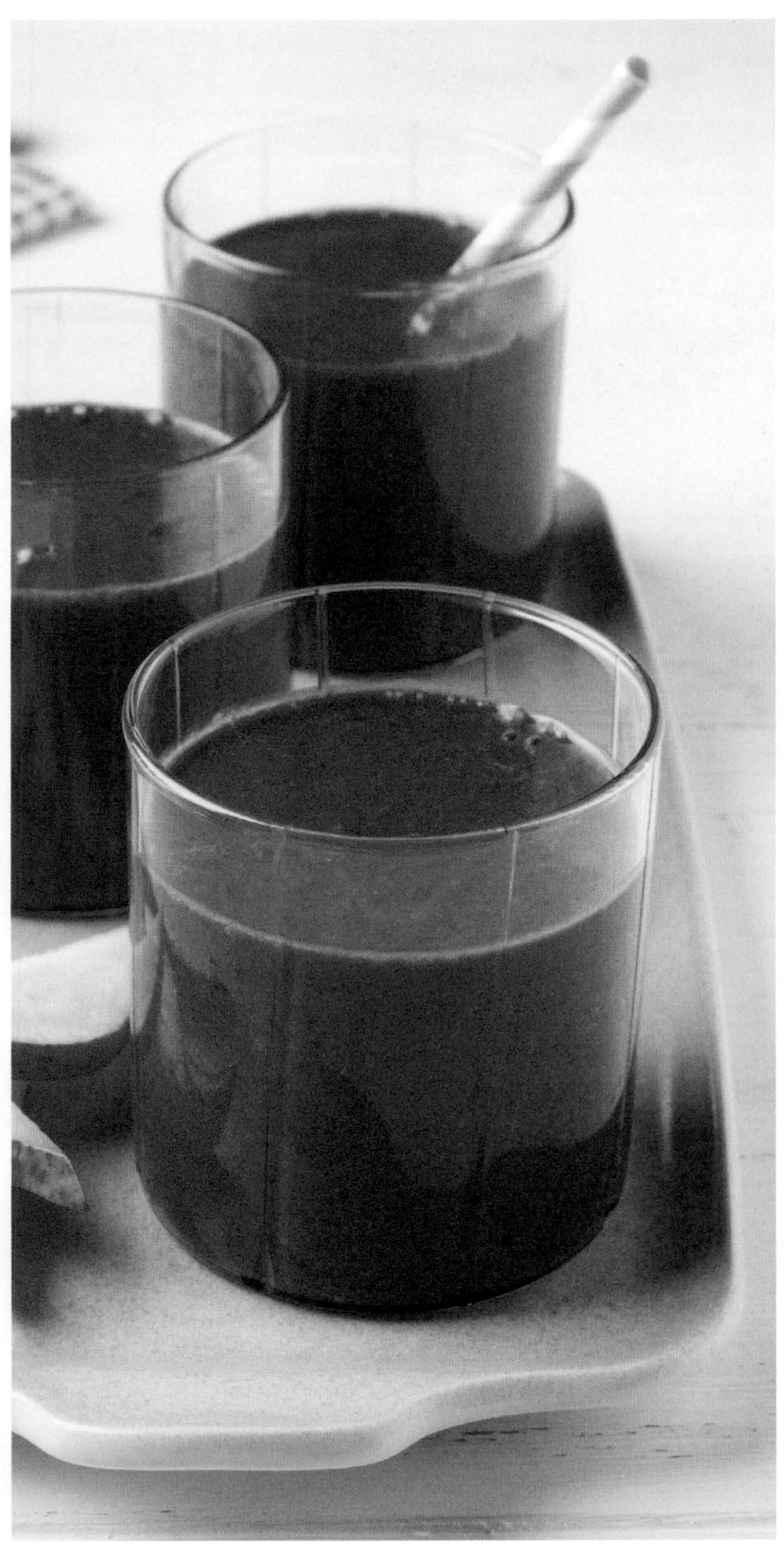

KALE SMOOTHIE

TAKES: 15 min.
MAKES: 4 servings

- 1 small bunch kale, chopped
- 1 medium pear, chopped
- 1 cup frozen sweetened mixed berries
- 1 medium banana, halved
- 1 cup unsweetened almond milk
- ½ cup low-fat vanilla almond milk yogurt
- 3 Tbsp. agave nectar

In a large bowl, mix kale and fruits. Pour in almond milk, yogurt and agave nectar; stir to combine. Process in batches in a blender until smooth. Serve immediately or refrigerate.

1 CUP *184 cal., 3g fat (0 sat. fat), 0 chol., 86mg sod., 40g carb. (23g sugars, 6g fiber), 4g pro.*

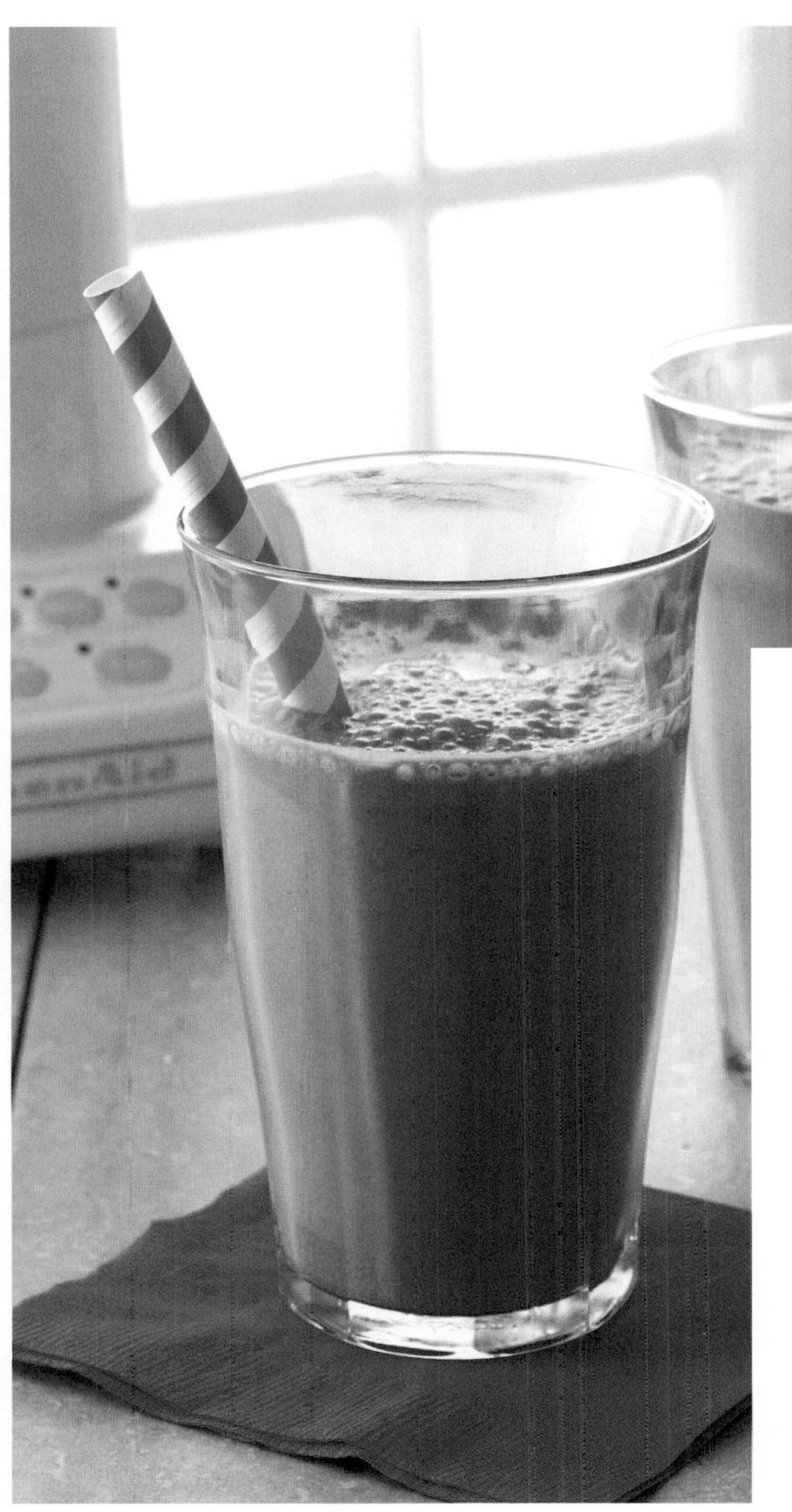

BERRY-CARROT SMOOTHIE

TAKES: 5 min.
MAKES: 5 servings

- 2 cups reduced-fat plain dairy or vegan Greek yogurt
- 1 cup carrot juice
- 1 cup orange juice
- 1 cup frozen pineapple chunks
- 1 cup frozen unsweetened sliced strawberries

Place all ingredients in a blender; cover and process until smooth.

1 CUP *141 cal., 2g fat (1g sat. fat), 5mg chol., 79mg sod., 20g carb. (15g sugars, 1g fiber), 10g pro.* ***Diabetic exchanges:*** *1 fruit, ½ reduced-fat milk*

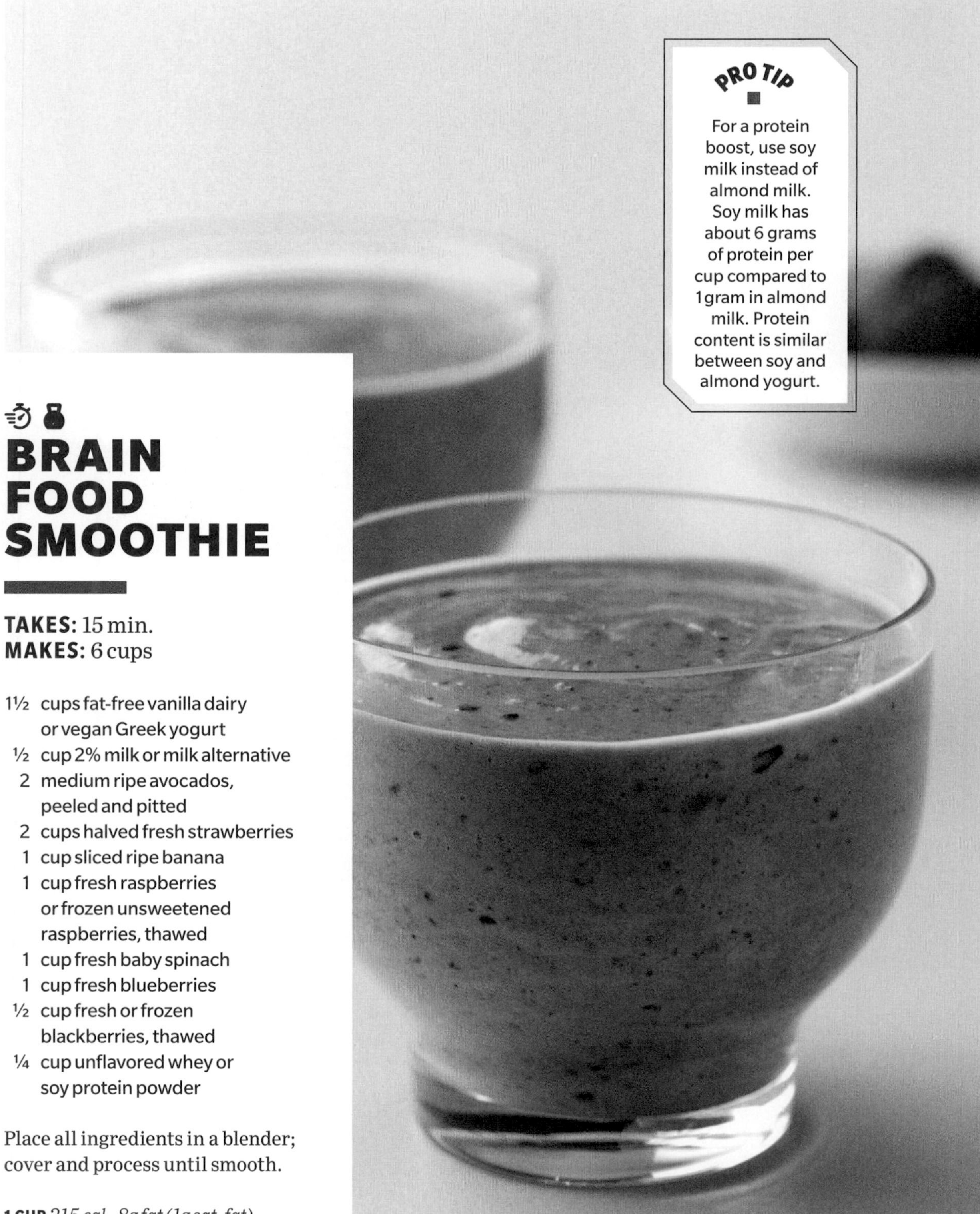

PRO TIP

For a protein boost, use soy milk instead of almond milk. Soy milk has about 6 grams of protein per cup compared to 1 gram in almond milk. Protein content is similar between soy and almond yogurt.

BRAIN FOOD SMOOTHIE

TAKES: 15 min.
MAKES: 6 cups

- 1½ cups fat-free vanilla dairy or vegan Greek yogurt
- ½ cup 2% milk or milk alternative
- 2 medium ripe avocados, peeled and pitted
- 2 cups halved fresh strawberries
- 1 cup sliced ripe banana
- 1 cup fresh raspberries or frozen unsweetened raspberries, thawed
- 1 cup fresh baby spinach
- 1 cup fresh blueberries
- ½ cup fresh or frozen blackberries, thawed
- ¼ cup unflavored whey or soy protein powder

Place all ingredients in a blender; cover and process until smooth.

1 CUP *215 cal., 8g fat (1g sat. fat), 3mg chol., 65mg sod., 29g carb. (17g sugars, 7g fiber), 10g pro.*

BLUEBERRY PANCAKE SMOOTHIE

TAKES: 5 min.
MAKES: 2 servings

- 1 cup unsweetened almond milk
- 1 medium banana
- ½ cup frozen unsweetened blueberries
- ¼ cup instant plain oatmeal
- 1 tsp. maple syrup
- ½ tsp. ground cinnamon
- Dash sea salt

Place the first 6 ingredients in a blender; cover and process until smooth. Pour into 2 chilled glasses; sprinkle with sea salt. Serve immediately.

1 CUP *153 cal., 3g fat (0 sat. fat), 0 chol., 191mg sod., 31g carb. (13g sugars, 5g fiber), 3g pro.* ***Diabetic exchanges:*** *2 starch*

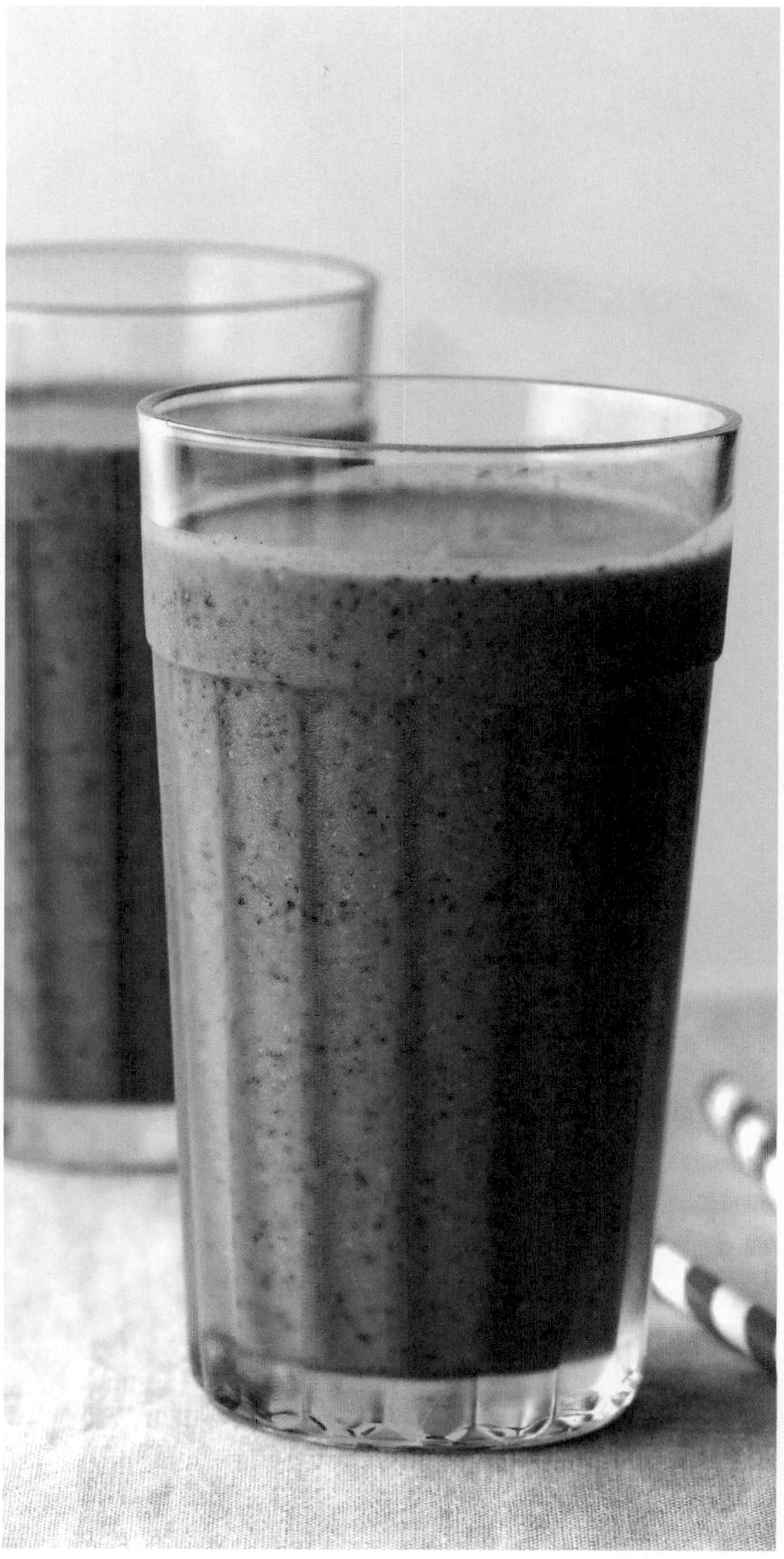

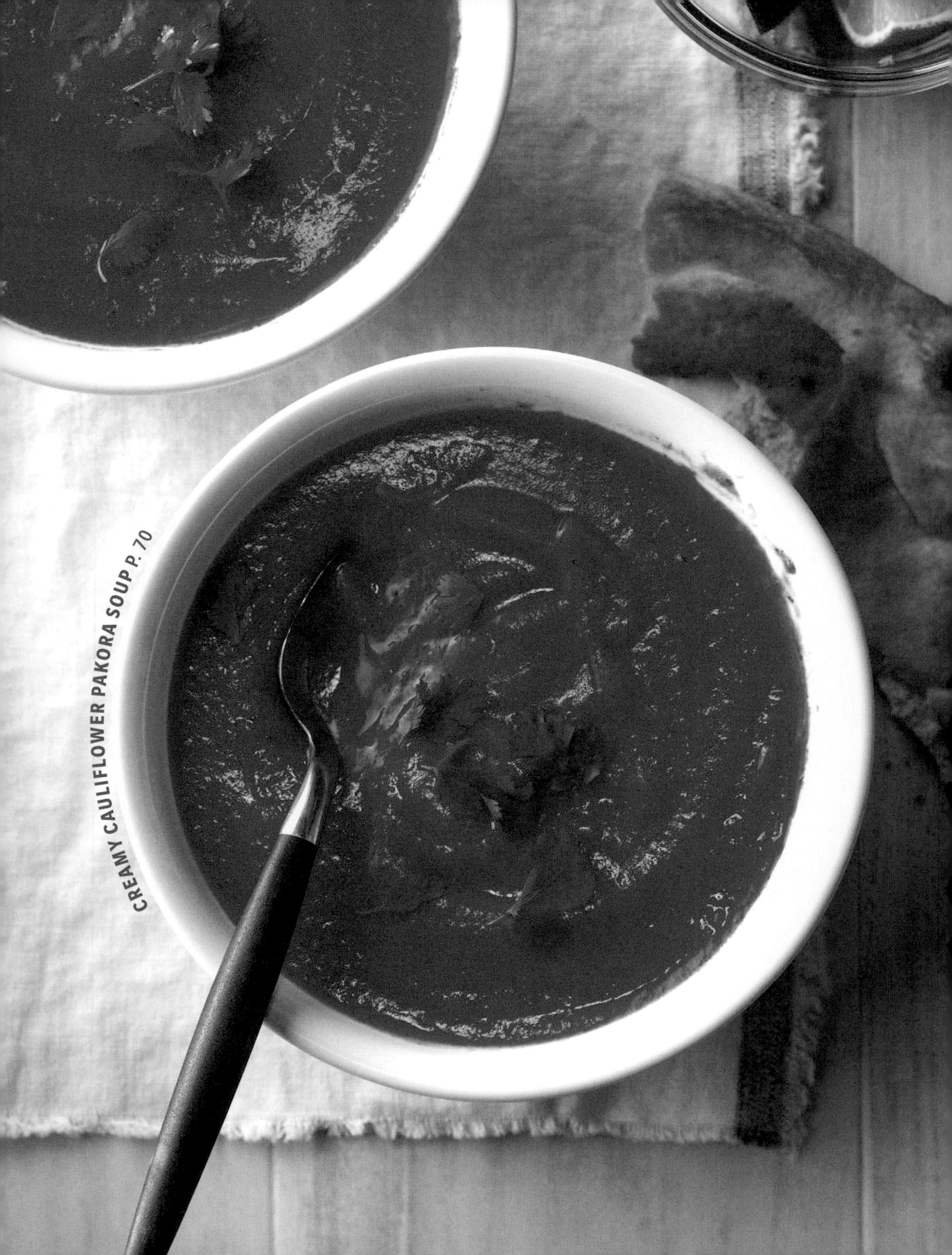

CREAMY CAULIFLOWER PAKORA SOUP P. 70

CHAPTER 5

SOUPS, STEWS & CHILIS

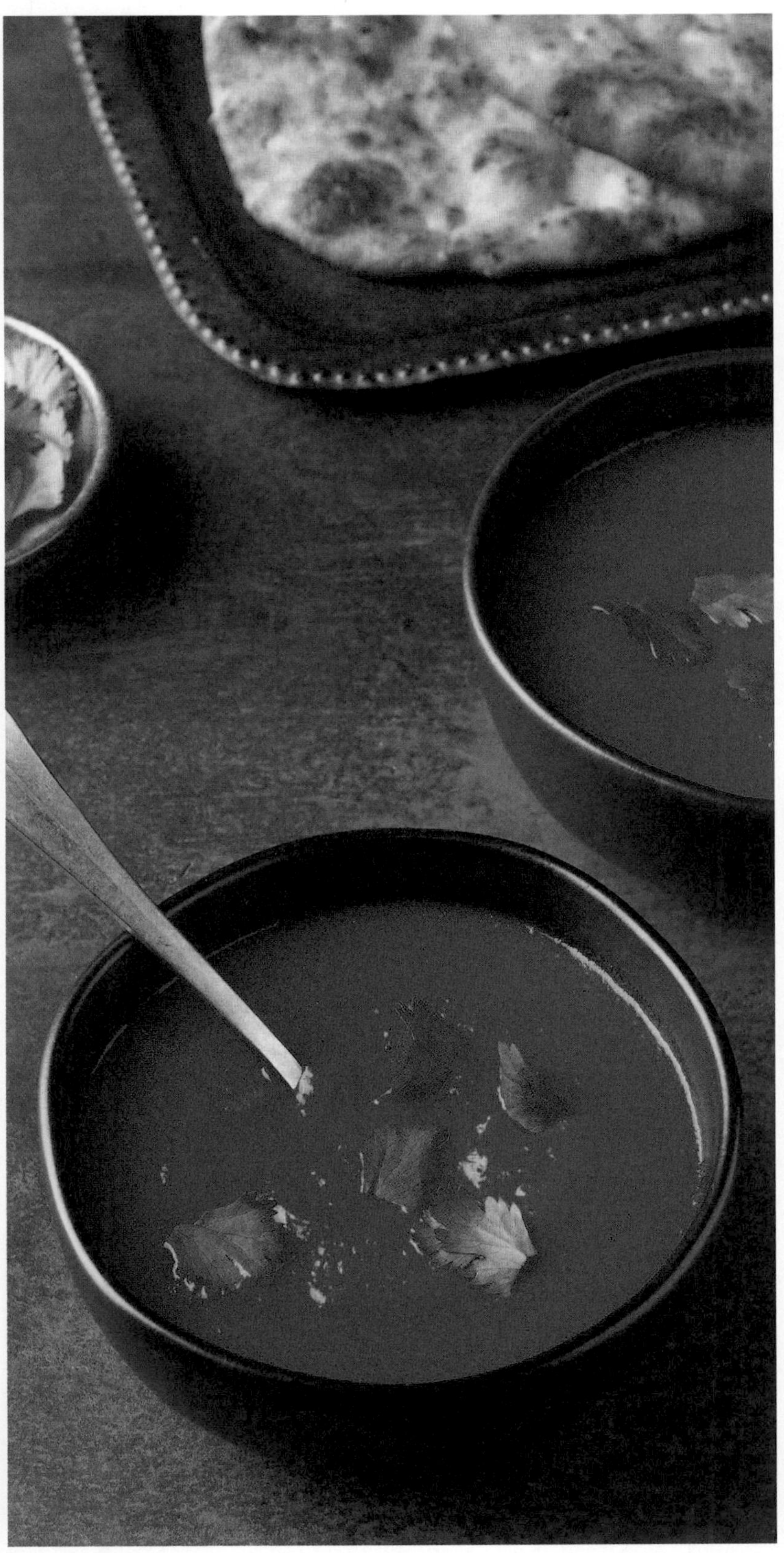

QUICK CARROT SOUP

TAKES: 30 min.
MAKES: 6 servings

- 1 medium onion, chopped
- 2 celery ribs, chopped
- 1 Tbsp. canola oil
- 4 cups vegetable broth
- 1 lb. carrots, sliced
- 2 large Yukon Gold potatoes, peeled and cubed
- 1 tsp. salt
- ¼ tsp. pepper
- Fresh cilantro leaves, optional

1 In a large saucepan, saute onion and celery in oil until tender. Add the broth, carrots and potatoes; bring to a boil. Reduce heat; cover and simmer for 15-20 minutes or until the vegetables are tender. Remove from heat; cool slightly.

2 Transfer to a blender; cover and process until blended. Return to pan; stir in salt and pepper. Heat through. If desired, sprinkle with cilantro.

1 CUP *176 cal., 3g fat (0 sat. fat), 0 chol., 710mg sod., 35g carb. (7g sugars, 4g fiber), 4g pro.* ***Diabetic exchanges:*** *2 starch, ½ fat*

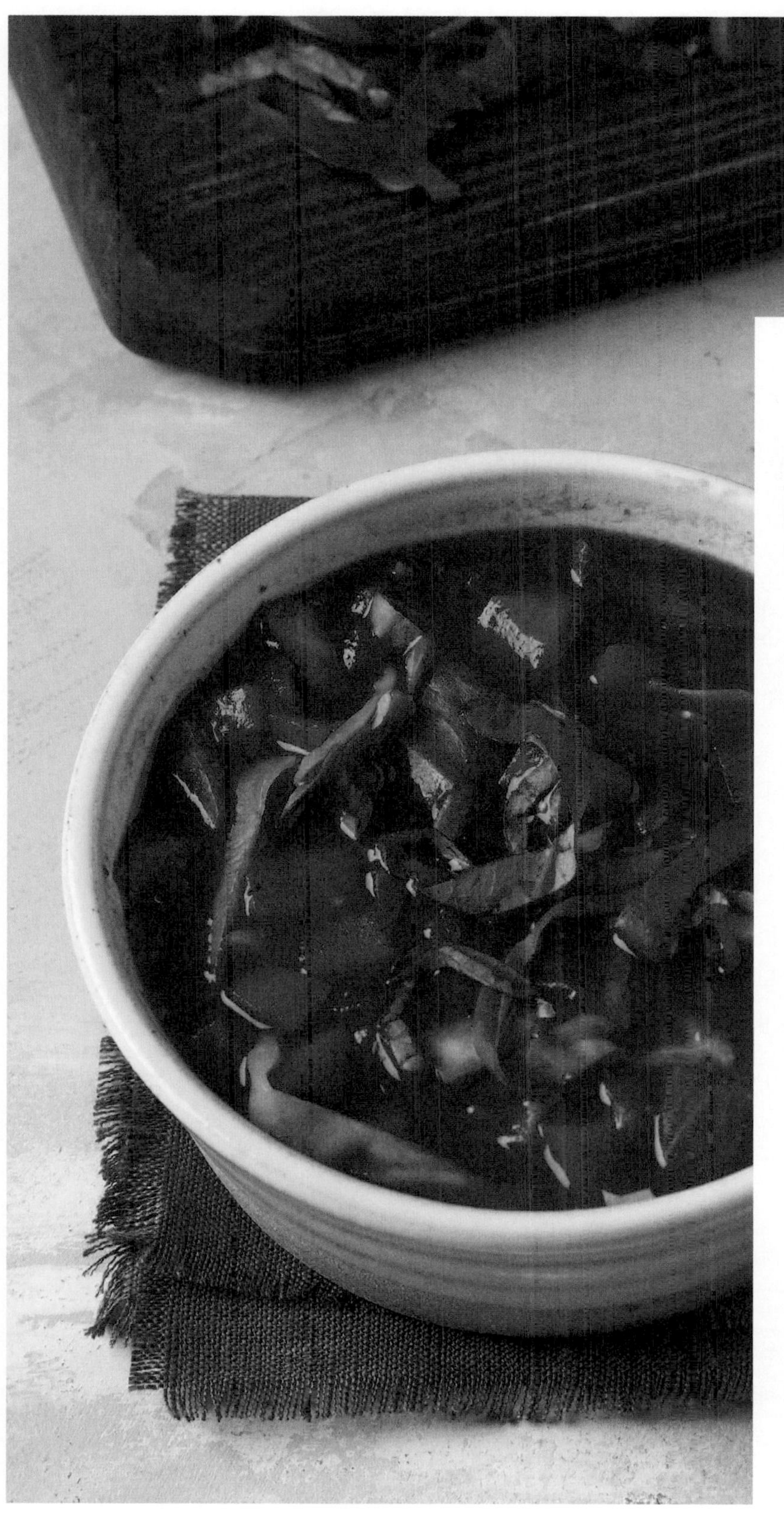

ITALIAN CABBAGE SOUP

PREP: 15 min.
COOK: 6 hours
MAKES: 10 servings (2½ qt.)

- 4 cups vegetable stock
- 1 can (14 oz.) Italian diced tomatoes
- 1 can (6 oz.) tomato paste
- 1 small head cabbage (about 1½ lbs.), shredded
- 4 celery ribs, chopped
- 2 large carrots, chopped
- 1 medium onion, chopped
- 2 garlic cloves, minced
- 2 tsp. Italian seasoning
- ½ tsp. salt
- Fresh basil, optional

In a 5- or 6-qt. slow cooker, whisk together vegetable stock, diced tomatoes and tomato paste. Stir in the vegetables, garlic, Italian seasoning and salt. Cook, covered, on low until vegetables are tender, 6-8 hours. If desired, top with fresh basil.

1 CUP *110 cal., 0 fat (0 sat. fat), 0 chol., 866mg sod., 24g carb. (13g sugars, 6g fiber), 4g pro.*

CREAM OF BROCCOLI SOUP

PREP: 20 min. **COOK:** 25 min. **MAKES:** 8 servings (2 qt.)

- 3 medium onions, chopped
- 2 celery ribs, chopped
- 2 Tbsp. canola oil
- 4 cups plus ½ cup vegetable broth
- 4 medium russet potatoes, peeled and cubed (about 4 cups)
- 6 cups chopped fresh broccoli (about 3 small heads)
- 1 tsp. salt
- ¼ tsp. pepper

1 In a large saucepan, saute onions and celery in oil until tender. Add 4 cups broth and potatoes; bring to a boil. Reduce the heat; cover and simmer for 15-20 minutes or until potatoes are tender.

2 Cool slightly. In a blender, process soup in batches until smooth. Return to pan; add the remaining broth and bring to a boil. Add broccoli, salt and pepper. Reduce heat; simmer, uncovered, 8-10 minutes or until broccoli is tender.

1 CUP *142 cal., 4g fat (0 sat. fat), 0 chol., 409mg sod., 24g carb. (5g sugars, 4g fiber), 4g pro.* ***Diabetic exchanges:*** *1½ starch, 1 vegetable, ½ fat*

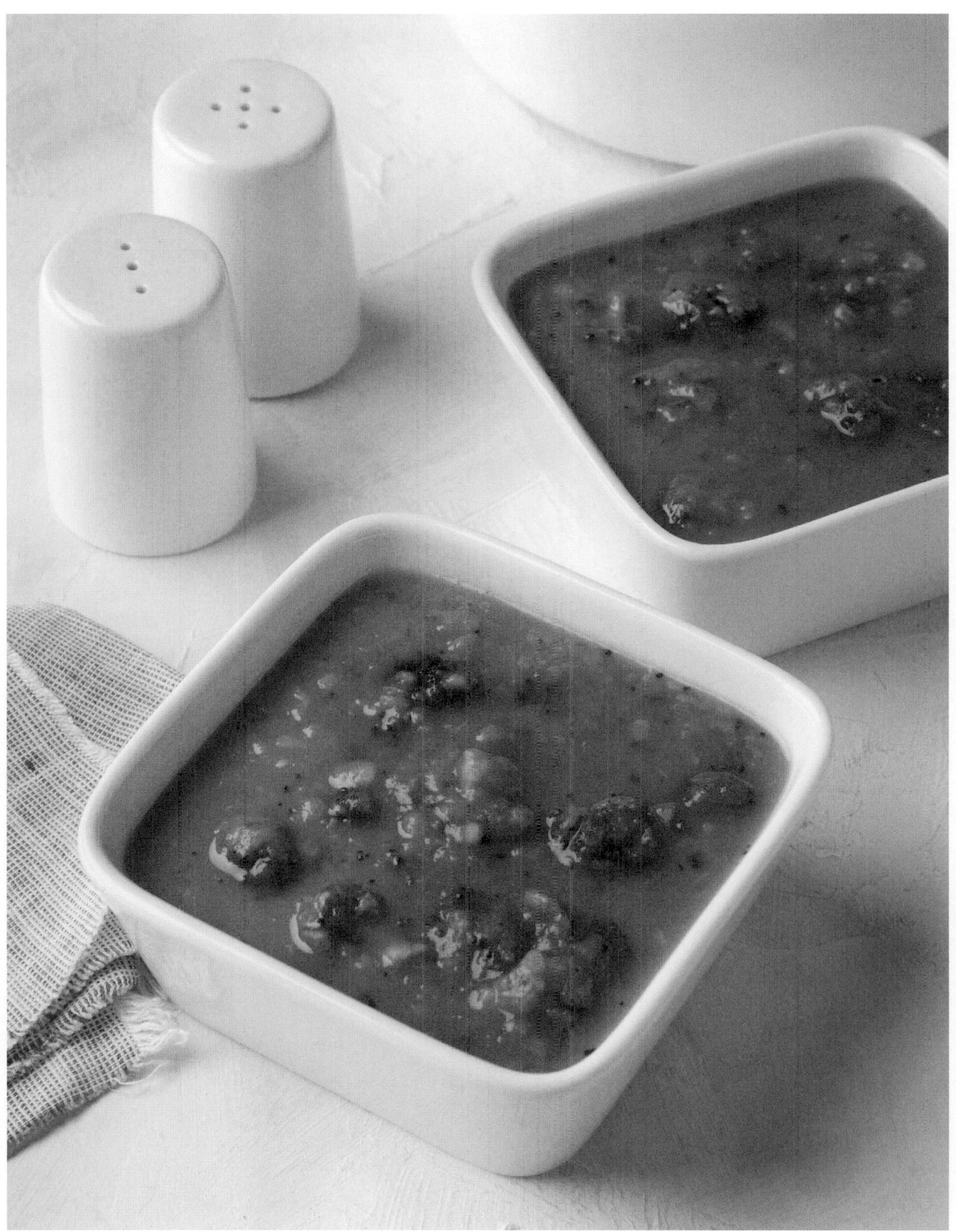

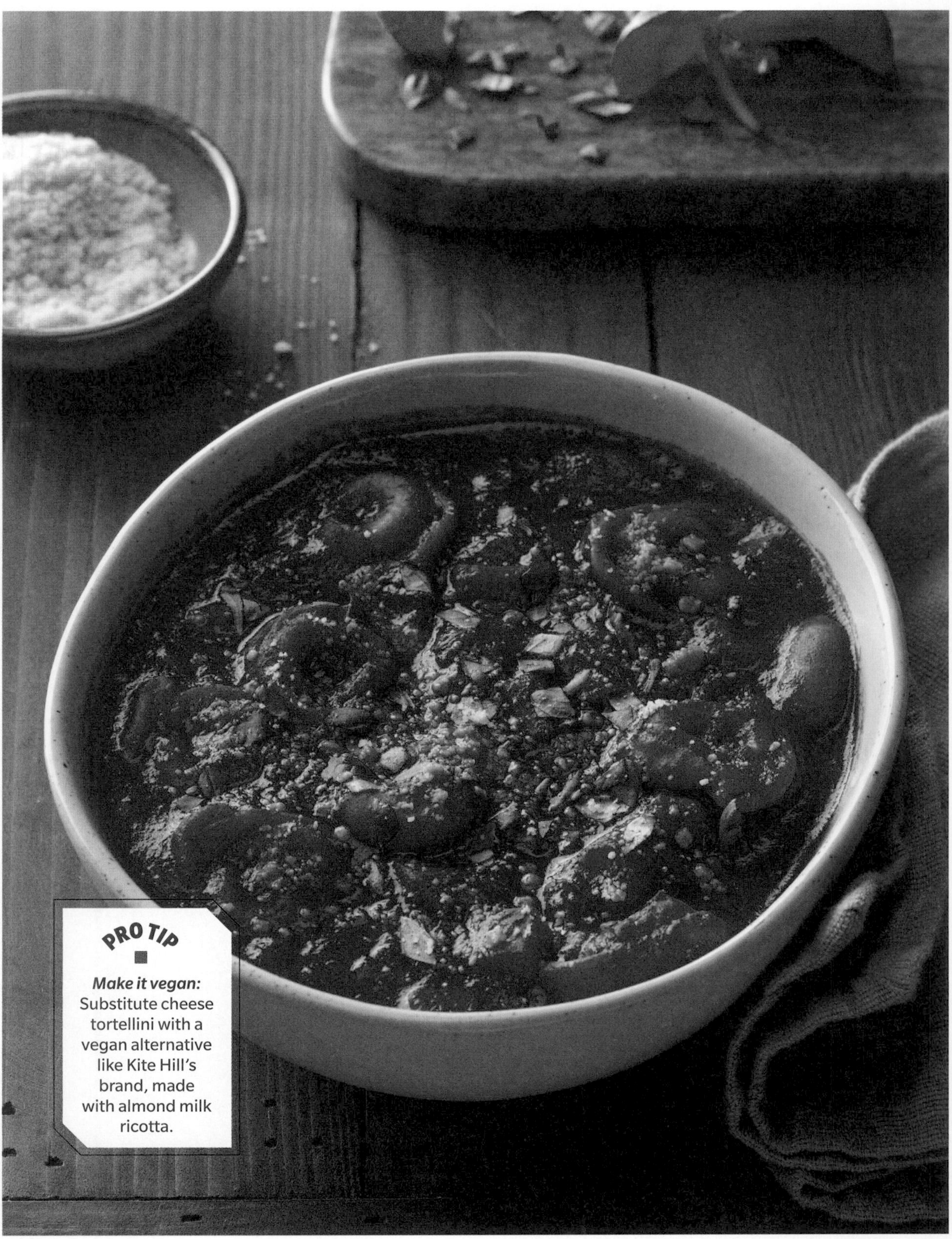

PRO TIP

Make it vegan: Substitute cheese tortellini with a vegan alternative like Kite Hill's brand, made with almond milk ricotta.

TOMATO BASIL TORTELLINI SOUP

PREP: 25 min. **COOK:** 6¼ hours **MAKES:** 18 servings (4½ qt.)

- 2 Tbsp. olive oil
- 1 medium onion, chopped
- 3 medium carrots, chopped
- 5 garlic cloves, minced
- 3 cans (28 oz. each) crushed tomatoes, undrained
- 1 carton (32 oz.) vegetable broth
- 1 Tbsp. sugar
- 1 tsp. dried basil
- 1 bay leaf
- 3 pkg. (9 oz. each) refrigerated dairy or vegan cheese tortellini
- ¾ cup dairy or vegan half-and-half cream
- Shredded Parmesan or vegan Parmesan-style cheese
- Minced fresh basil

1 In a large skillet, heat oil over medium-high heat. Add onion and carrots; cook and stir until crisp-tender, 5-6 minutes. Add garlic; cook 1 minute longer. Transfer to a 6- or 7-qt. slow cooker. Add the tomatoes, broth, sugar, basil and bay leaf. Cook, covered, on low until vegetables are tender, 6-7 hours.

2 Stir in tortellini. Cook, covered, on high 15 minutes. Reduce heat to low; stir in cream until heated through. Discard bay leaf. Serve with Parmesan cheese and basil.

TO FREEZE Before stirring in half-and-half, cool soup and freeze in freezer containers. To use, partially thaw in refrigerator overnight. Heat through in a saucepan, stirring occasionally; add half-and-half as directed.

1 CUP *214 cal., 7g fat (3g sat. fat), 23mg chol., 569mg sod., 32g carb. (9g sugars, 4g fiber), 9g pro.* ***Diabetic exchanges:*** *2 starch, 1 fat*

CREAMY CAULIFLOWER PAKORA SOUP

PREP: 20 min. **COOK:** 20 min. **MAKES:** 8 servings (3 qt.)

- 1 large head cauliflower, cut into small florets
- 5 medium potatoes, peeled and diced
- 1 large onion, diced
- 4 medium carrots, peeled and diced
- 2 celery ribs, diced
- 1 carton (32 oz.) vegetable stock
- 1 tsp. garam masala
- 1 tsp. garlic powder
- 1 tsp. ground coriander
- 1 tsp. ground turmeric
- 1 tsp. ground cumin
- 1 tsp. pepper
- 1 tsp. salt
- ½ tsp. crushed red pepper flakes
- Water or additional vegetable stock
- Fresh cilantro leaves
- Lime wedges, optional

In a Dutch oven over medium-high heat, combine the first 14 ingredients; bring to a boil. Cook and stir until vegetables are tender, about 20 minutes. Remove from heat; cool slightly. Process in batches in a blender or food processor until smooth. Adjust consistency as desired with water or additional stock. Sprinkle with fresh cilantro. Serve the soup hot, with lime wedges if desired.

TO FREEZE Before adding cilantro, freeze the cooled soup in freezer containers. To use, partially thaw soup in refrigerator overnight. Heat through in a saucepan, stirring occasionally; add water if necessary. Sprinkle with fresh cilantro. If desired, serve with lime wedges.

1½ CUPS *135 cal., 1g fat (0 sat. fat), 0 chol., 645mg sod., 30g carb. (6g sugars, 5g fiber), 4g pro.* ***Diabetic exchanges:*** *1½ starch, 1 vegetable*

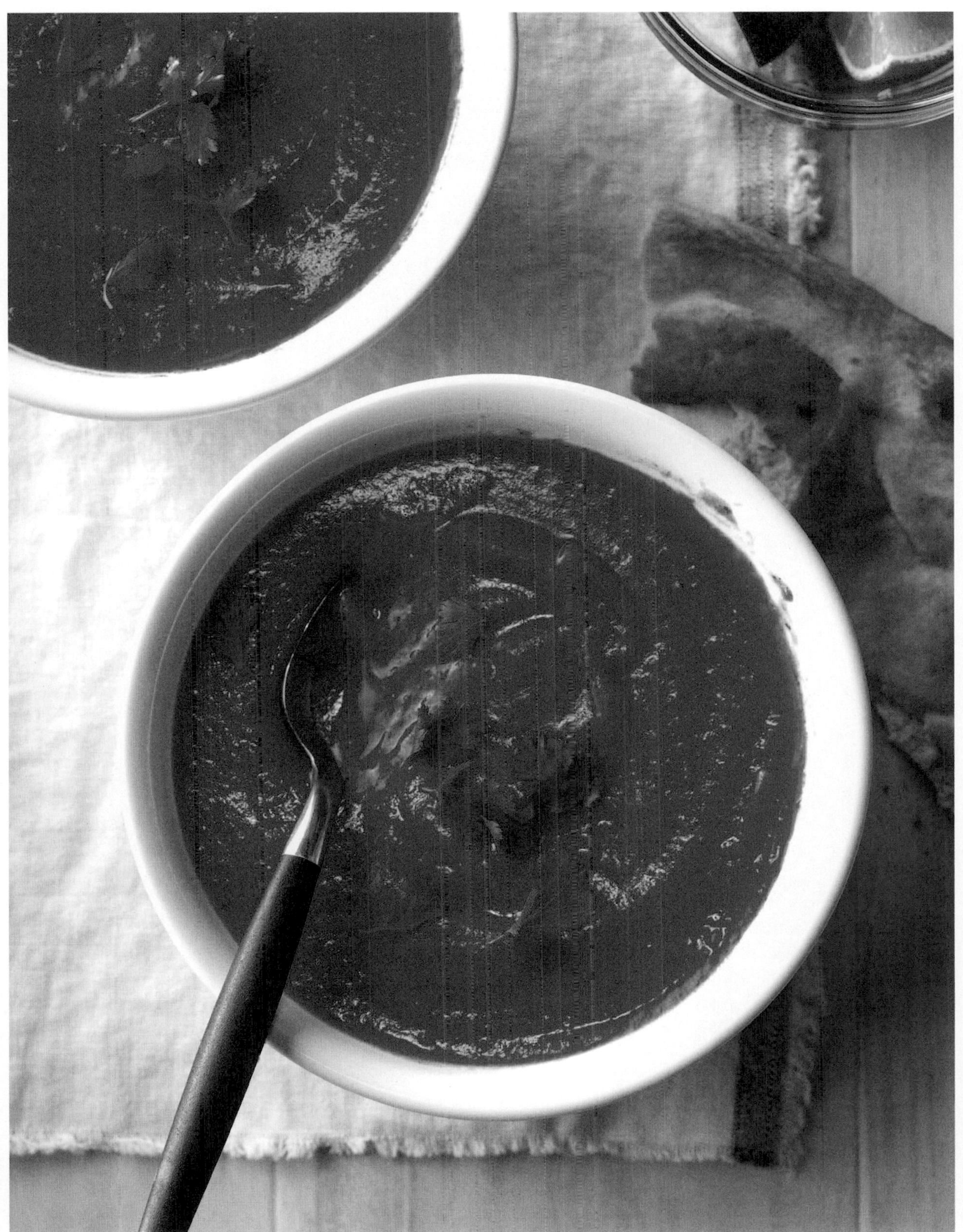

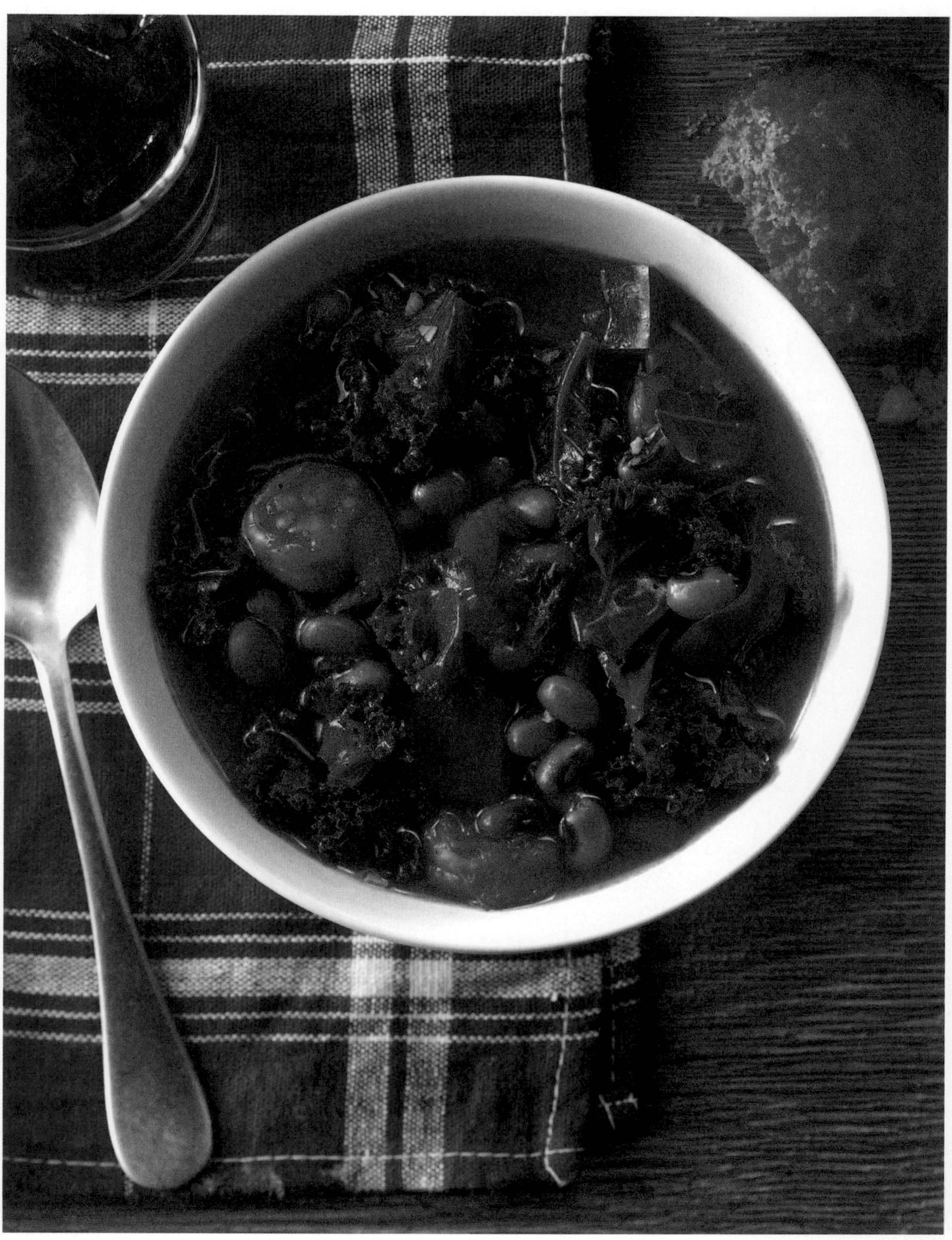

CAROLINA SHRIMP SOUP

TAKES: 25 min. **MAKES:** 6 servings

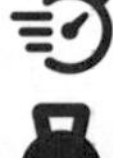

- 4 tsp. olive oil, divided
- 1 lb. uncooked shrimp (31-40 per lb.), peeled and deveined
- 5 garlic cloves, minced
- 1 bunch kale, trimmed and coarsely chopped (about 16 cups)
- 1 medium sweet red pepper, cut into ¾-in. pieces
- 3 cups reduced-sodium chicken or vegetable broth
- 1 can (15½ oz.) black-eyed peas, rinsed and drained
- ¼ tsp. salt
- ¼ tsp. pepper
- Minced fresh chives, optional

1 In a 6-qt. stockpot, heat 2 tsp. oil over medium-high heat. Add shrimp; cook and stir 2 minutes. Add garlic; cook just until shrimp turn pink, 1-2 minutes longer. Remove from pot.

2 In same pot, heat remaining oil over medium-high heat. Stir in the kale and red pepper; cook, covered, for 8-10 minutes or until the kale is tender, stirring occasionally. Add broth; bring to a boil. Stir in peas, salt, pepper and shrimp; heat through. If desired, sprinkle servings with minced chives.

1 CUP *188 cal., 5g fat (1g sat. fat), 92mg chol., 585mg sod., 18g carb. (2g sugars, 3g fiber), 19g pro.* ***Diabetic exchanges:*** *2 vegetable, 2 lean meat, ½ starch, ½ fat*

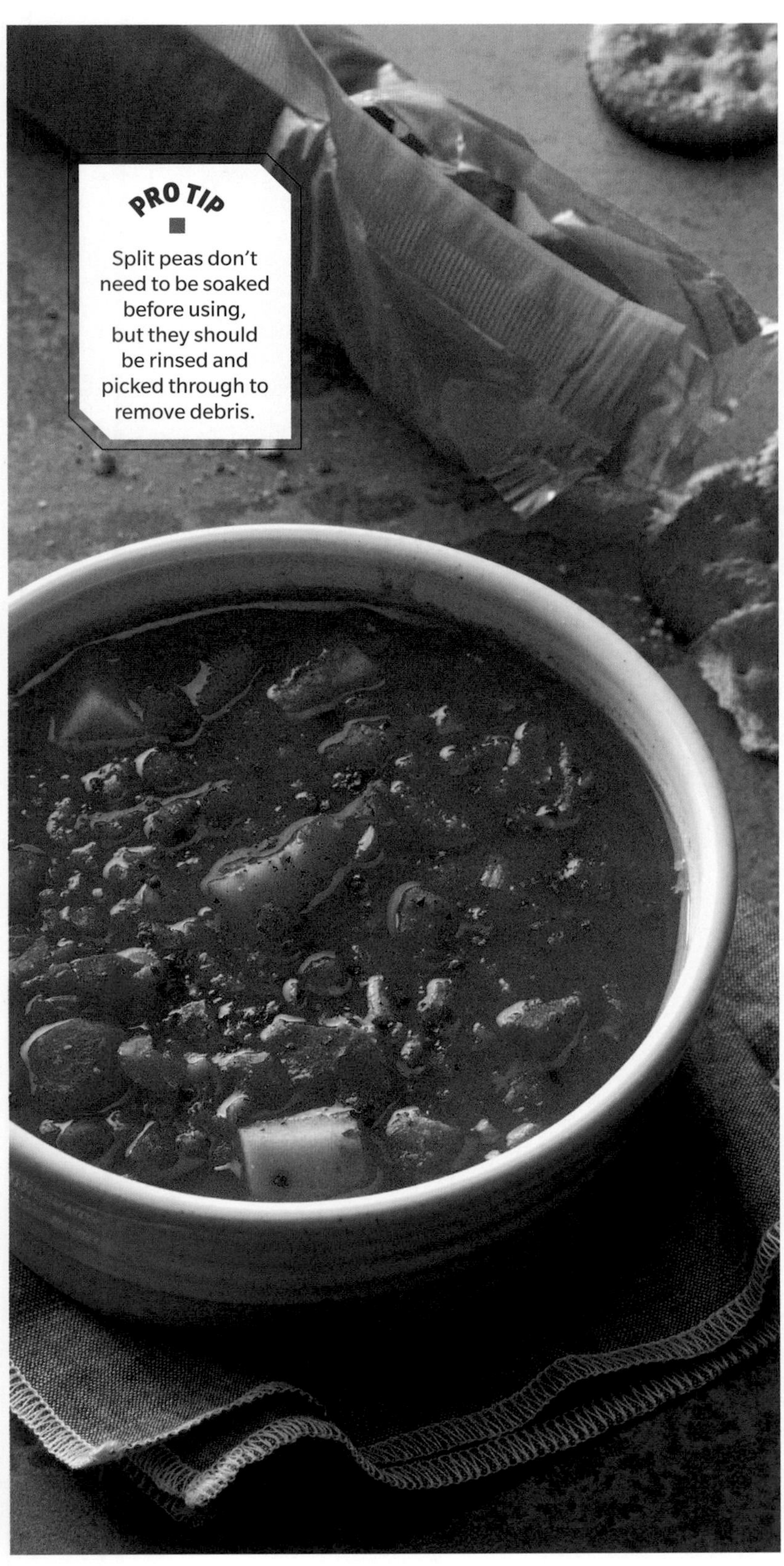

PRO TIP

Split peas don't need to be soaked before using, but they should be rinsed and picked through to remove debris.

CARROT SPLIT PEA SOUP

PREP: 15 min.
COOK: 7 hours
MAKES: 8 servings (2 qt.)

- 1 pkg. (16 oz.) dried green split peas, rinsed
- 1 medium leek (white portion only), chopped
- 3 celery ribs, chopped
- 1 medium potato, peeled and chopped
- 2 medium carrots, chopped
- 1 garlic clove, minced
- ¼ cup minced fresh parsley
- 2 cartons (32 oz. each) reduced-sodium vegetable broth
- 1½ tsp. ground mustard
- ½ tsp. pepper
- ½ tsp. dried oregano
- 1 bay leaf

In a 5-qt. slow cooker, combine all ingredients. Cover and cook on low for 7-8 hours or until the peas are tender. Discard bay leaf. Stir before serving.

1 CUP *248 cal., 1g fat (0 sat. fat), 0 chol., 702mg sod., 46g carb. (7g sugars, 16g fiber), 15g pro.*

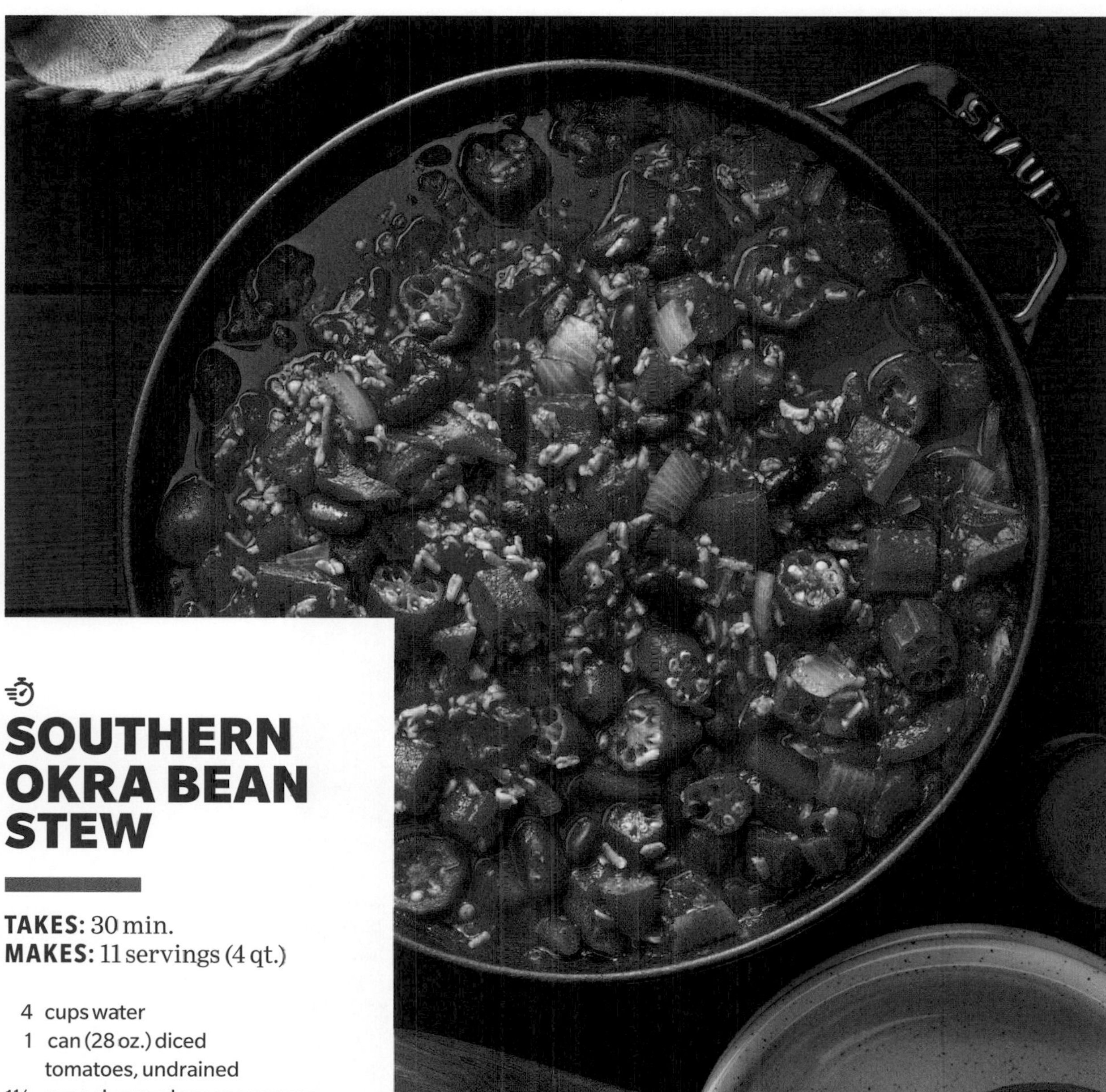

SOUTHERN OKRA BEAN STEW

TAKES: 30 min.
MAKES: 11 servings (4 qt.)

- 4 cups water
- 1 can (28 oz.) diced tomatoes, undrained
- 1½ cups chopped green peppers
- 1 large onion, chopped
- 3 garlic cloves, minced
- 1 tsp. Italian seasoning
- 1 tsp. chili powder
- ½ to 1 tsp. hot pepper sauce
- ¾ tsp. salt
- 1 bay leaf
- 4 cups cooked brown rice
- 2 cans (16 oz. each) kidney beans, rinsed and drained
- 3 cans (8 oz. each) tomato sauce
- 1 pkg. (16 oz.) frozen sliced okra

1 In a large Dutch oven or soup kettle, combine the first 10 ingredients. Bring to a boil. Reduce heat; simmer, uncovered, for 5 minutes.

2 Add the rice, beans, tomato sauce and sliced okra. Simmer, uncovered, for 8-10 minutes or until the vegetables are tender. Discard bay leaf.

1½ CUPS *198 cal., 1g fat (0 sat. fat), 0 chol., 926mg sod., 41g carb. (0 sugars, 7g fiber), 8g pro.*

PRESSURE-COOKER LENTIL STEW

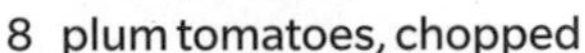

PREP: 45 min. **COOK:** 15 min. + releasing **MAKES:** 8 servings (2¾ qt.)

- 2 Tbsp. canola oil
- 2 large onions, thinly sliced, divided
- 8 plum tomatoes, chopped
- 2 Tbsp. minced fresh gingerroot
- 3 garlic cloves, minced
- 2 tsp. ground coriander
- 1½ tsp. ground cumin
- ¼ tsp. cayenne pepper
- 3 cups vegetable broth
- 2 cups dried lentils, rinsed
- 2 cups water
- 1 can (4 oz.) chopped green chiles
- ¾ cup dairy or vegan heavy whipping cream
- 2 Tbsp. butter or canola oil
- 1 tsp. cumin seeds
- 6 cups hot cooked basmati or jasmine rice
- Optional toppings: Sliced green onions or minced fresh cilantro

1 Select saute setting on a 6-qt. electric pressure cooker. Adjust for medium heat; add oil. When oil is hot, cook and stir half the onions 2-3 minutes or until crisp-tender. Add tomatoes, ginger, garlic, coriander, cumin and cayenne; cook and stir for 1 minute longer. Press cancel. Stir in the broth, lentils, water, green chiles and remaining onion.

2 Lock lid; close pressure-release valve. Adjust to pressure-cook on high for 15 minutes. Allow the pressure to release naturally. Just before serving, stir in cream. In a small skillet, heat butter over medium heat. Add cumin seeds; cook and stir until golden brown, 1-2 minutes. Add cumin seeds to lentil mixture.

3 Serve with rice. If desired, sprinkle with green onions or fresh cilantro.

1⅓ CUPS STEW WITH ¾ CUP RICE *497 cal., 16g fat (8g sat. fat), 33mg chol., 345mg sod., 73g carb. (5g sugars, 8g fiber), 17g pro.*

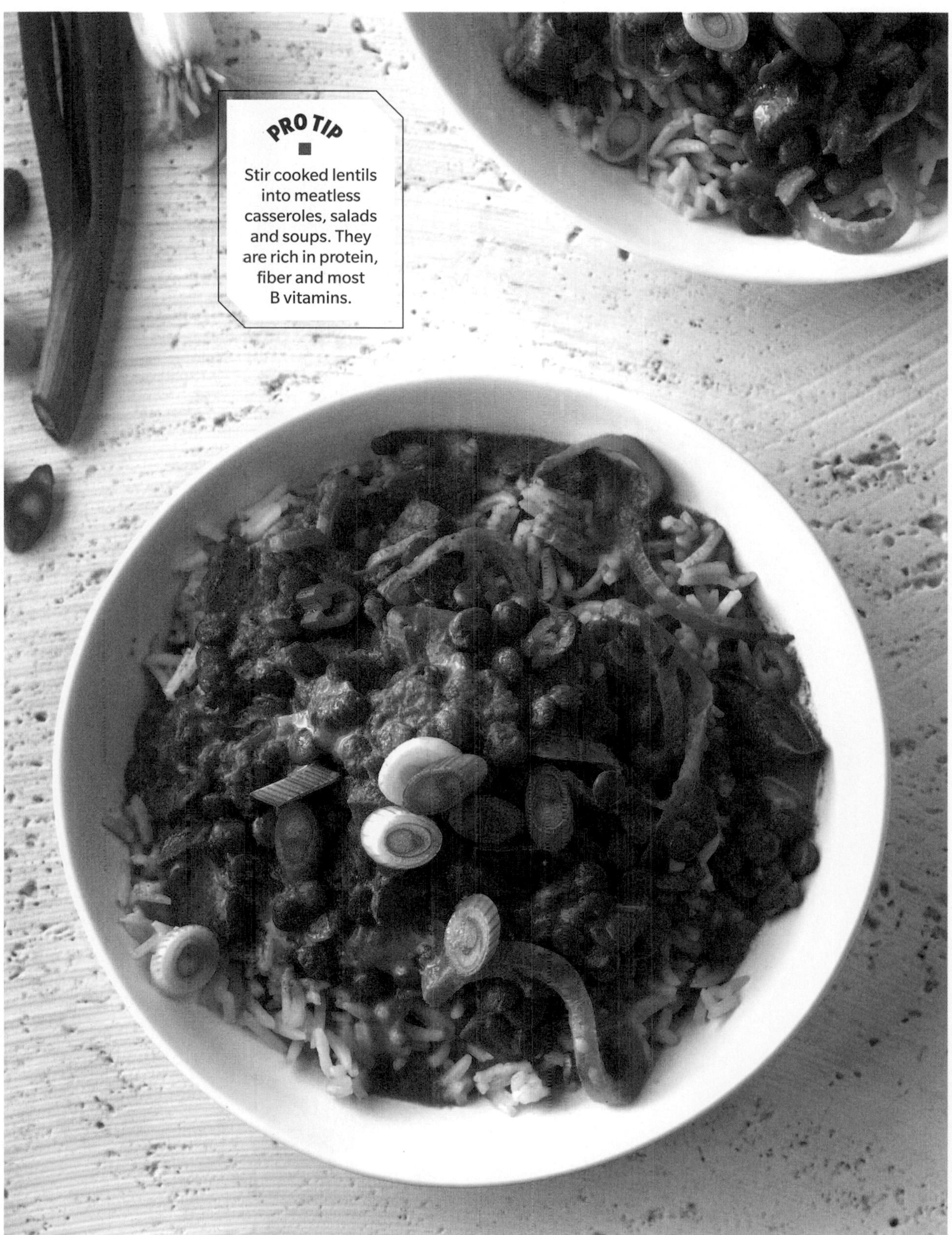
PRO TIP
Stir cooked lentils into meatless casseroles, salads and soups. They are rich in protein, fiber and most B vitamins.

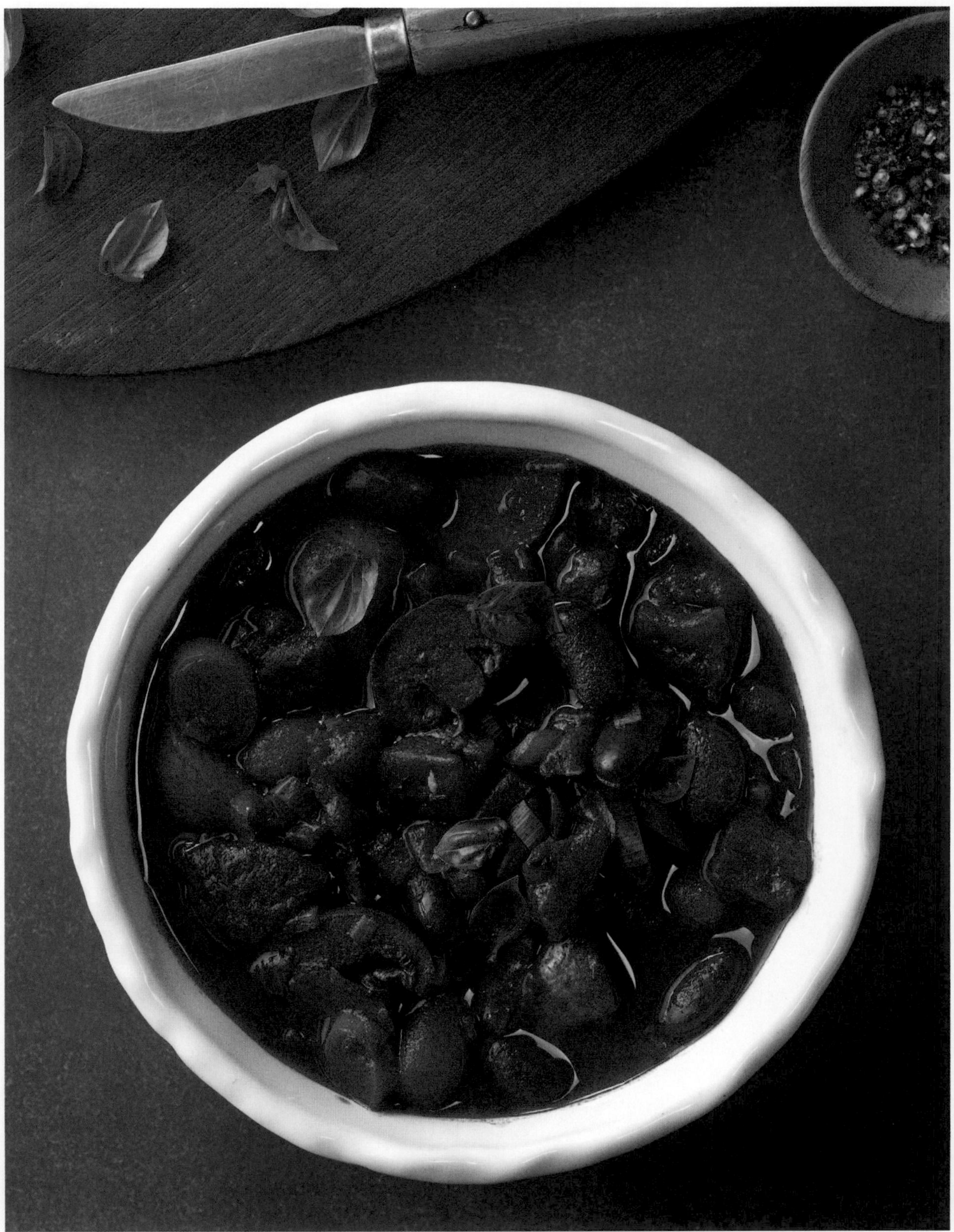

PRESSURE-COOKER MANCHESTER STEW

PREP: 25 min. **COOK:** 5 min. + releasing **MAKES:** 6 servings (2½ qt.)

- 2 Tbsp. olive oil
- 2 medium onions, chopped
- 2 garlic cloves, minced
- 1 tsp. dried oregano
- 1 cup dry red wine
- 1 lb. small red potatoes, quartered
- 1 can (16 oz.) kidney beans, rinsed and drained
- ½ lb. sliced fresh mushrooms
- 2 medium leeks (white portions only), sliced
- 1 cup fresh baby carrots
- 2½ cups water
- 1 can (14½ oz.) no-salt-added diced tomatoes
- 1 tsp. dried thyme
- ½ tsp. salt
- ¼ tsp. pepper
- Fresh basil leaves

1 Select saute setting on a 6-qt. electric pressure cooker. Adjust for medium heat; add oil. When oil is hot, cook and stir onions until crisp-tender, 2-3 minutes. Add garlic and oregano; cook and stir 1 minute longer. Stir in wine. Bring to a boil; cook until liquid is reduced by half, 3-4 minutes. Press cancel.

2 Add the red potatoes, beans, mushrooms, leeks and carrots. Stir in water, tomatoes, thyme, salt and pepper. Lock lid; close pressure-release valve. Adjust to pressure-cook on high for 3 minutes. Allow pressure to release naturally for 10 minutes, then quick-release any remaining pressure. Top with basil.

1⅔ CUPS *221 cal., 5g fat (1g sat. fat), 0 chol., 354mg sod., 38g carb. (8g sugars, 8g fiber), 8g pro.* ***Diabetic exchanges:*** *2 starch, 1 vegetable, 1 fat*

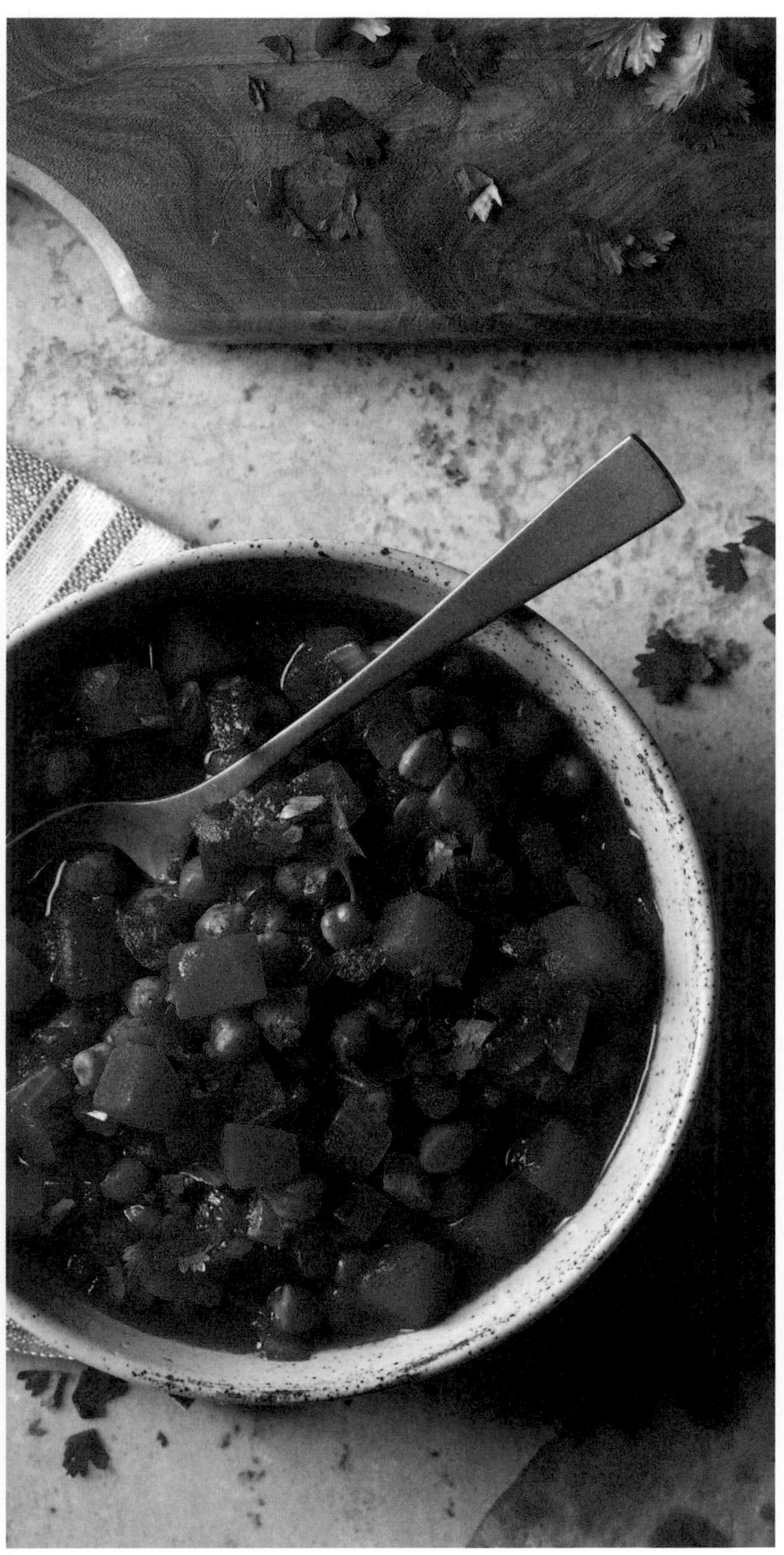

EASY MOROCCAN CHICKPEA STEW

TAKES: 30 min.
MAKES: 4 servings

- 1 Tbsp. olive oil
- 2 cups cubed peeled butternut squash (½-in. cubes)
- 1 large onion, chopped
- 1 large sweet red pepper, chopped
- 1 tsp. ground cinnamon
- ½ tsp. pepper
- ¼ tsp. ground ginger
- ¼ tsp. ground cumin
- ¼ tsp. salt
- 1 can (15 oz.) chickpeas or garbanzo beans, rinsed and drained
- 1 can (14½ oz.) diced tomatoes, undrained
- 1 cup water
- Chopped cilantro, optional

1 In a Dutch oven, heat oil over medium-high heat. Add squash, onion and red pepper; cook and stir until onion is translucent and red pepper is crisp-tender, about 5 minutes. Stir in seasonings until blended.

2 Add chickpeas, tomatoes and water; bring to a boil. Reduce heat; cover and simmer until squash is tender, about 8 minutes. If desired, top with cilantro.

1½ CUPS *217 cal., 6g fat (1g sat. fat), 0 chol., 455mg sod., 38g carb. (11g sugars, 9g fiber), 7g pro.*

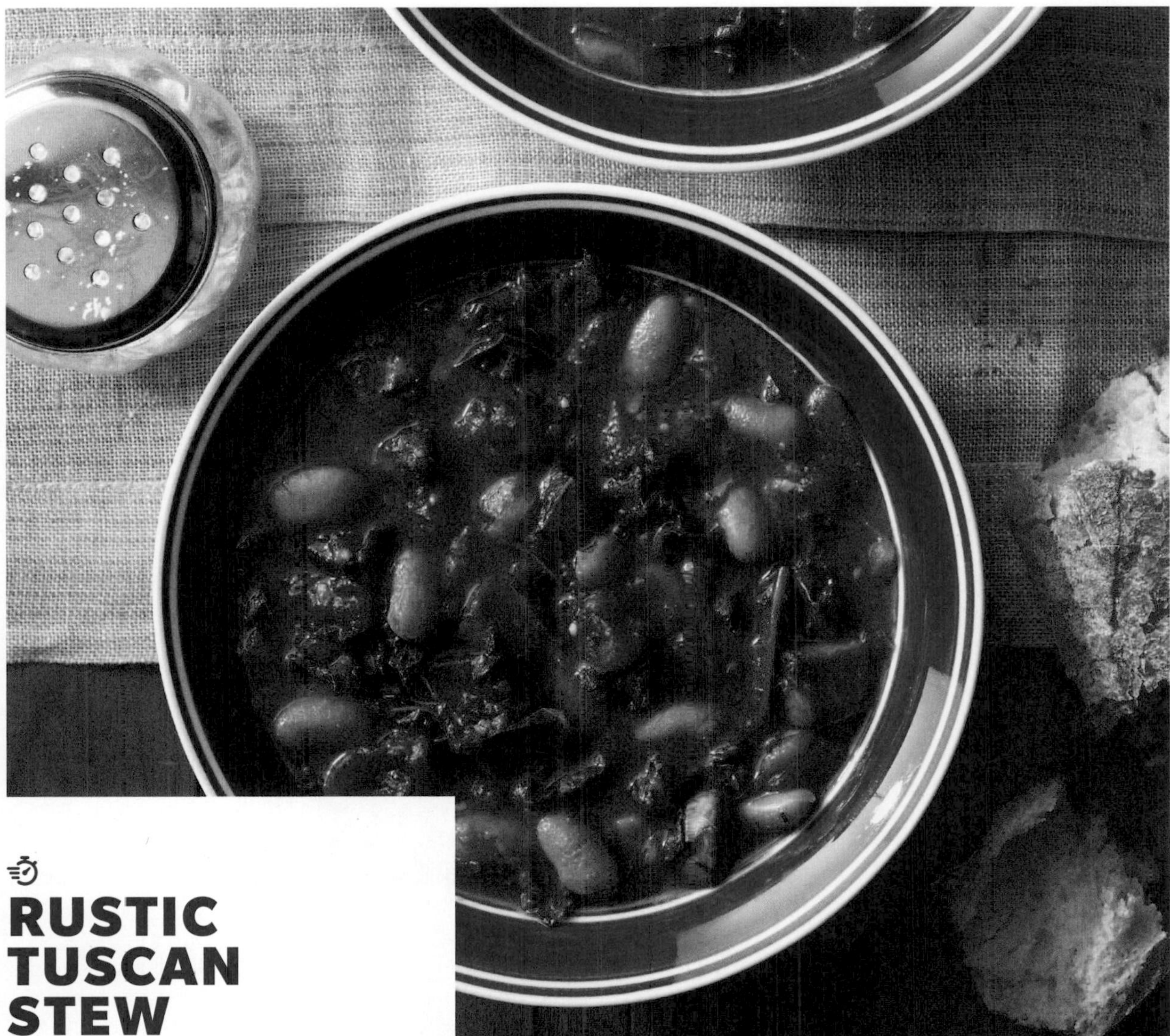

RUSTIC TUSCAN STEW

PREP: 20 min.
COOK: 20 min.
MAKES: 4 servings

- 2 large portobello mushrooms, coarsely chopped
- 1 medium onion, chopped
- 3 garlic cloves, minced
- 2 Tbsp. olive oil
- ½ cup white wine or vegetable broth
- 1 can (28 oz.) diced tomatoes, undrained
- 2 cups chopped fresh kale
- 1 bay leaf
- 1 tsp. dried thyme
- ½ tsp. dried basil
- ½ tsp. dried rosemary, crushed
- ¼ tsp. salt
- ¼ tsp. pepper
- 2 cans (15 oz. each) cannellini beans, rinsed and drained

1 In a large skillet, saute the mushrooms, onion and garlic in oil until tender. Add wine. Bring to a boil; cook until liquid is reduced by half. Stir in the tomatoes, kale and seasonings. Bring to a boil. Reduce heat; cover and simmer for 8-10 minutes.

2 Add beans; heat through. Discard bay leaf.

1¼ CUPS *309 cal., 8g fat (1g sat. fat), 0 chol., 672mg sod., 46g carb. (9g sugars, 13g fiber), 12g pro.* ***Diabetic exchanges:*** *2 starch, 2 vegetable, 1½ fat, 1 lean meat*

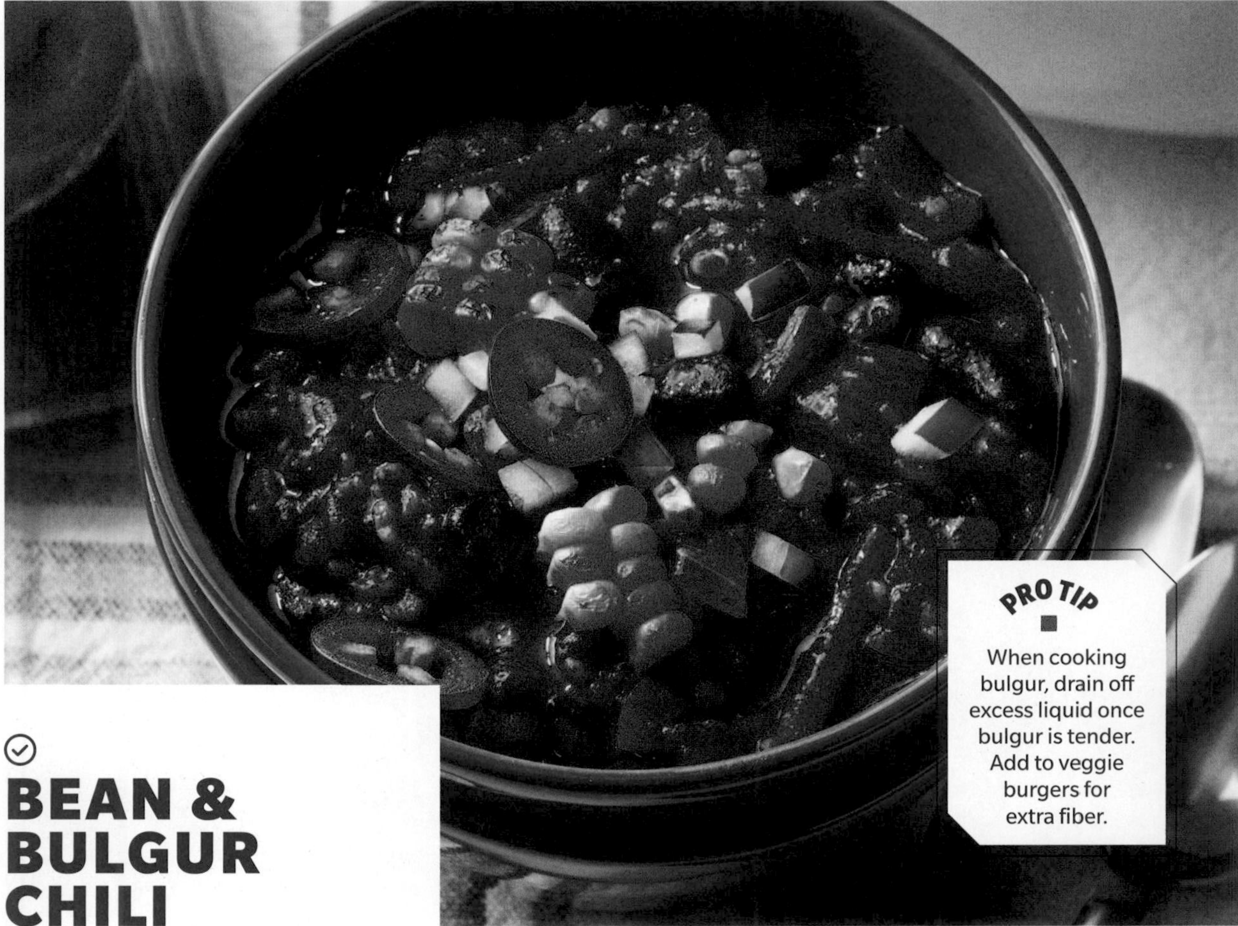

PRO TIP

When cooking bulgur, drain off excess liquid once bulgur is tender. Add to veggie burgers for extra fiber.

BEAN & BULGUR CHILI

PREP: 25 min.
COOK: 40 min.
MAKES: 10 servings (3½ qt.)

- 2 large onions, chopped
- 2 celery ribs, chopped
- 1 large green pepper, chopped
- 4 tsp. olive oil
- 4 garlic cloves, minced
- 1 large carrot, shredded
- 2 Tbsp. chili powder
- 1 tsp. dried oregano
- ½ tsp. coarsely ground pepper
- ½ tsp. ground cumin
- ⅛ tsp. ground cinnamon
- ⅛ tsp. ground allspice
- 2 cans (14½ oz. each) no-salt-added diced tomatoes, undrained
- 1 can (14½ oz.) fire-roasted diced tomatoes, undrained
- 1 can (16 oz.) kidney beans, rinsed and drained
- 1 can (15 oz.) pinto beans, rinsed and drained
- 1 can (15 oz.) black beans, rinsed and drained
- 1 can (14 oz.) vegetable broth
- ⅓ cup tomato paste
- 1 cup bulgur
- Optional toppings: Vegan sour cream, fresh corn, chopped red onion and sliced jalapeno peppers

1 In a Dutch oven over medium heat, cook the onions, celery and green pepper in oil until tender. Add garlic; cook 1 minute longer. Stir in carrot and seasonings; cook and stir 1 minute longer.

2 Stir in the tomatoes, beans, broth and tomato paste. Bring to a boil. Reduce heat; cover and simmer for 30 minutes.

3 Meanwhile, cook the bulgur according to package directions. Stir into chili; heat through. Garnish with desired toppings.

1⅓ CUPS *240 cal., 3g fat (0 sat. fat), 0 chol., 578mg sod., 45g carb. (9g sugars, 12g fiber), 11g pro.* ***Diabetic exchanges:*** *2 starch, 2 vegetable, 1 lean meat*

PRO TIP

Frozen vegetarian crumbles are pre-cooked. Just heat through and use in place of cooked meat in tacos and other dishes.

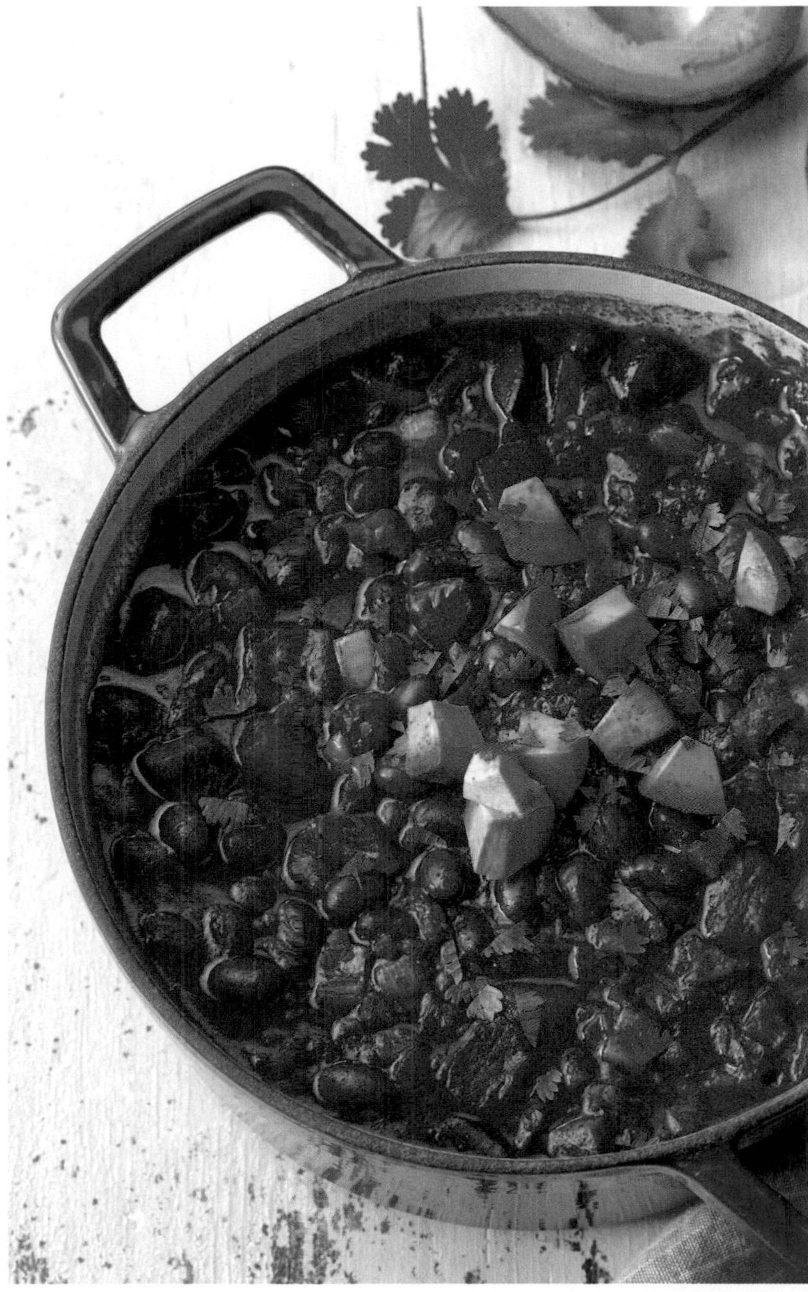

MUSHROOM CHILI

TAKES: 30 min.
MAKES: 9 servings (2¼ qt.)

1¾ cups chopped baby portobello mushrooms
1 medium onion, finely chopped
½ cup chopped sun-dried tomatoes (not packed in oil)
2 Tbsp. olive oil
2 garlic cloves, minced
1 pkg. (12 oz.) frozen vegetarian meat crumbles
2 cans (16 oz. each) chili beans, undrained
2 cans (14½ oz. each) no-salt-added diced tomatoes
½ cup water
½ cup vegetable broth
4½ tsp. chili powder
2 tsp. brown sugar
½ tsp. celery salt
½ tsp. ground cumin
1 medium ripe avocado, peeled and finely chopped
Vegan sour cream, optional

1 In a Dutch oven, saute the mushrooms, onion and sun-dried tomatoes in oil until tender. Add garlic; cook 1 minute longer. Add meat crumbles; heat through.

2 Stir in beans, tomatoes, water, broth, chili powder, brown sugar, celery salt and cumin. Bring to a boil. Reduce the heat; simmer, uncovered, for 10 minutes. Ladle chili into bowls. Top each with avocado and, if desired, vegan sour cream.

1 CUP *238 cal., 8g fat (1g sat. fat), 0 chol., 611mg sod., 34g carb. (9g sugars, 12g fiber), 14g pro.* ***Diabetic exchanges:*** *2 vegetable, 2 lean meat, 1½ starch, 1 fat*

WHITE CHICKEN CHILI

PREP: 15 min. **COOK:** 25 min. **MAKES:** 10 servings (2½ qt.)

- 1 lb. boneless skinless chicken breasts, chopped
- 1 medium onion, chopped
- 1 Tbsp. olive oil
- 2 garlic cloves, minced
- 2 cans (14 oz. each) chicken or vegetable broth
- 1 can (4 oz.) chopped green chiles
- 2 tsp. ground cumin
- 2 tsp. dried oregano
- 1½ tsp. cayenne pepper
- 3 cans (14½ oz. each) great northern beans, drained, divided
- 1 cup shredded Monterey Jack or vegan Monterey Jack-style cheese
- Sliced jalapeno pepper, optional

1 In a Dutch oven over medium heat, cook chicken and onion in oil until lightly browned. Add garlic; cook 1 minute longer. Stir in broth, chiles, cumin, oregano and cayenne; bring to a boil.

2 Reduce heat to low. With a potato masher, mash 1 can of beans until smooth. Add to saucepan. Add the remaining beans to saucepan. Simmer until chicken is no longer pink and onion is tender, 20-30 minutes.

3 Top each serving with cheese and, if desired, jalapeno pepper.

TO FREEZE Freeze cooled chili in freezer containers. To use, partially thaw in refrigerator overnight. Heat through in a saucepan, stirring occasionally; add broth or water if necessary.

1 CUP *219 cal., 7g fat (3g sat. fat), 37mg chol., 644mg sod., 21g carb. (1g sugars, 7g fiber), 19g pro.* ***Diabetic exchanges:*** *2 lean meat, 1½ starch, 1 fat*

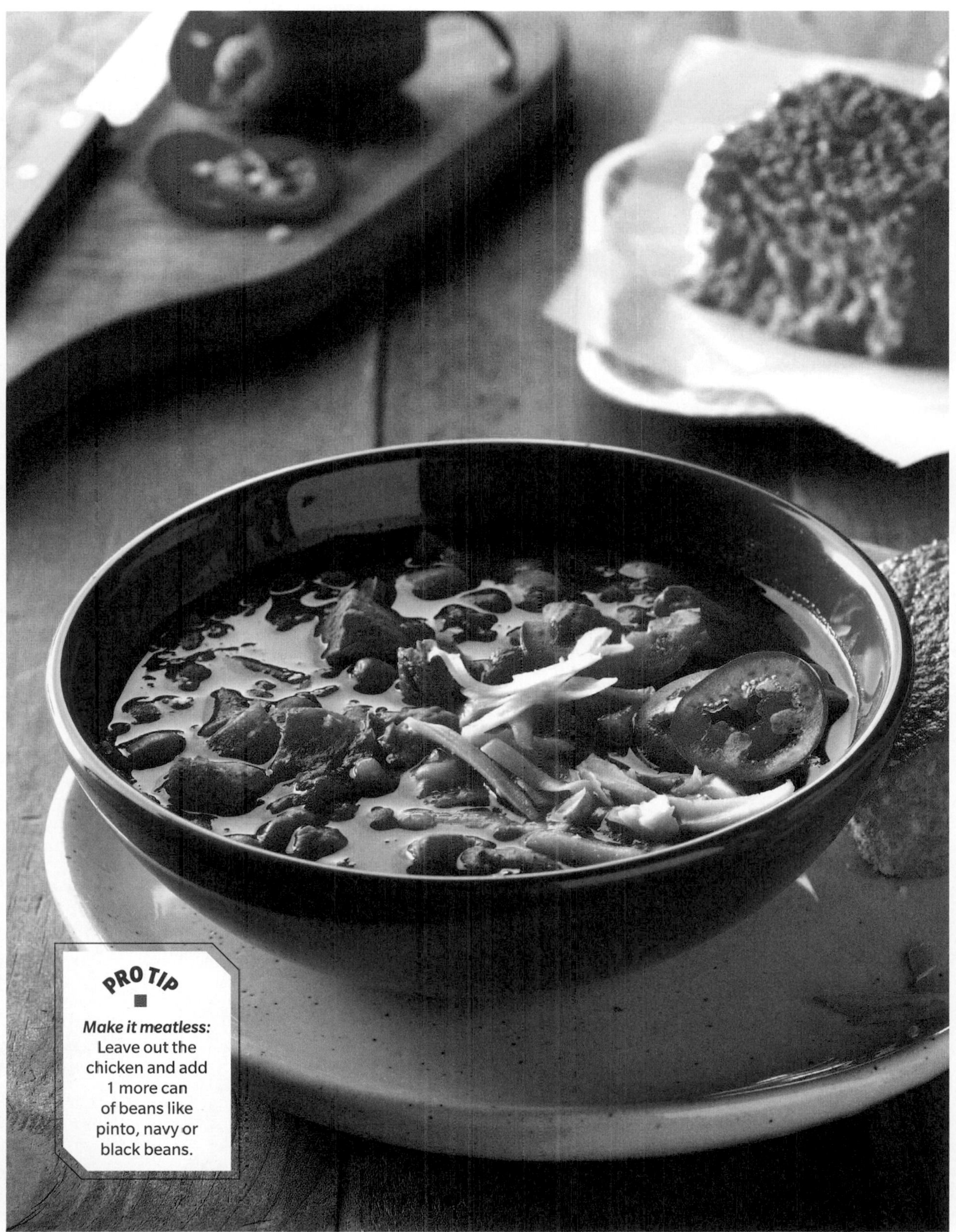

PRO TIP

Make it meatless: Leave out the chicken and add 1 more can of beans like pinto, navy or black beans.

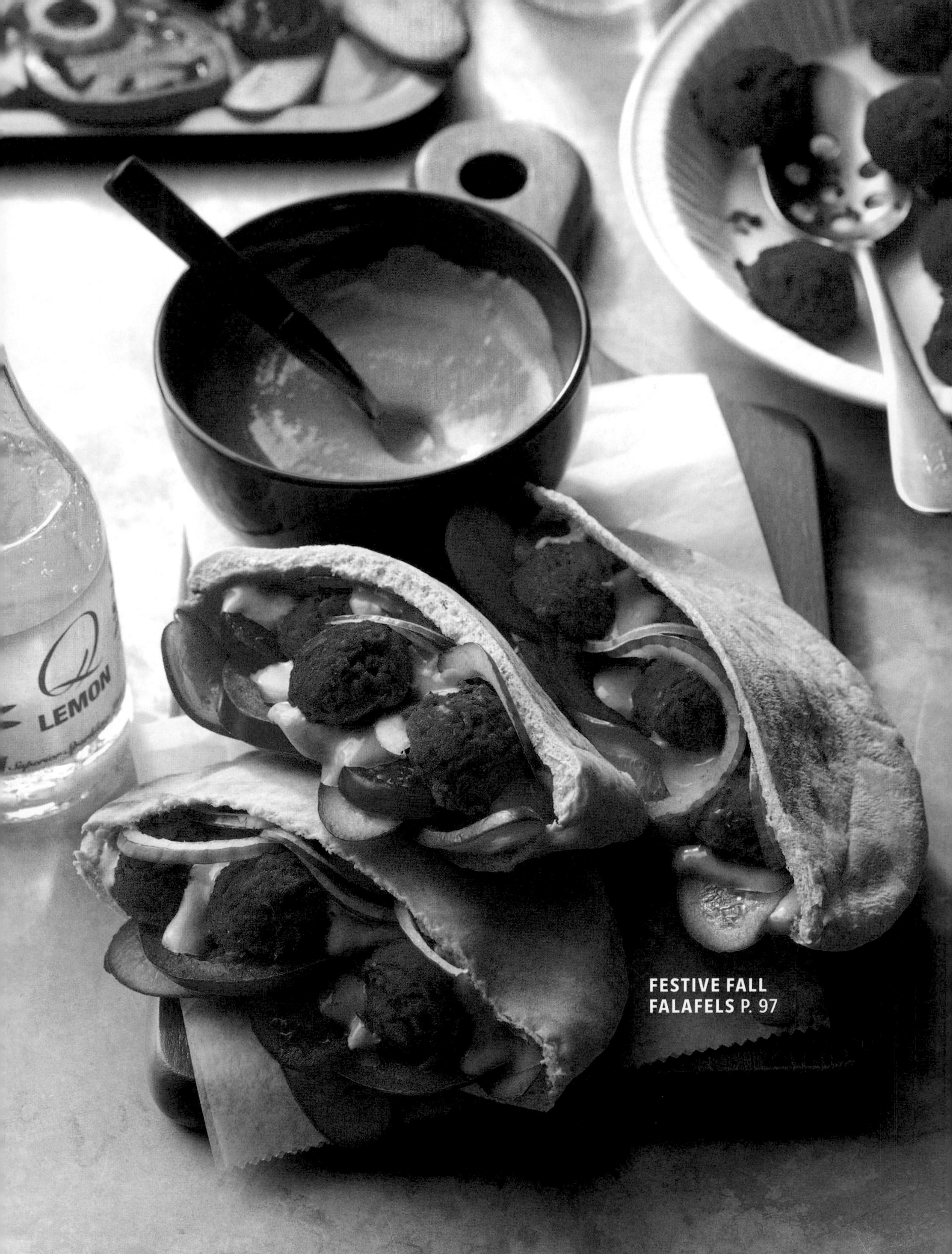

FESTIVE FALL FALAFELS P. 97

CHAPTER 6

BURGERS, SANDWICHES & WRAPS

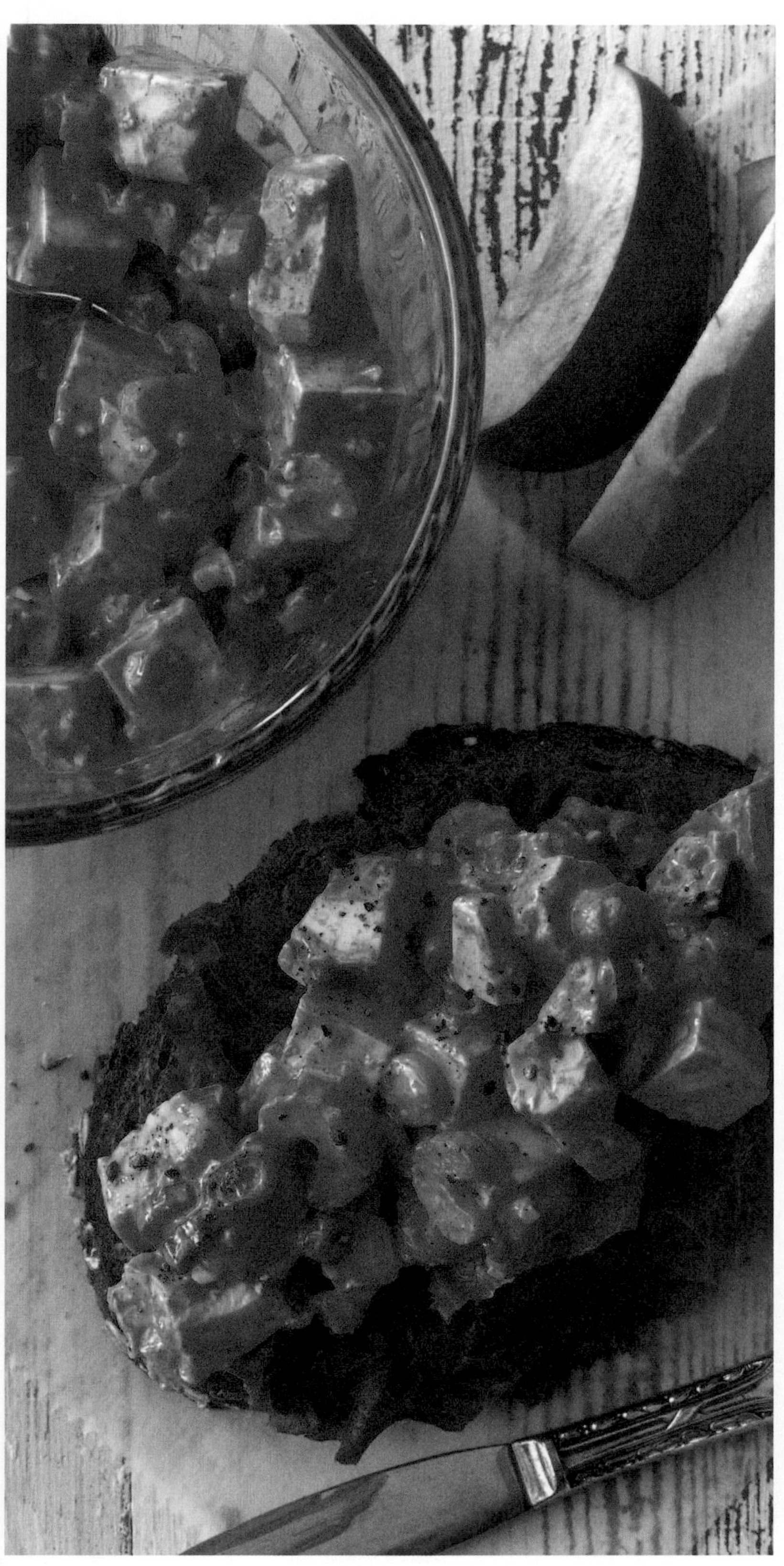

BETTER THAN EGG SALAD

TAKES: 20 min.
MAKES: 4 servings

- ¼ cup vegan mayonnaise
- ¼ cup chopped celery
- 2 green onions, chopped
- 2 Tbsp. sweet pickle relish
- 1 Tbsp. Dijon mustard
- ¼ tsp. ground turmeric
- ¼ tsp. salt
- ⅛ tsp. cayenne pepper
- 1 pkg. (12.3 oz.) silken firm tofu, cubed
- 8 slices whole wheat bread
- 4 lettuce leaves
- Coarsely ground pepper, optional

Mix first 8 ingredients; stir in tofu. Line 4 slices of bread with lettuce. Top with tofu mixture. If desired, sprinkle with pepper; close sandwiches.

1 SANDWICH *310 cal., 14g fat (2g sat. fat), 0 chol., 680mg sod., 30g carb. (6g sugars, 4g fiber), 14g pro.*
Diabetic exchanges: *2 starch, 2 fat, 1 lean meat*

PRO TIP
Chickpeas are a good source of protein at 6 grams per half cup. Try adding these nutty legumes to salads and soups.

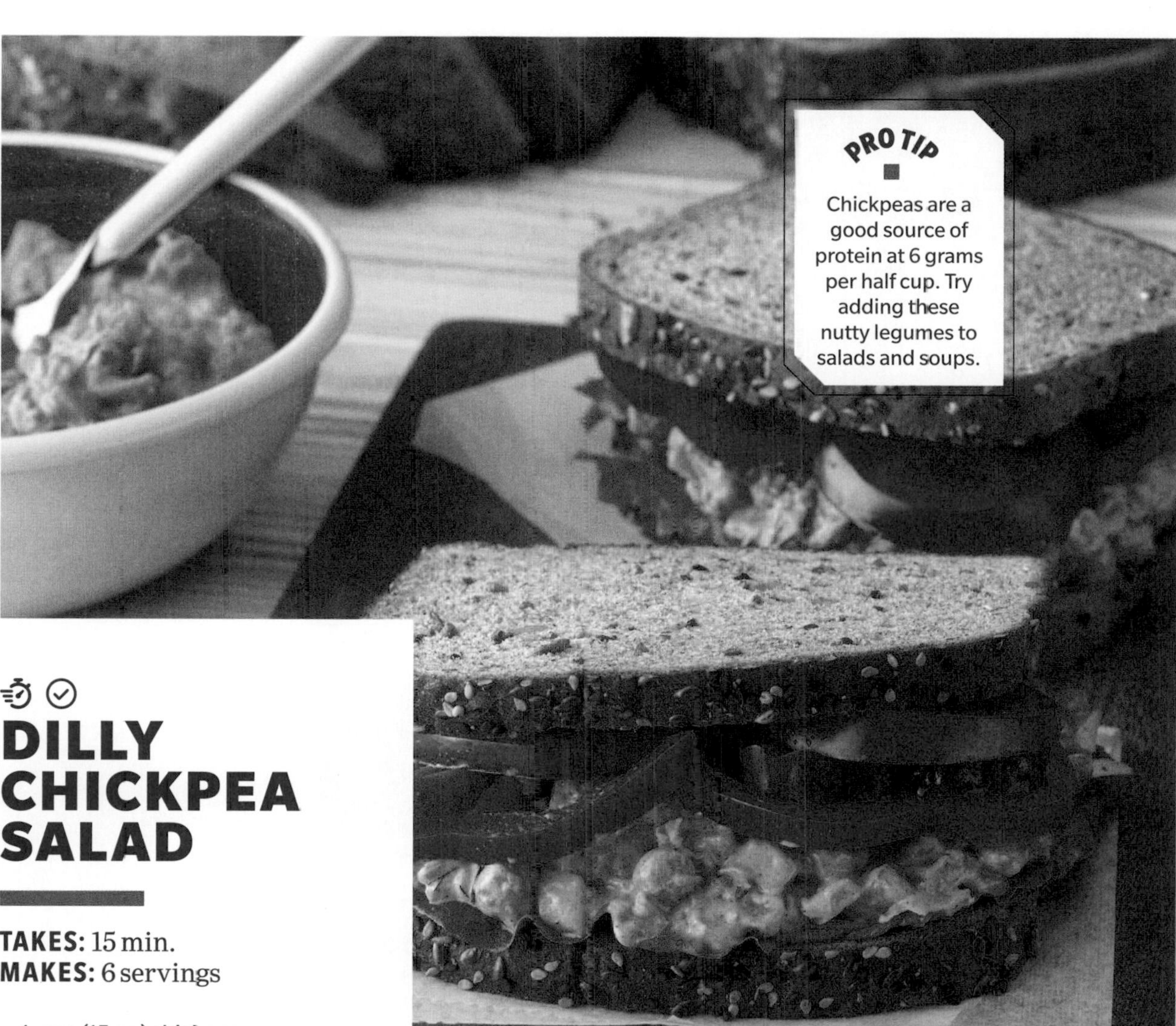

DILLY CHICKPEA SALAD

TAKES: 15 min.
MAKES: 6 servings

- 1 can (15 oz.) chickpeas or garbanzo beans, rinsed and drained
- ½ cup finely chopped onion
- ½ cup finely chopped celery
- ½ cup reduced-fat mayonnaise or vegan mayonnaise
- 3 Tbsp. honey mustard or Dijon mustard
- 2 Tbsp. snipped fresh dill
- 1 Tbsp. red wine vinegar
- ¼ tsp. salt
- ¼ tsp. paprika
- ¼ tsp. pepper
- 12 slices multigrain bread
  Optional toppings: Romaine leaves, tomato slices, dill pickle slices and red pepper rings

Place chickpeas in a large bowl; mash to desired consistency. Stir in onion, celery, mayonnaise, mustard, dill, vinegar, salt, paprika and pepper. Spread over each of 6 bread slices; layer with toppings of your choice and remaining bread.

1 SANDWICH *295 cal., 11g fat (2g sat. fat), 7mg chol., 586mg sod., 41g carb. (9g sugars, 7g fiber), 10g pro.*

GRILLED VEGGIE SANDWICHES WITH CILANTRO PESTO

PREP: 20 min. **GRILL:** 20 min. + standing **MAKES:** 4 servings

- 2/3 cup packed fresh cilantro sprigs
- 1/4 cup packed fresh parsley sprigs
- 2 Tbsp. grated Parmesan or vegan Parmesan-style cheese
- 2 garlic cloves, peeled
- 2 Tbsp. water
- 1 Tbsp. pine nuts
- 1 Tbsp. olive oil

SANDWICHES

- 2 large sweet red peppers
- 4 slices eggplant (1/2 in. thick) Cooking spray
- 1/2 tsp. salt
- 1/4 tsp. pepper
- 1/2 cup shredded part-skim mozzarella or vegan mozzarella-style cheese
- 4 kaiser rolls, split

1 For pesto, place cilantro, parsley, Parmesan cheese and garlic in a small food processor; pulse until chopped. Add water and pine nuts; process until blended. While processing, slowly add oil.

2 Grill peppers, covered, over medium heat until skins are blistered and blackened, turning occasionally, 10-15 minutes. Immediately place peppers in a large bowl; let stand, covered, for 20 minutes. Peel off and discard charred skin. Cut peppers in half; remove stems and seeds.

3 Lightly spritz both sides of eggplant slices with cooking spray; sprinkle with salt and pepper. Grill, covered, over medium heat 3-5 minutes on each side or until tender. Top with the peppers; sprinkle with mozzarella cheese. Grill, covered, for 2-3 minutes or until cheese is melted; remove from grill.

4 Spread roll bottoms with pesto. Top with the eggplant stacks and roll tops.

1 SANDWICH *310 cal., 12g fat (3g sat. fat), 11mg chol., 755mg sod., 40g carb. (6g sugars, 4g fiber), 12g pro.* ***Diabetic exchanges:*** *2 starch, 1 vegetable, 1 lean meat, 1 fat*

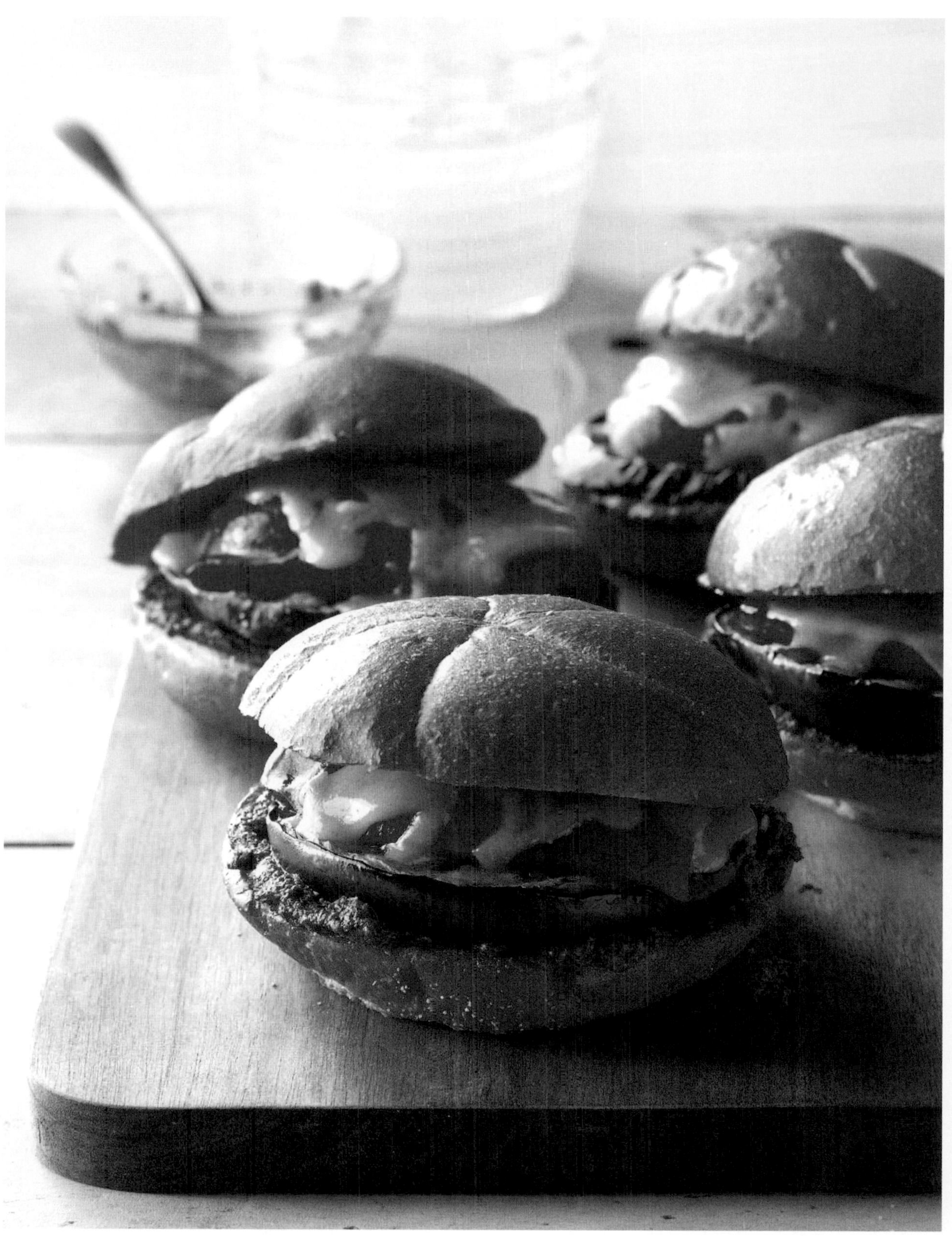

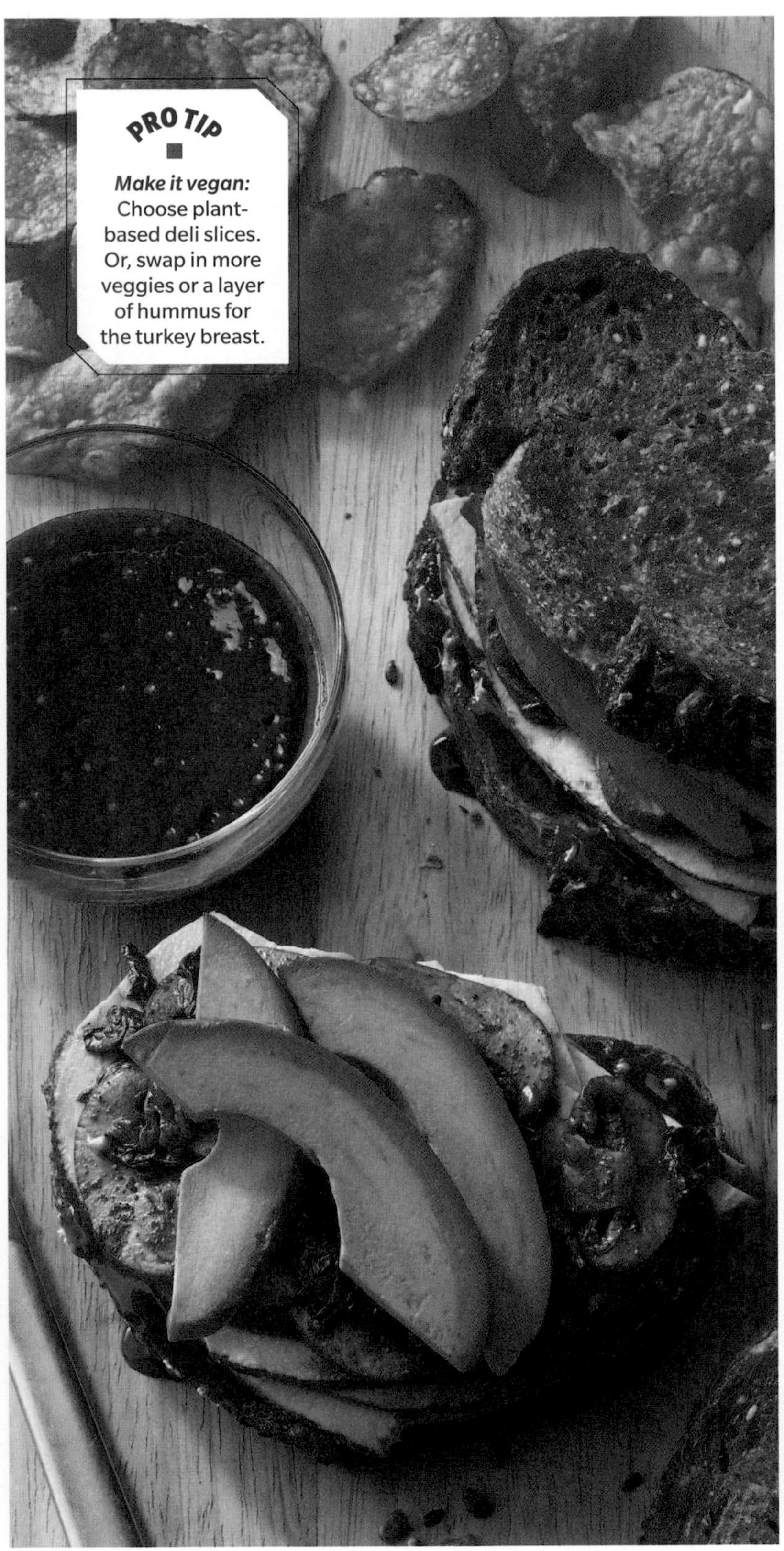

PRO TIP

Make it vegan: Choose plant-based deli slices. Or, swap in more veggies or a layer of hummus for the turkey breast.

TURKEY SANDWICHES WITH BERRY MUSTARD

TAKES: 25 min.
MAKES: 2 servings

- 1 Tbsp. agave nectar
- 1 Tbsp. spicy brown mustard
- 1 tsp. red raspberry preserves
- ¼ tsp. mustard seed
- 1 Tbsp. olive oil
- 4 oz. fresh mushrooms, thinly sliced
- 1 cup fresh baby spinach, coarsely chopped
- 1 garlic clove, minced
- ½ tsp. chili powder
- 4 slices multigrain bread, toasted
- 6 oz. sliced cooked turkey breast or vegan turkey-style deli slices
- ½ medium ripe avocado, sliced

1 Combine the agave, mustard, preserves and mustard seed; set aside. In a large skillet, heat oil over medium-high heat. Add the mushrooms; cook and stir until tender, 4-5 minutes. Add spinach, garlic and chili powder; cook and stir 3-4 minutes or until spinach is wilted.

2 Spread the mustard mixture over the toast. Layer 2 slices of toast with turkey, mushroom mixture and avocado. Place the remaining toast on top.

1 SANDWICH *449 cal., 16g fat (3g sat. fat), 68mg chol., 392mg sod., 40g carb. (14g sugars, 7g fiber), 35g pro.*

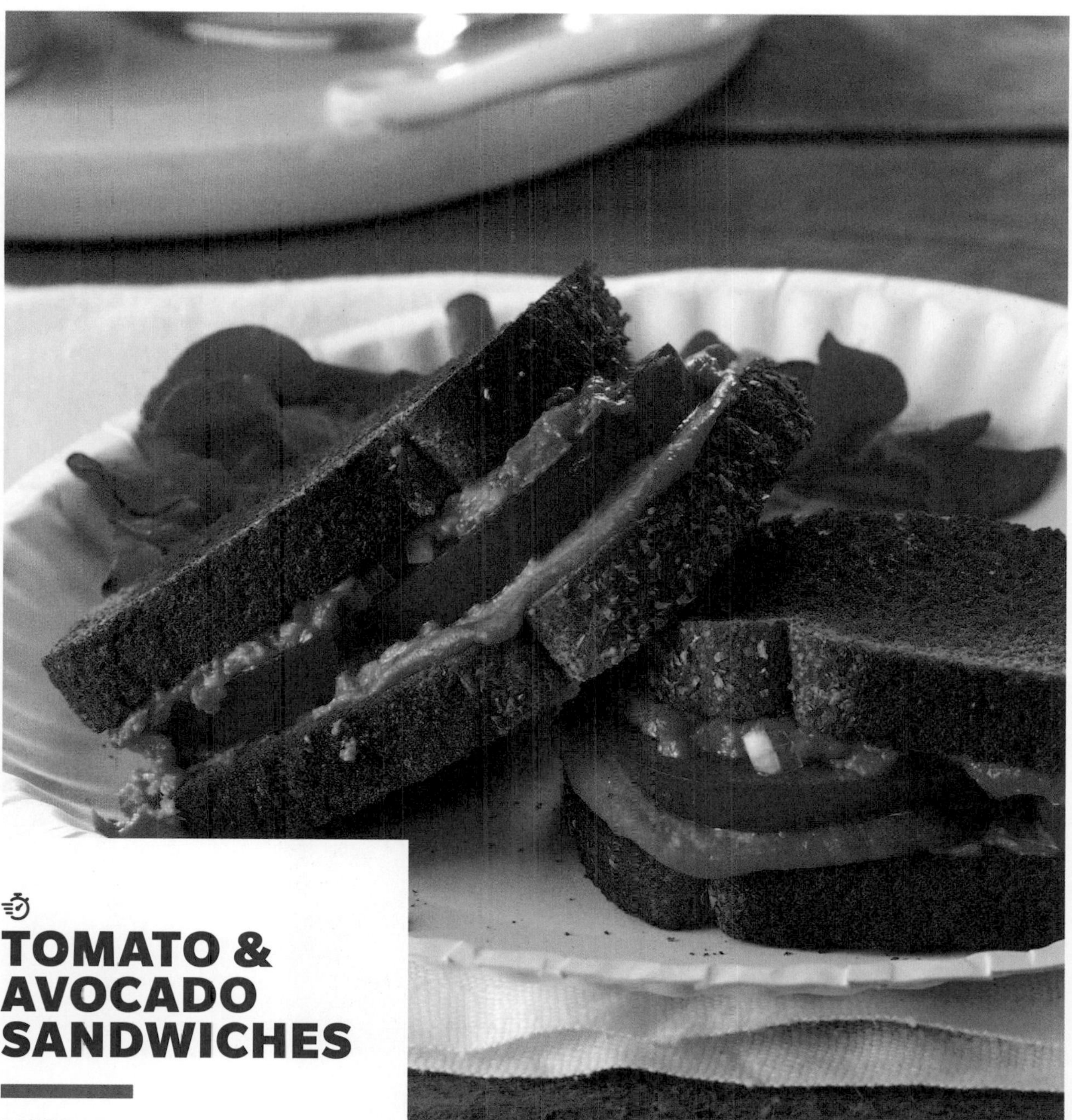

TOMATO & AVOCADO SANDWICHES

TAKES: 10 min.
MAKES: 2 servings

- ½ medium ripe avocado, peeled and mashed
- 4 slices whole wheat bread, toasted
- 1 medium tomato, sliced
- 2 Tbsp. finely chopped shallot
- ¼ cup hummus

Spread avocado over 2 slices of toast. Top with tomato and shallot. Spread hummus over remaining toast slices; place on top of avocado toast, facedown on top of tomato layer.

1 SANDWICH *278 cal., 11g fat (2g sat. fat), 0 chol., 379mg sod., 35g carb. (6g sugars, 9g fiber), 11g pro.* ***Diabetic exchanges:*** *2 starch, 2 fat*

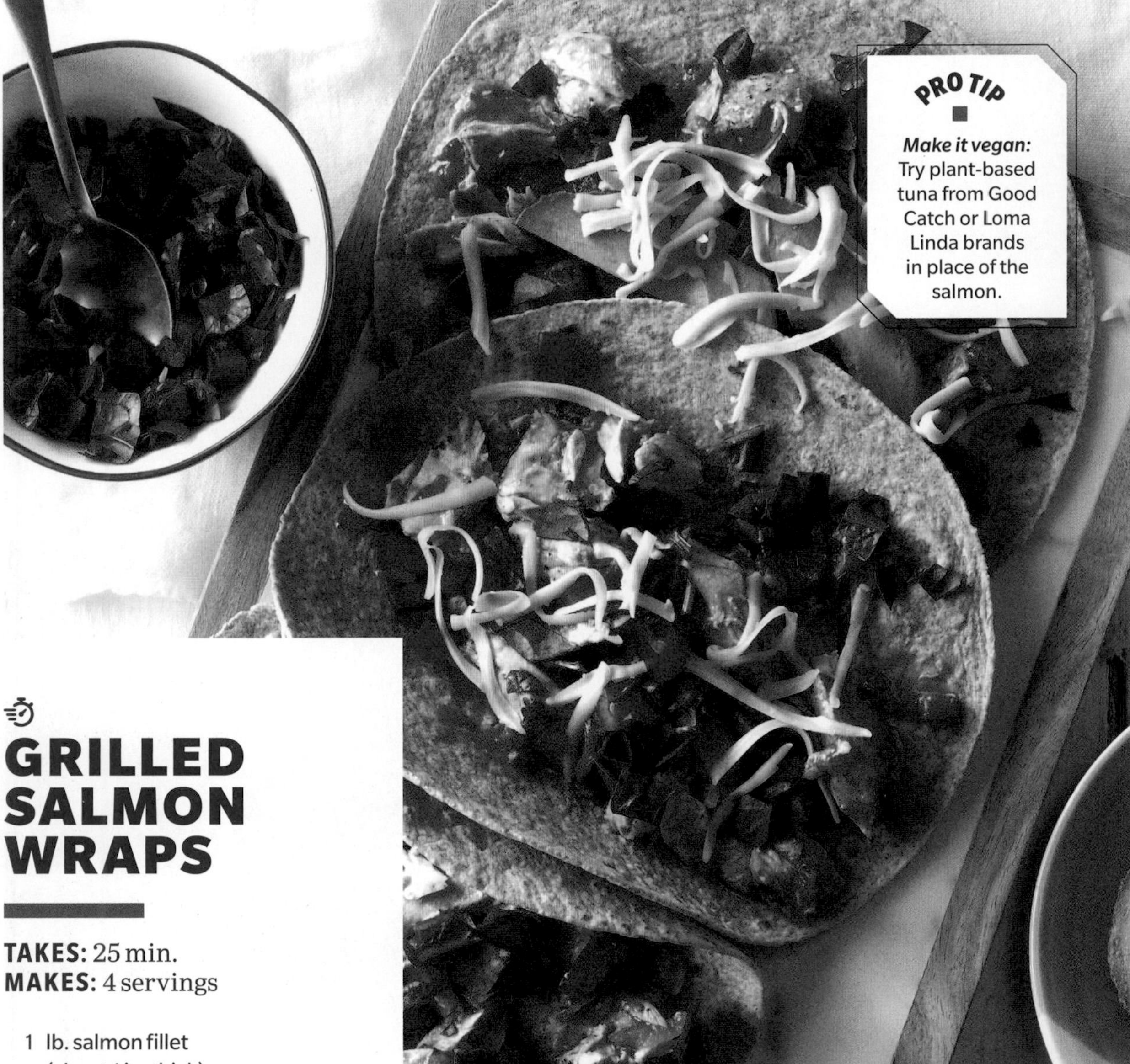

PRO TIP

Make it vegan: Try plant-based tuna from Good Catch or Loma Linda brands in place of the salmon.

GRILLED SALMON WRAPS

TAKES: 25 min.
MAKES: 4 servings

- 1 lb. salmon fillet (about 1 in. thick)
- ½ tsp. salt
- ¼ tsp. pepper
- ½ cup salsa verde
- 4 whole wheat tortillas (8 in.), warmed
- 1 cup chopped fresh spinach
- 1 medium tomato, seeded and chopped
- ½ cup shredded Monterey Jack or vegan Monterey Jack-style cheese
- ½ medium ripe avocado, peeled and thinly sliced

1 Sprinkle salmon with salt and pepper; place on an oiled grill rack over medium heat, skin side down. Grill, covered, until fish just begins to flake easily with a fork, 8-10 minutes.

2 Remove from grill. Break salmon into bite-sized pieces, removing skin if desired. Toss gently with the salsa; serve in tortillas. Top with remaining ingredients.

1 WRAP *380 cal., 18g fat (5g sat. fat), 69mg chol., 745mg sod., 27g carb. (2g sugars, 5g fiber), 27g pro.* ***Diabetic exchanges:*** *3 lean meat, 2 starch, 2 fat*

CALIFORNIA ROLL WRAPS

TAKES: 20 min.
MAKES: 6 wraps

- ½ cup wasabi mayonnaise or ½ cup vegan mayonnaise plus ½ teaspoon wasabi
- 6 whole wheat tortillas (8 in.)
- 2 pkg. (8 oz. each) imitation crabmeat or vegan crab-style shreds
- 1 medium ripe avocado, peeled and thinly sliced
- 1½ cups julienned peeled jicama
- 1 medium sweet red pepper, julienned
- 1 small cucumber, seeded and julienned
- ¾ cup bean sprouts

Divide the wasabi mayonnaise evenly among the 6 tortillas and spread to within ½ in. of edges. Layer with crabmeat, avocado, jicama, red pepper, cucumber and bean sprouts. Roll up tightly.

1 WRAP *365 cal., 18g fat (3g sat. fat), 10mg chol., 647mg sod., 39g carb. (2g sugars, 7g fiber), 13g pro.* ***Diabetic exchanges:*** *2 starch, 2 fat, 1 vegetable, 1 lean meat,*

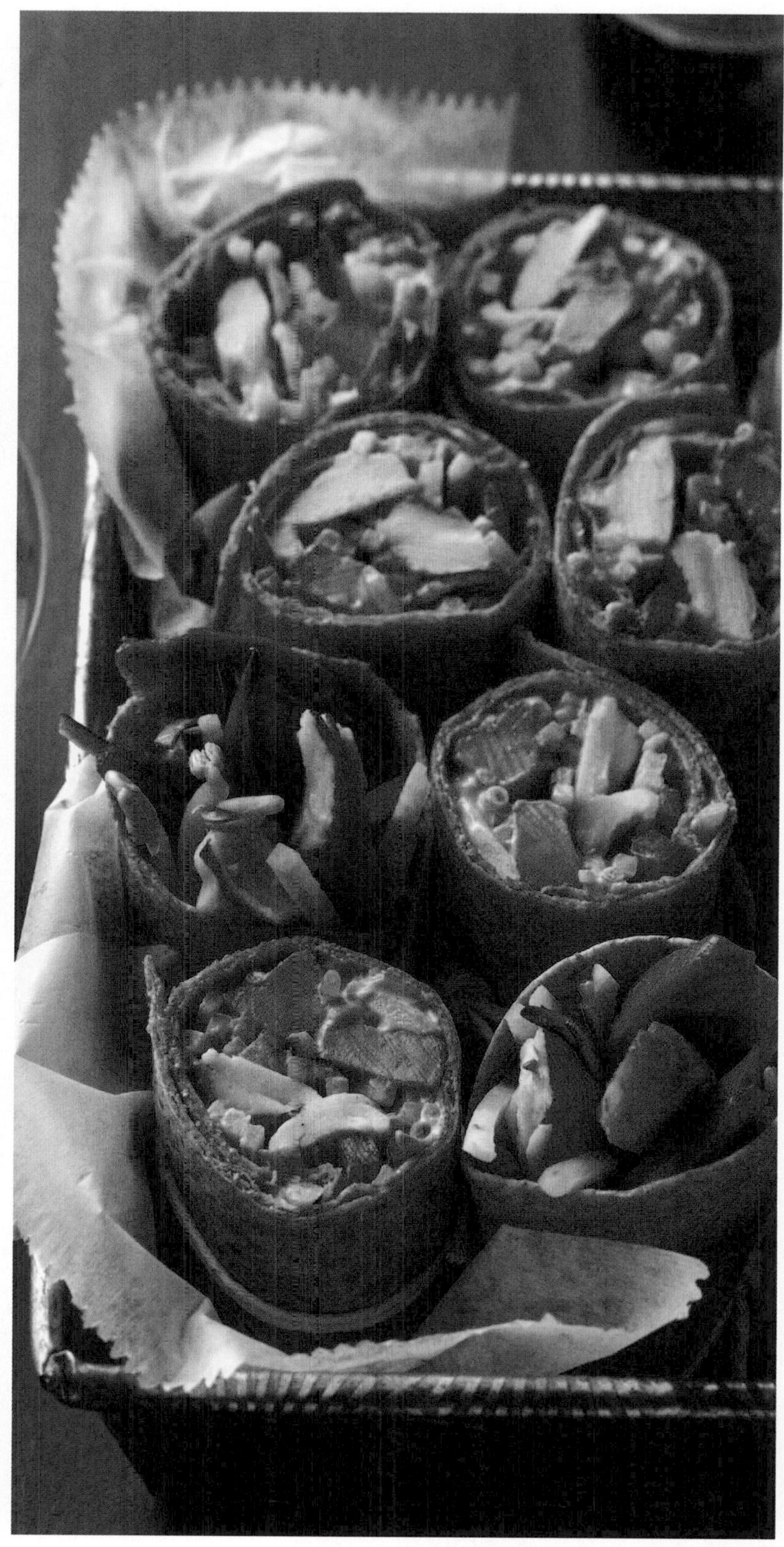

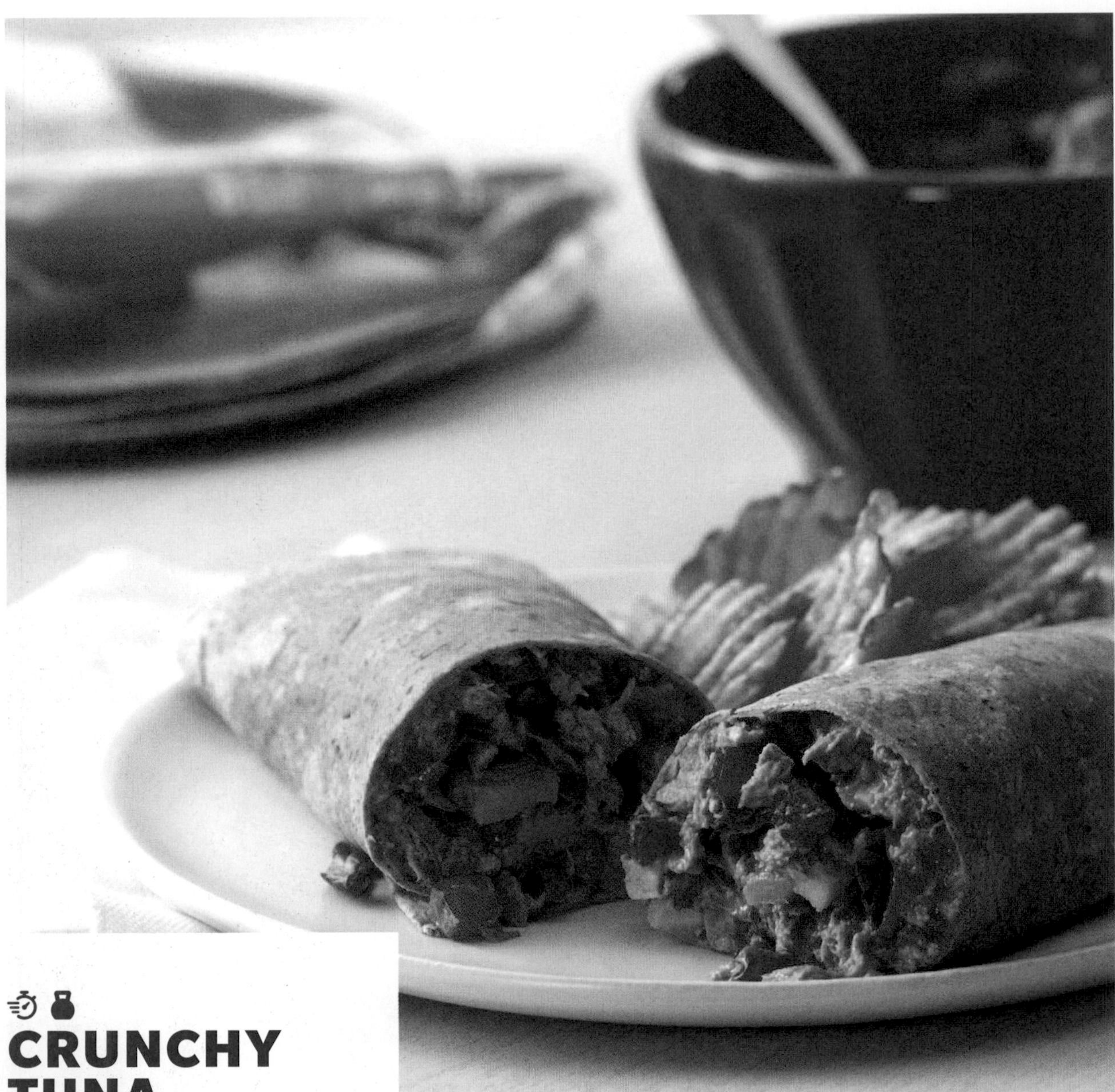

CRUNCHY TUNA WRAPS

TAKES: 10 min.
MAKES: 2 servings

- 1 pouch (6.4 oz.) light tuna in water or vegan tuna-style chunks
- ¼ cup finely chopped celery
- ¼ cup chopped green onions
- ¼ cup sliced water chestnuts, chopped
- 3 Tbsp. chopped sweet red pepper
- 2 Tbsp. reduced-fat mayonnaise or vegan mayonnaise
- 2 tsp. prepared mustard
- 2 spinach tortillas (8 in.), room temperature
- 1 cup shredded lettuce

In a small bowl, mix the first 7 ingredients until blended. Spread over tortillas; sprinkle with lettuce. Roll up tightly.

1 WRAP *312 cal., 10g fat (2g sat. fat), 38mg chol., 628mg sod., 34g carb. (2g sugars, 3g fiber), 23g pro.* ***Diabetic exchanges:*** *3 lean meat, 2 starch, ½ fat*

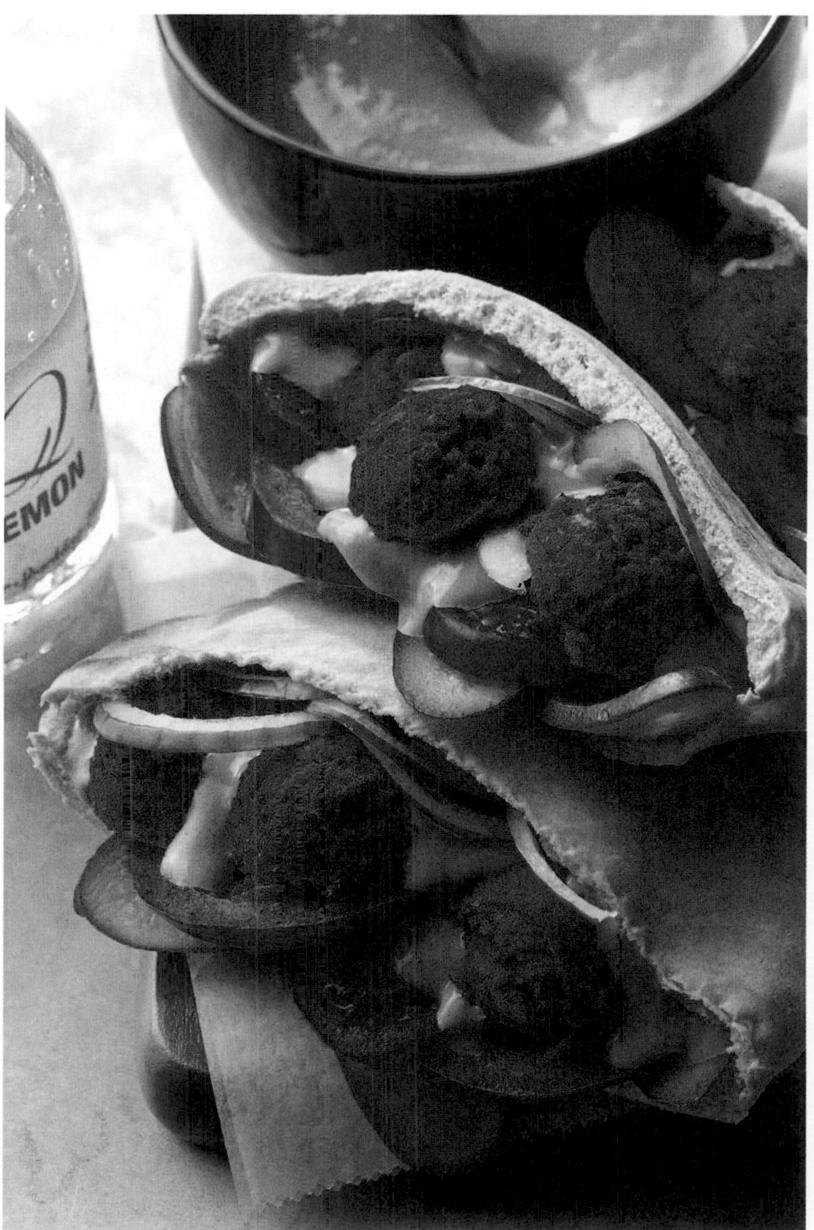

FESTIVE FALL FALAFELS

PREP: 20 min. **BAKE:** 30 min.
MAKES: 4 servings

- 1 cup canned garbanzo beans or chickpeas, rinsed and drained
- ½ cup canned pumpkin
- ½ cup fresh cilantro leaves
- ¼ cup chopped onion
- 1 garlic clove, halved
- ¾ tsp. salt
- ½ tsp. ground ginger
- ½ tsp. ground cumin
- ¼ tsp. ground coriander
- ¼ tsp. cayenne pepper

MAPLE TAHINI SAUCE

- ½ cup tahini
- ¼ cup water
- 2 Tbsp. maple syrup
- 1 Tbsp. cider vinegar
- ½ tsp. salt
- 8 pita pocket halves
  Optional toppings: Sliced cucumber, onions and tomatoes

1 Preheat oven to 400°. Place the first 10 ingredients in a food processor; pulse until combined. Drop by tablespoonfuls onto a greased baking sheet. Bake for 30-35 minutes or until firm and golden brown.

2 Meanwhile, in a small bowl, combine tahini, water, syrup, vinegar and salt. Serve falafel in pita halves with maple tahini sauce and optional toppings as desired.

2 FILLED PITA HALVES *469 cal., 21g fat (3g sat. fat), 0 chol., 1132mg sod., 57g carb. (10g sugars, 8g fiber), 14g pro.*

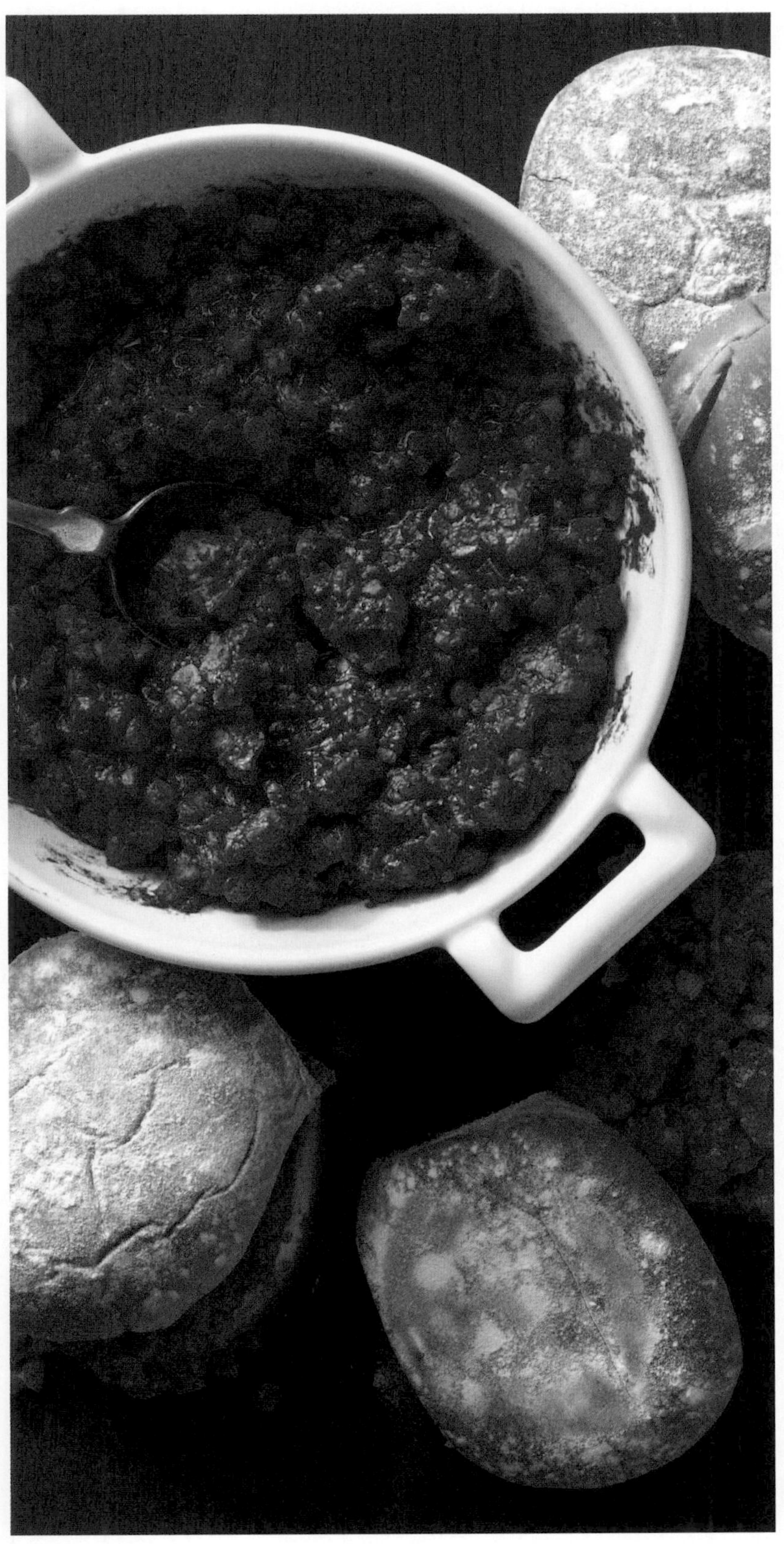

SAUCY TEMPEH SLOPPY JOES

PREP: 15 min. **COOK:** 25 min.
MAKES: 10 servings

- 2 Tbsp. olive oil
- 1 medium onion, chopped
- ½ medium green pepper, chopped
- 2 garlic cloves, minced
- 2 pkg. (8 oz. each) tempeh
- 1 can each (15 oz. and 8 oz.) tomato sauce
- 3 Tbsp. packed brown sugar
- 1 Tbsp. soy sauce
- ½ tsp. dried oregano
- ½ tsp. dried thyme
- ¼ tsp. salt
- ⅛ tsp. cayenne pepper
- 10 hamburger buns, split

In a large skillet, heat oil over medium-high heat. Add onion and green pepper; cook and stir until tender, 6-8 minutes. Add the garlic; cook 1 minute longer. Crumble tempeh into skillet; cook and stir for 5 minutes. Add the tomato sauce, brown sugar, soy sauce and seasonings; cook and stir over medium heat until thickened, 10-15 minutes. Serve on buns.

1 SANDWICH *273 cal., 10g fat (2g sat. fat), 0 chol., 674mg sod., 34g carb. (9g sugars, 2g fiber), 15g pro.*

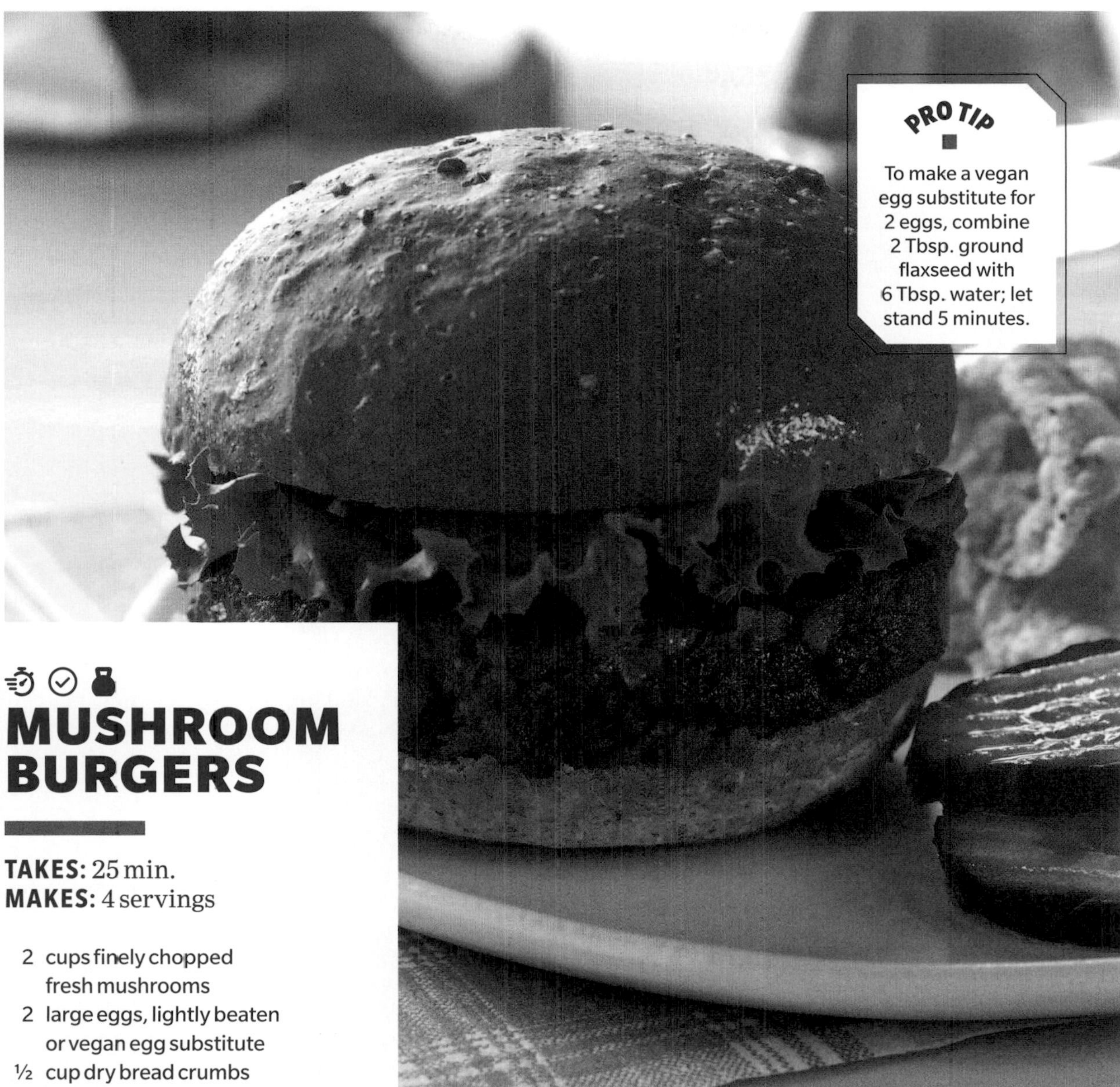

PRO TIP

To make a vegan egg substitute for 2 eggs, combine 2 Tbsp. ground flaxseed with 6 Tbsp. water; let stand 5 minutes.

MUSHROOM BURGERS

TAKES: 25 min.
MAKES: 4 servings

- 2 cups finely chopped fresh mushrooms
- 2 large eggs, lightly beaten or vegan egg substitute
- ½ cup dry bread crumbs
- ½ cup shredded cheddar or vegan cheddar-style cheese
- ½ cup finely chopped onion
- ¼ cup all-purpose flour
- ½ tsp. salt
- ¼ tsp. dried thyme
- ¼ tsp. pepper
- 1 Tbsp. canola oil
- 4 whole wheat hamburger buns, split
- 4 lettuce leaves
- Optional: Sliced tomatoes and vegan mayonnaise

1 In a large bowl, combine the first 9 ingredients. Shape into four ¾-in.-thick patties.

2 In a large cast-iron or other heavy skillet, heat the oil over medium heat. Add burgers; cook until crisp and lightly browned, 3-4 minutes on each side. Serve on buns with lettuce leaves and, if desired, tomato and mayonnaise.

1 BURGER *330 cal., 13g fat (5g sat. fat), 121mg chol., 736mg sod., 42g carb. (4g sugars, 5g fiber), 14g pro.* ***Diabetic exchanges:*** *3 starch, 1 medium-fat meat, ½ fat*

CUMIN-SPICED LENTIL BURGERS

PREP: 30 min. **COOK:** 10 min./batch **MAKES:** 8 servings

- 2¼ cups water, divided
- 1 cup dried red lentils, rinsed
- 1 cup bulgur (fine grind)
- 1½ tsp. salt, divided
- 6 Tbsp. canola oil, divided
- 1 large onion, chopped
- 1 Tbsp. ground cumin
- 1 Tbsp. chili powder
- 1 large egg, lightly beaten or vegan egg substitute
- 6 green onions, sliced
- 3 Tbsp. chopped fresh parsley
- 8 flatbreads wraps
- 8 Tbsp. Sriracha mayonnaise or 8 Tbsp. vegan mayonnaise plus 2 tsp. Sriracha chili sauce
- Optional toppings: Lettuce leaves, sliced tomato and sliced onions

1 Place 2 cups water and lentils in a large saucepan. Bring to a boil. Reduce heat; simmer, uncovered, until lentils are tender, 15-20 minutes, stirring occasionally. Remove from heat; stir in bulgur and 1 tsp. salt. Cover and let stand until tender and the liquid is absorbed, 15-20 minutes.

2 Meanwhile, in a large nonstick skillet, heat 2 Tbsp. oil over medium-high heat. Add onion; cook and stir 8-10 minutes or until tender. Add cumin and chili powder; cook 1 minute longer. Remove from heat. Add onion mixture to lentil mixture. Stir in egg, green onions, parsley and remaining ½ tsp. salt, mixing lightly but thoroughly. If needed, add the remaining ¼ cup water, 1 Tbsp. at a time, to help mixture stay together when squeezed; shape into eight ½-in.-thick patties.

3 In the same skillet, heat remaining 4 Tbsp. oil over medium heat. Add burgers in batches; cook until golden brown, 3-5 minutes on each side. Serve in wraps with Sriracha mayonnaise and desired toppings.

1 BURGER *434 cal., 23g fat (2g sat. fat), 1mg chol., 780mg sod., 54g carb. (2g sugars, 16g fiber), 16g pro.*

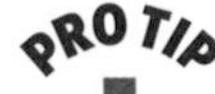

To make a vegan egg substitute, combine 1 Tbsp. ground flaxseed with 3 Tbsp. water; let stand 5 minutes to thicken.

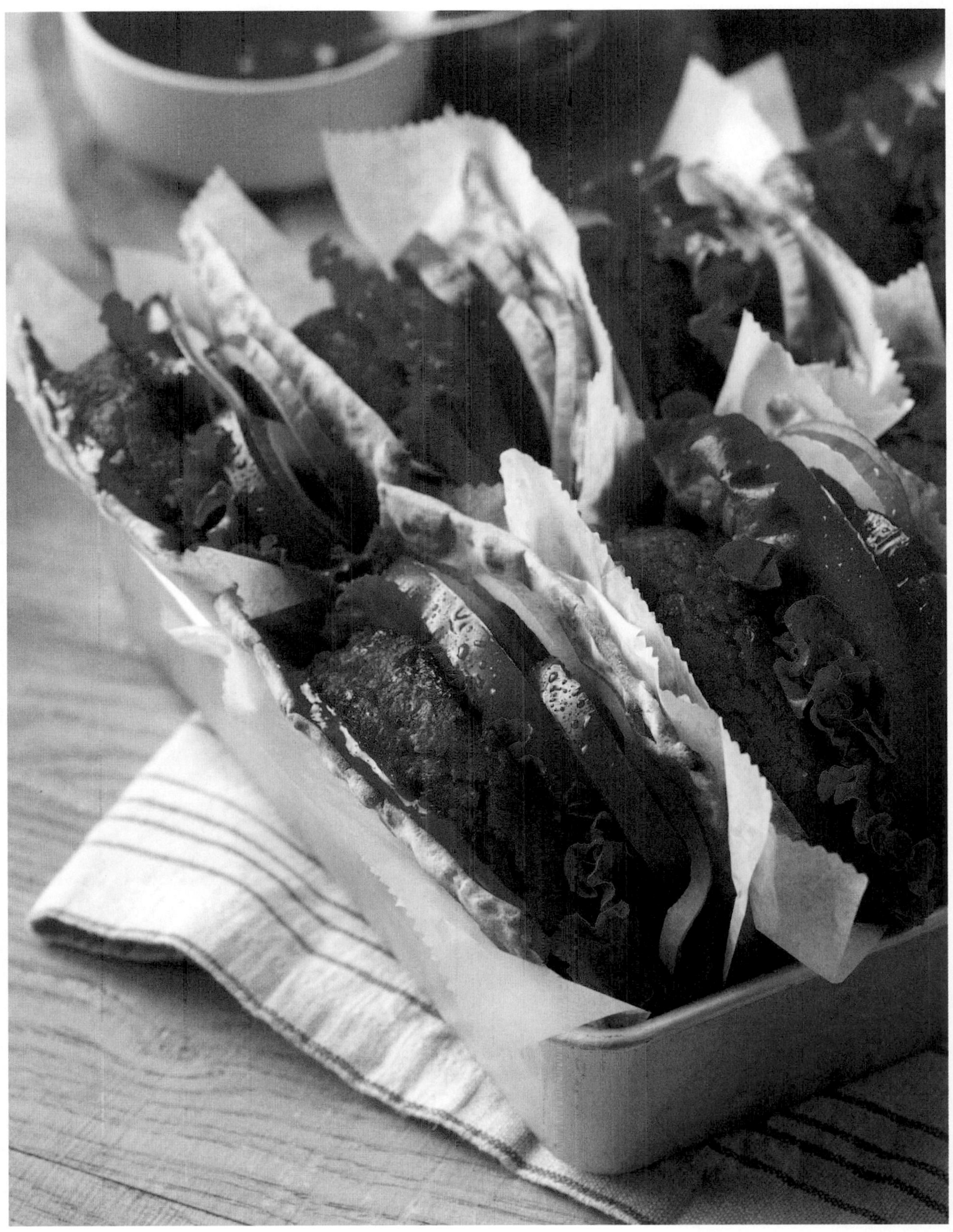

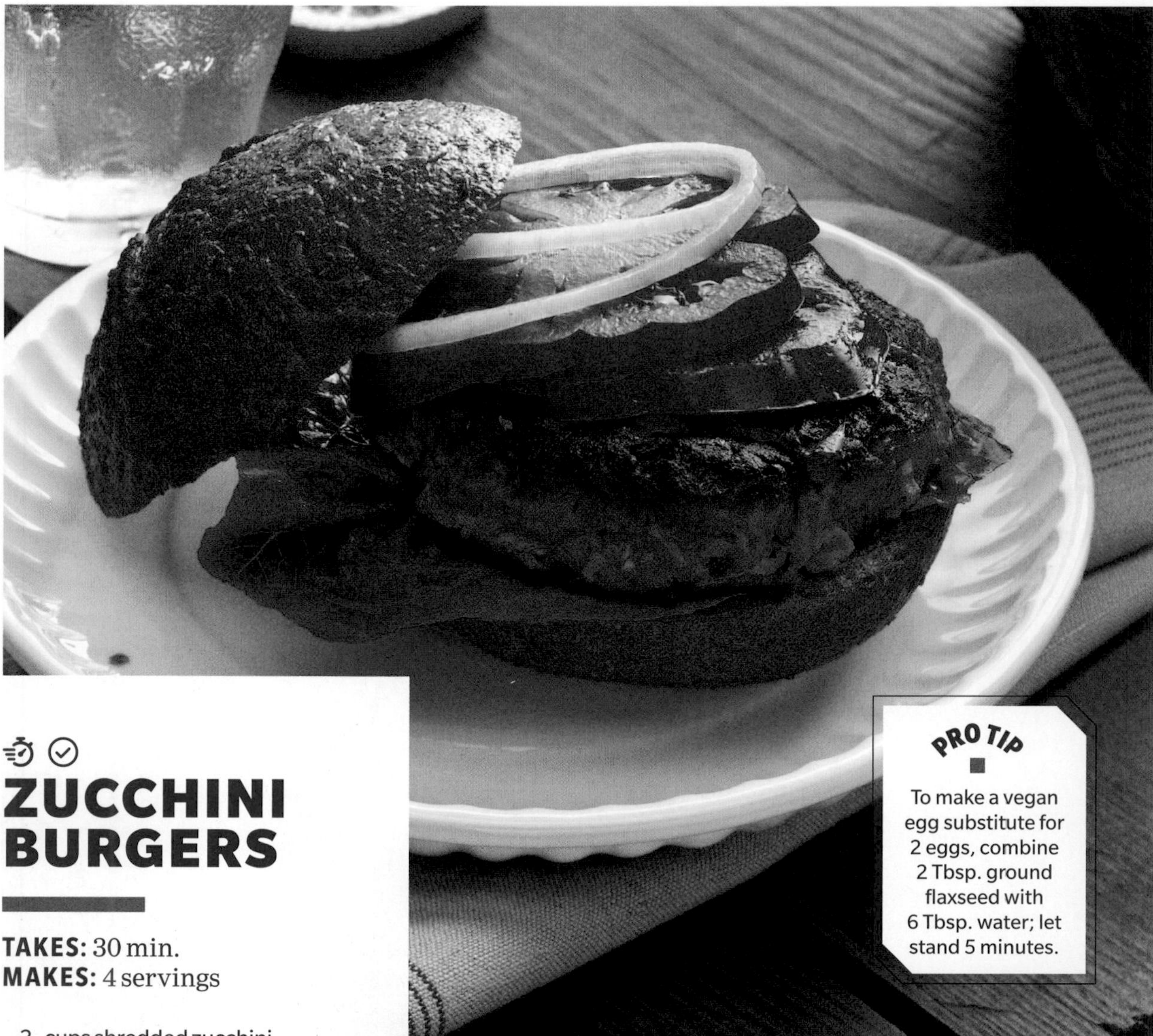

PRO TIP

To make a vegan egg substitute for 2 eggs, combine 2 Tbsp. ground flaxseed with 6 Tbsp. water; let stand 5 minutes.

ZUCCHINI BURGERS

TAKES: 30 min.
MAKES: 4 servings

- 2 cups shredded zucchini
- 1 medium onion, finely chopped
- ½ cup dry bread crumbs
- 2 large eggs, lightly beaten or vegan egg substitute
- ⅛ tsp. salt
- Dash cayenne pepper
- 3 hard-boiled large egg whites, chopped or ⅓ cup additional shredded zucchini
- 2 Tbsp. canola oil
- 4 whole wheat hamburger buns, split
- 4 lettuce leaves
- 4 slices tomato
- 4 slices onion

1 In a sieve or colander, drain zucchini, squeezing to remove excess liquid. Pat dry. In a small bowl, combine the zucchini, onion, bread crumbs, eggs, salt and cayenne. Gently stir in chopped egg whites.

2 Heat 1 Tbsp. oil in a large nonstick skillet over medium-low heat. Drop the batter by scant ⅔ cupfuls into oil; press lightly to flatten. Fry in batches until golden brown on both sides, using remaining oil as needed.

3 Serve on buns with lettuce, tomato and onion.

1 BURGER *314 cal., 12g fat (2g sat. fat), 106mg chol., 467mg sod., 40g carb. (9g sugars, 6g fiber), 13g pro.*
Diabetic exchanges: *2 starch, 1½ fat, 1 vegetable, 1 lean meat*

SALSA BLACK BEAN BURGERS

TAKES: 20 min.
MAKES: 4 servings

- 1 can (15 oz.) black beans, rinsed and drained
- ⅔ cup dry bread crumbs
- 1 small tomato, seeded and finely chopped
- 1 jalapeno pepper, seeded and finely chopped
- 1 large egg or vegan egg substitute
- 1 tsp. minced fresh cilantro
- 1 garlic clove, minced
- 1 Tbsp. olive oil
- 4 whole wheat hamburger buns, split
- Optional toppings: Spicy or vegan ranch salad dressing, lettuce, sliced tomato and sliced red onions

1 Place beans in a food processor; cover and process until blended. Transfer to a large bowl. Add the bread crumbs, tomato, jalapeno, egg, cilantro and garlic. Mix until combined. Shape into 4 patties.

2 In a large nonstick skillet, cook patties in oil over medium heat 4-6 minutes on each side or until lightly browned. Serve on buns with desired toppings.

1 BURGER: *323 cal., 8g fat (1g sat. fat), 53mg chol., 557mg sod., 51g carb. (6g sugars, 9g fiber), 13g pro.*

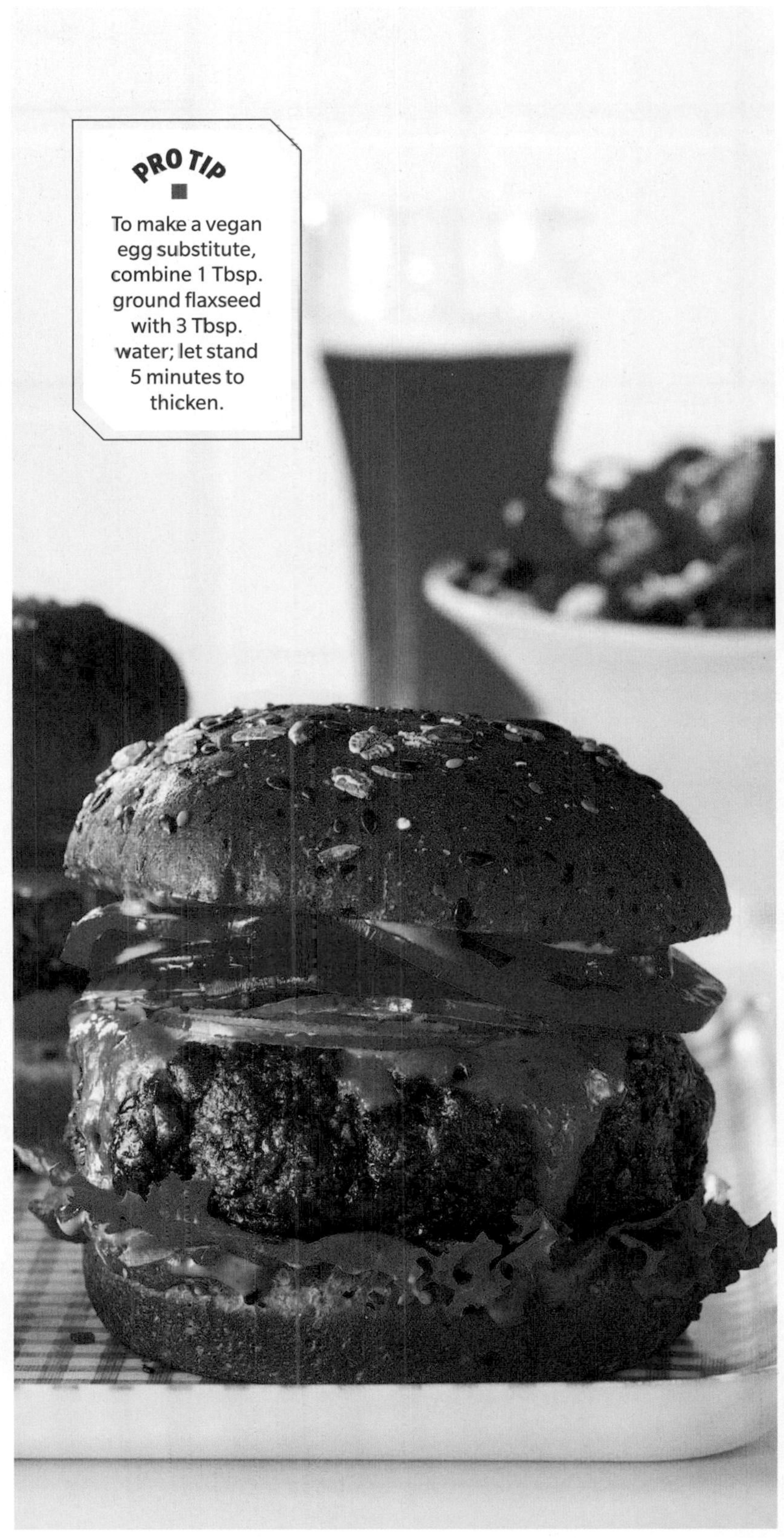

PRO TIP

To make a vegan egg substitute, combine 1 Tbsp. ground flaxseed with 3 Tbsp. water; let stand 5 minutes to thicken.

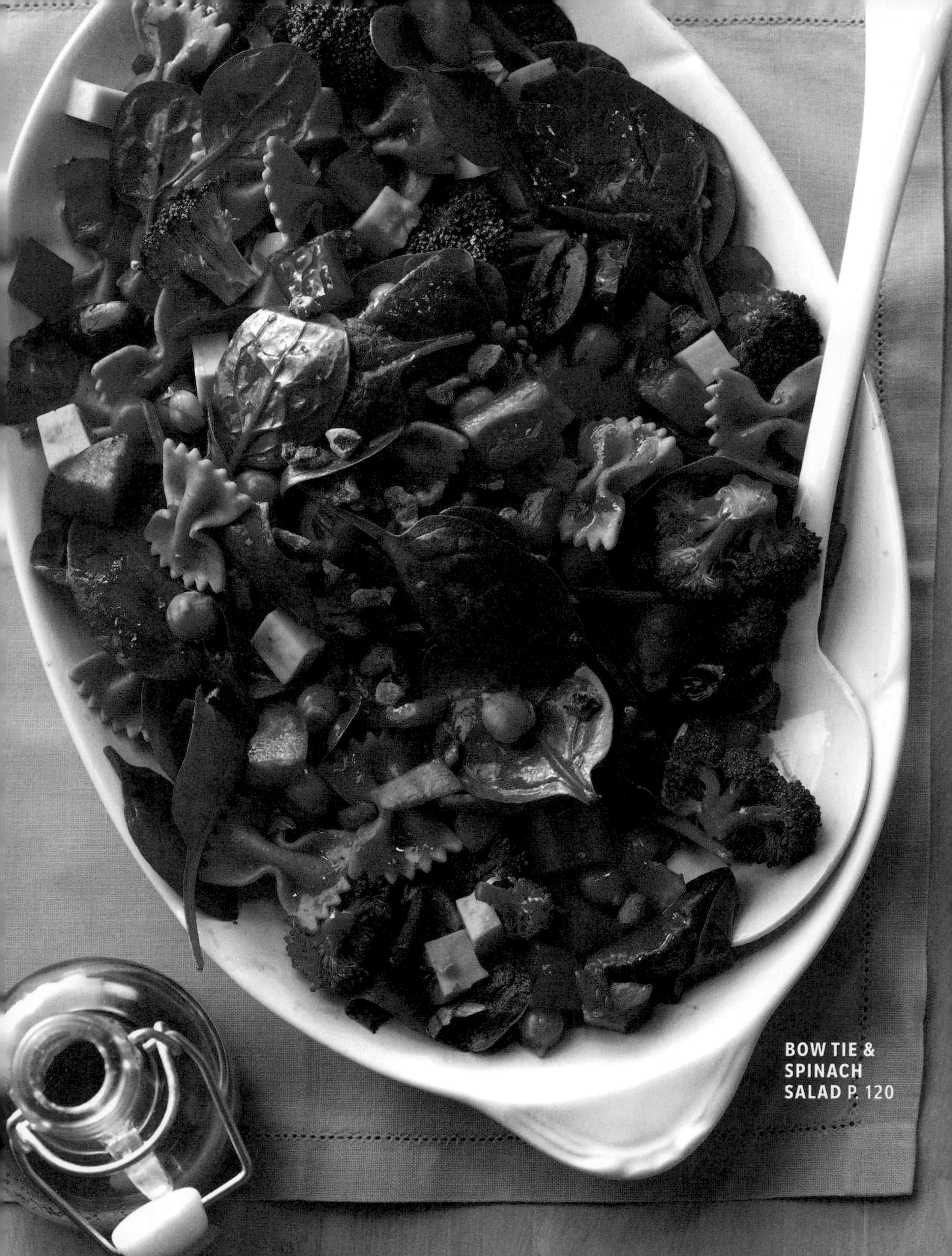

BOW TIE & SPINACH SALAD P. 120

CHAPTER 7

SALADS & BOWLS

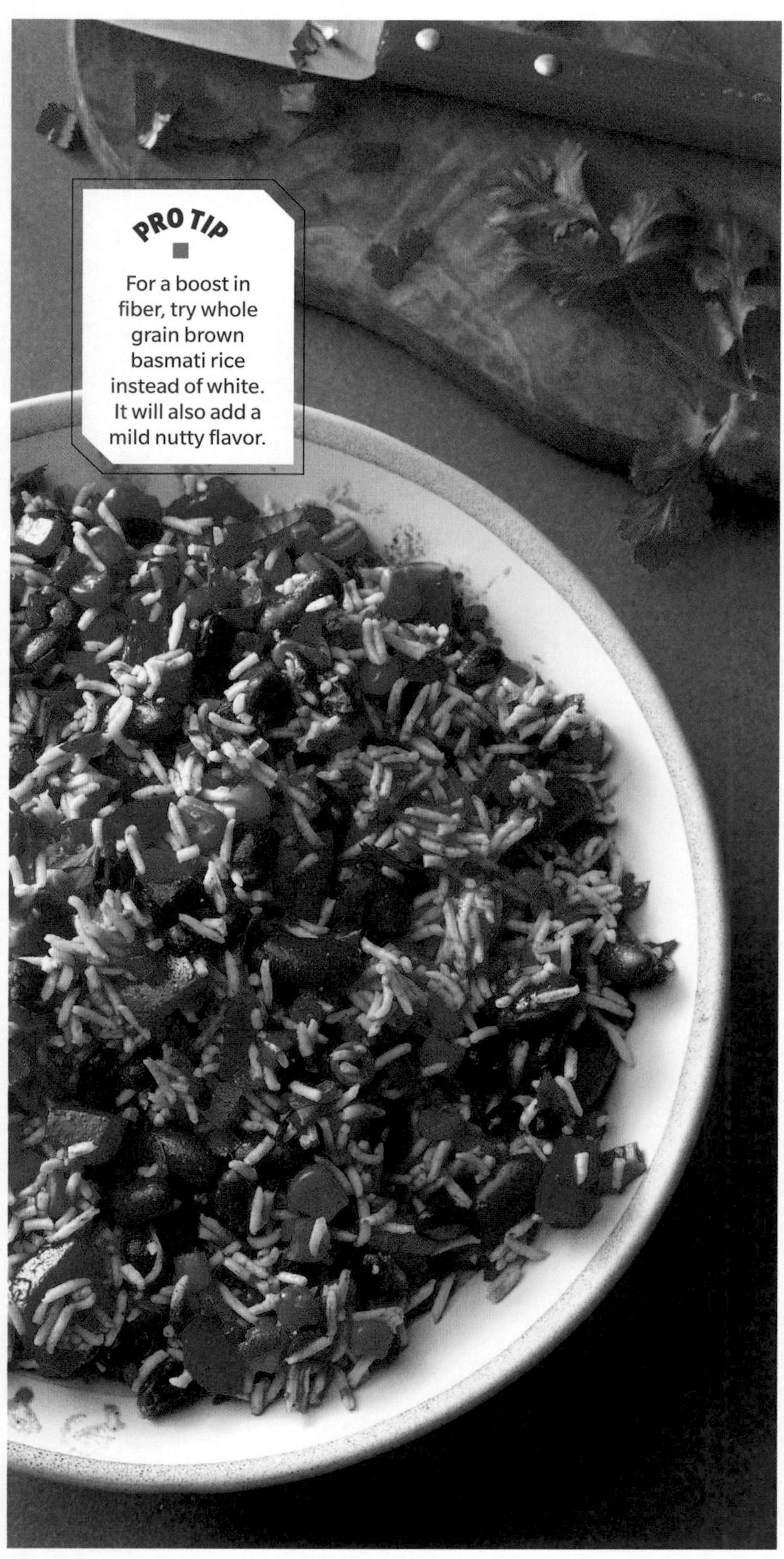

PRO TIP

For a boost in fiber, try whole grain brown basmati rice instead of white. It will also add a mild nutty flavor.

COOL BEANS SALAD

TAKES: 20 min.
MAKES: 6 servings

- ½ cup olive oil
- ¼ cup red wine vinegar
- 1 Tbsp. sugar
- 1 garlic clove, minced
- 1 tsp. salt
- 1 tsp. ground cumin
- 1 tsp. chili powder
- ¼ tsp. pepper
- 3 cups cooked basmati rice
- 1 can (16 oz.) kidney beans, rinsed and drained
- 1 can (15 oz.) black beans, rinsed and drained
- 1½ cups frozen corn, thawed
- 4 green onions, sliced
- 1 small sweet red pepper, chopped
- ¼ cup minced fresh cilantro

In a large bowl, whisk the first 8 ingredients. Add the remaining ingredients; toss to coat. Chill until serving.

1⅓ CUPS *440 cal., 19g fat (3g sat. fat), 0 chol., 659mg sod., 58g carb. (5g sugars, 8g fiber), 12g pro.*

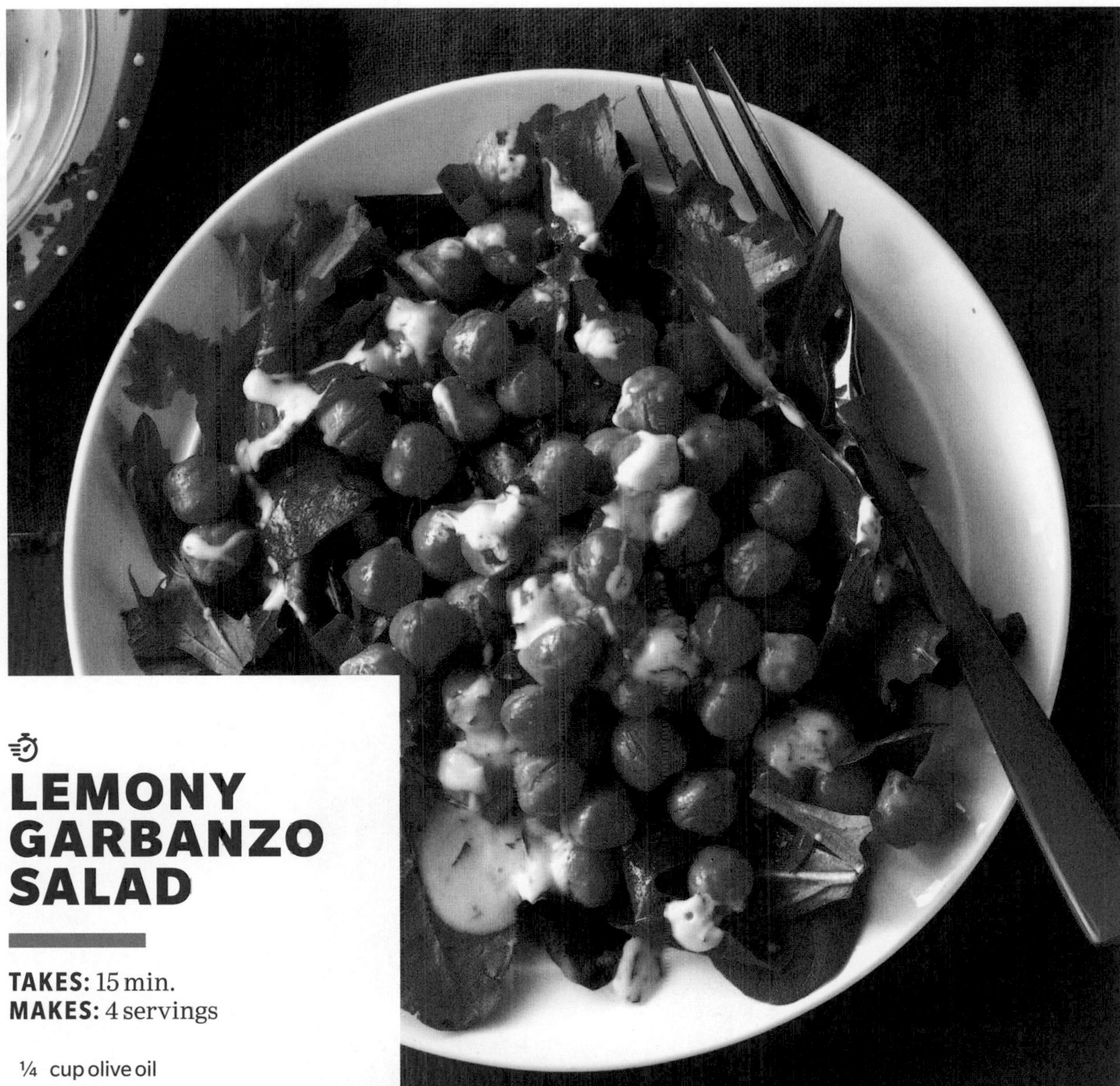

LEMONY GARBANZO SALAD

TAKES: 15 min.
MAKES: 4 servings

- ¼ cup olive oil
- 3 Tbsp. lemon juice
- ¾ tsp. ground cumin
- ¼ tsp. salt
- ¼ tsp. ground coriander
- ¼ tsp. pepper
- 2 cans (15 oz. each) garbanzo beans or chickpeas, rinsed and drained
- 3 green onions, chopped
- ½ cup plain vegan yogurt
- 1 Tbsp. minced fresh parsley
- 1 Tbsp. orange marmalade
- 4 cups spring mix salad greens

1 In a large bowl, whisk together first 6 ingredients; stir in beans and green onions. In another bowl, mix yogurt, parsley and marmalade.

2 To serve, divide greens among 4 plates; top with bean mixture. Serve with yogurt sauce.

1 SERVING *363 cal., 18g fat (2g sat. fat), 0 chol., 478mg sod., 41g carb. (9g sugars, 10g fiber), 11g pro.*

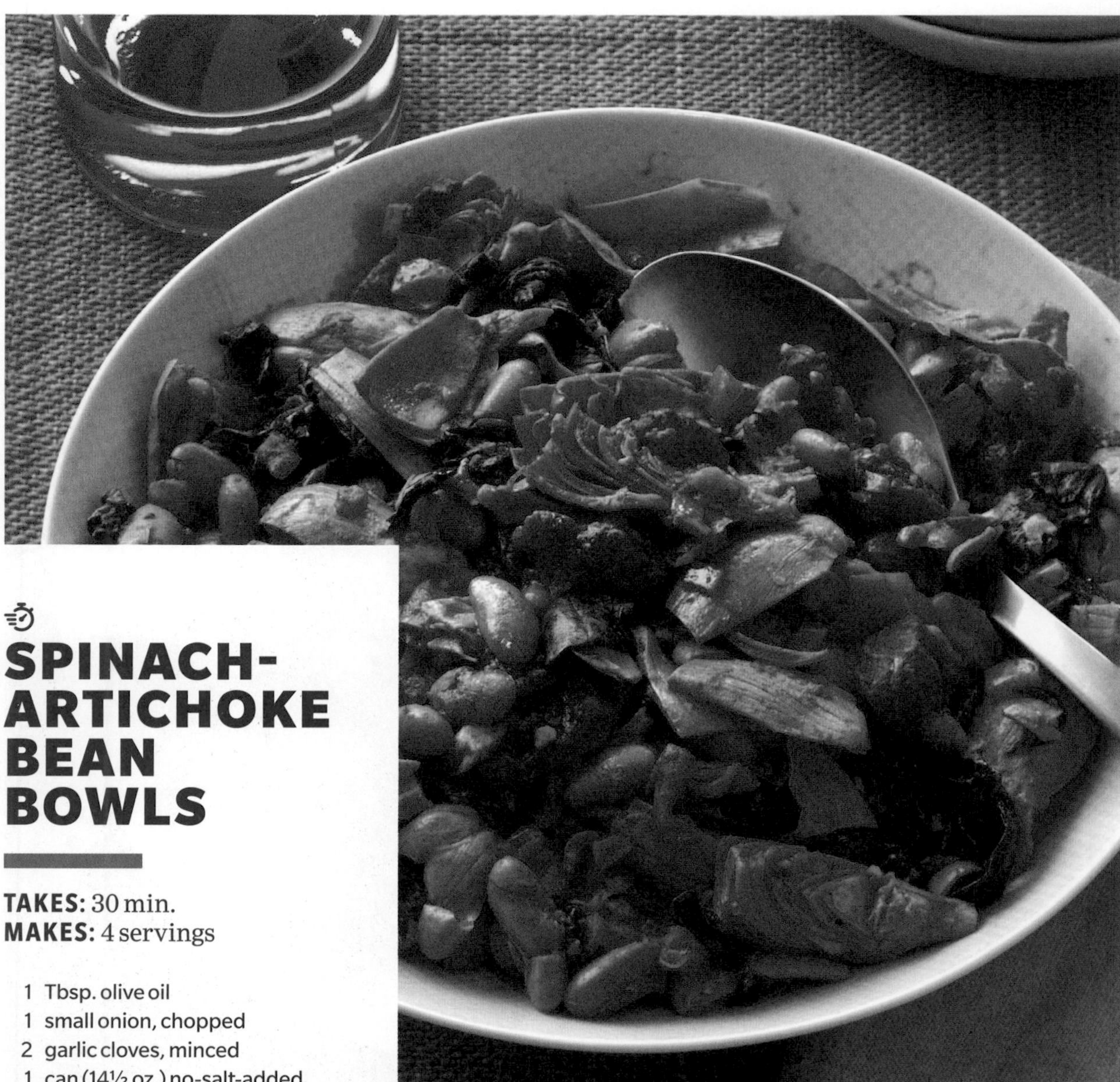

SPINACH-ARTICHOKE BEAN BOWLS

TAKES: 30 min.
MAKES: 4 servings

- 1 Tbsp. olive oil
- 1 small onion, chopped
- 2 garlic cloves, minced
- 1 can (14½ oz.) no-salt-added diced tomatoes, undrained
- 2 Tbsp. vegan Worcestershire sauce
- ¼ tsp. salt
- ¼ tsp. pepper
- ⅛ tsp. crushed red pepper flakes
- 1 can (15 oz.) cannellini beans, rinsed and drained
- 1 can (14 oz.) water-packed artichoke hearts, rinsed, drained and quartered
- 6 oz. fresh baby spinach (about 8 cups)

1 In a 12-in. skillet, heat oil over medium-high heat; saute onion until tender, 3-5 minutes. Add garlic; cook and stir 1 minute. Stir in the tomatoes, Worcestershire sauce and seasonings; bring to a boil. Reduce the heat; simmer, uncovered, until liquid is almost evaporated, 6-8 minutes.

2 Add beans, artichoke hearts and spinach; cook and stir until spinach is wilted, 3-5 minutes.

1½ CUPS *187 cal., 4g fat (1g sat. fat), 0 chol., 650mg sod., 30g carb. (4g sugars, 6g fiber), 8g pro.* ***Diabetic exchanges:*** *2 vegetable, 1 starch, 1 lean meat, 1 fat*

EDAMAME SALAD WITH SESAME GINGER DRESSING

TAKES: 15 min.
MAKES: 6 servings

- 6 cups baby kale salad blend (about 5 oz.)
- 1 can (15 oz.) garbanzo beans or chickpeas, rinsed and drained
- 2 cups frozen shelled edamame (about 10 oz.), thawed
- 3 clementines, peeled and segmented
- 1 cup fresh bean sprouts
- ½ cup salted peanuts
- 2 green onions, diagonally sliced
- ½ cup sesame ginger salad dressing

Divide the salad blend among 6 bowls. Top with all remaining ingredients except the salad dressing. Serve with dressing.

1 SERVING *317 cal., 17g fat (2g sat. fat), 0 chol., 355mg sod., 32g carb. (14g sugars, 8g fiber), 13g pro.*

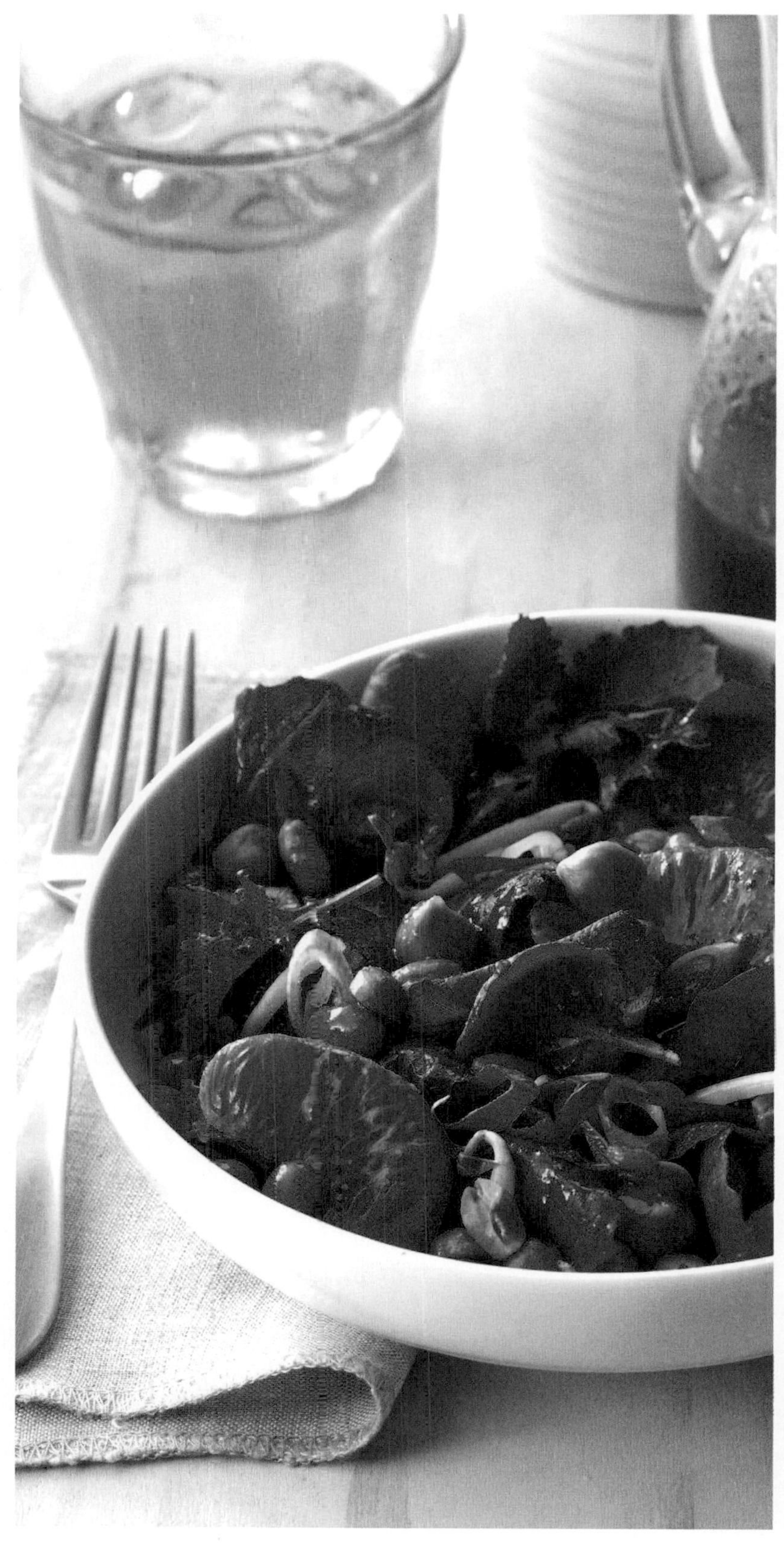

COLORFUL TACO SALAD

TAKES: 30 min. **MAKES:** 6 servings

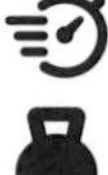

- 1 Tbsp. canola oil
- 1 medium sweet red pepper, chopped
- 1 small onion, chopped
- 3 garlic cloves, minced
- 1 pkg. (12 oz.) frozen vegetarian meat crumbles
- 1½ cups salsa, divided
- 1 Tbsp. chili powder
- 1 tsp. ground cumin
- 8 cups torn romaine
- 1 can (15 oz.) black beans, rinsed and drained
- 1 cup coarsely crushed tortilla chips
- 1 cup frozen corn, thawed
- 2 roma tomatoes, chopped
- 1 medium ripe avocado, peeled and cubed
- ¼ cup chopped fresh cilantro
- ¼ cup vegan ranch salad dressing
- Lime wedges, optional

1 In a large skillet, heat oil over medium heat. Add pepper and onion; cook and stir until tender, 5-7 minutes. Add the garlic; cook 1 minute longer. Stir in crumbles, ¾ cup salsa, chili powder and cumin; cook and stir until heated through, 3-5 minutes.

2 In a large bowl, combine lettuce, beans, tortilla chips, corn, tomato, avocado, cilantro and crumble mixture. Combine remaining salsa and vegan ranch, pore over salad and toss to coat. If desired, serve with lime wedges.

2 CUPS *354 cal., 15g fat (2g sat. fat), 1mg chol., 807mg sod., 40g carb. (7g sugars, 11g fiber), 17g pro.* ***Diabetic exchanges:*** *2½ starch, 2 lean meat, 2 fat*

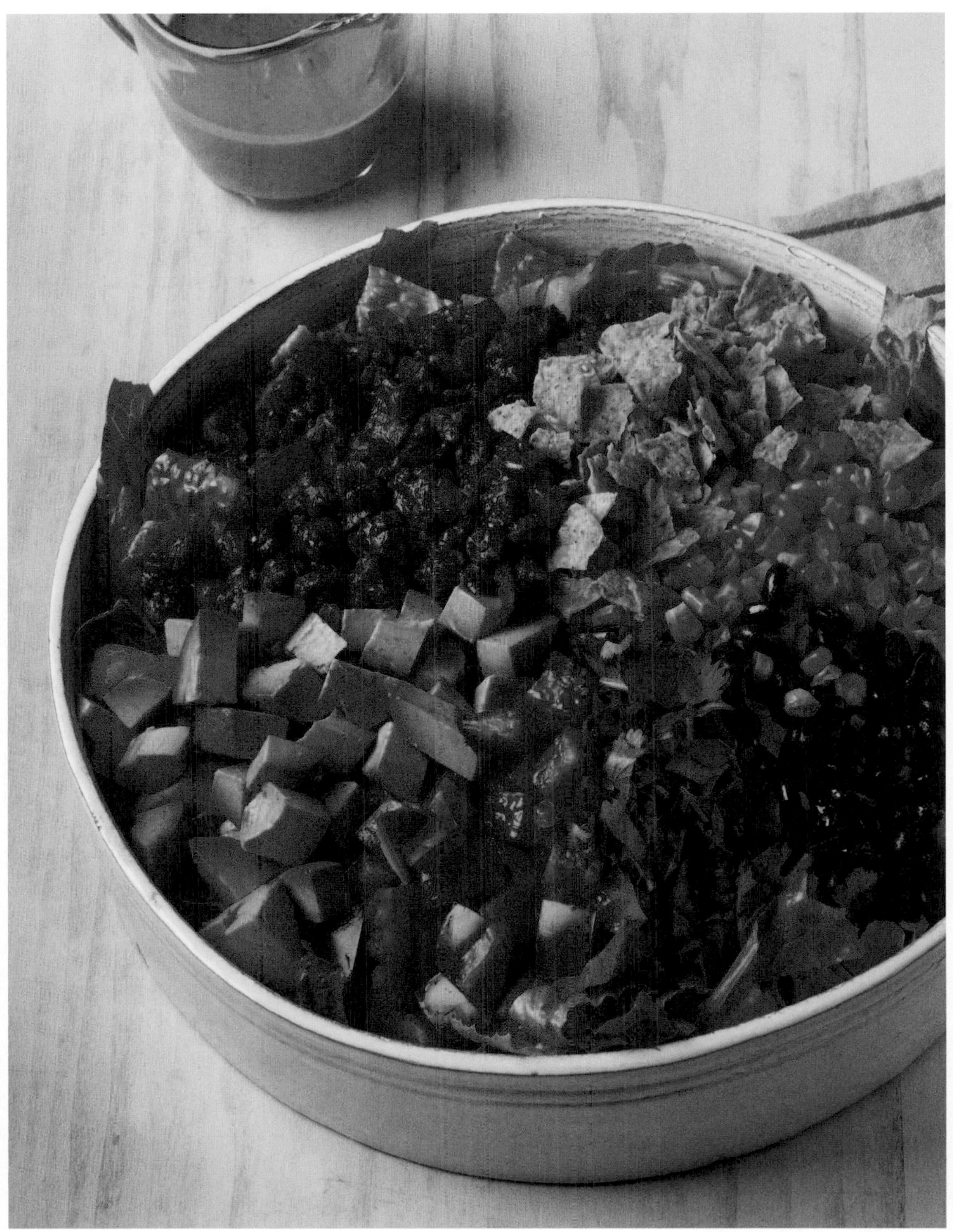

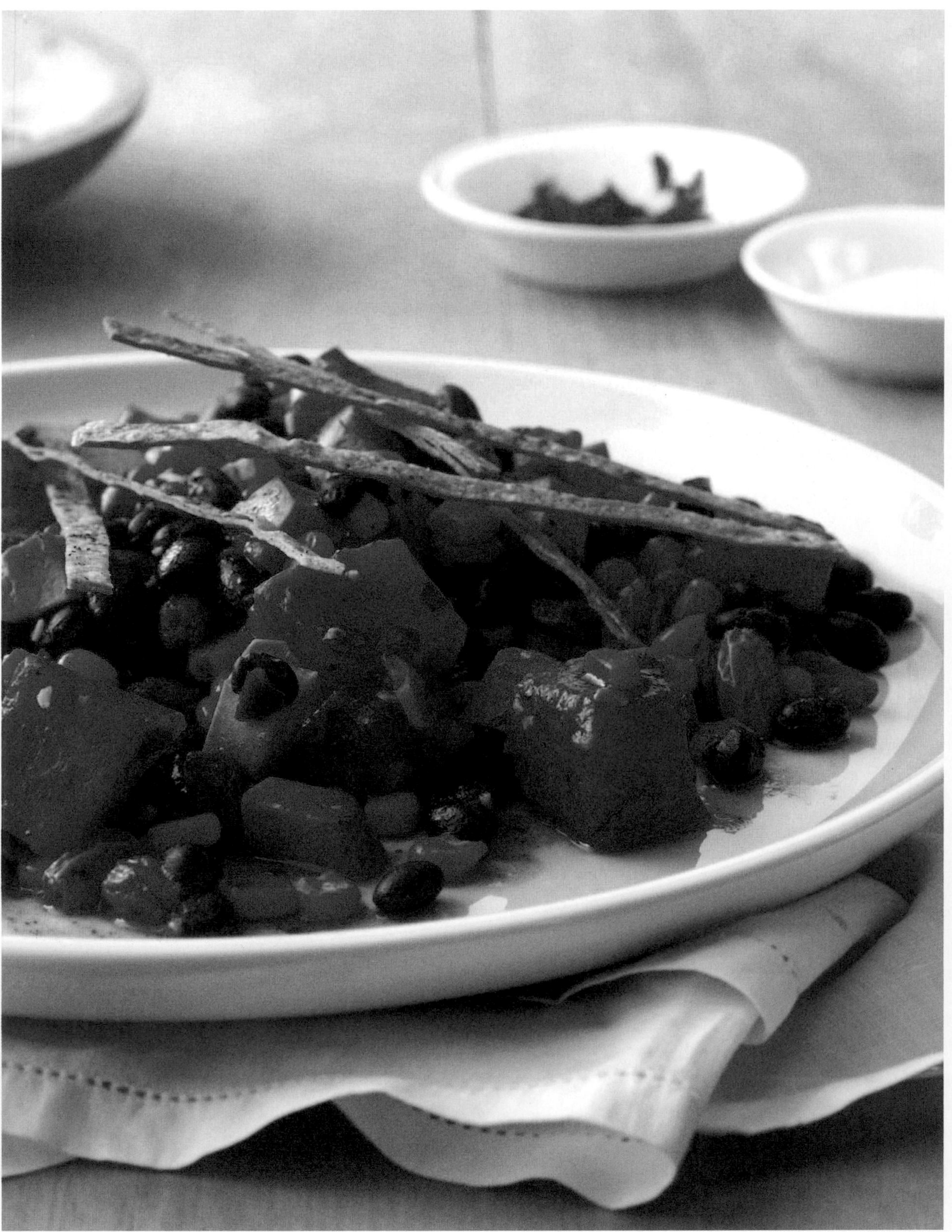

TROPICAL FUSION SALAD WITH SPICY TORTILLA RIBBONS

TAKES: 30 min. **MAKES:** 4 servings

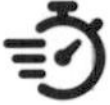

- 2 cups cubed peeled papaya
- 1 can (15 oz.) black beans, rinsed and drained
- 1 medium ripe avocado, peeled and cubed
- 1 cup frozen corn, thawed
- ½ cup golden raisins
- ¼ cup minced fresh cilantro
- ¼ cup orange juice
- 2 serrano peppers, seeded and chopped
- 2 Tbsp. lime juice
- 1 Tbsp. cider vinegar
- 2 garlic cloves, minced
- 2 tsp. ground ancho chile pepper, divided
- ¼ tsp. sugar
- ¼ tsp. salt
- 2 corn tortillas (6 in.), cut into ¼-in. strips
- Cooking spray

1 Preheat oven to 350°. In a large bowl, combine papaya, beans, avocado, corn, raisins, cilantro, orange juice, peppers, lime juice, vinegar, garlic, ½ teaspoon chili pepper, sugar and salt.

2 Place the tortilla strips on a greased baking sheet; spritz with cooking spray. Sprinkle with the remaining chili pepper. Bake for 8-10 minutes or until crisp. Top salad with tortilla strips.

1 SERVING *321 cal., 8g fat (1g sat. fat), 0 chol., 380mg sod., 58g carb. (20g sugars, 11g fiber), 9g pro.*

VEGGIE NICOISE SALAD

PREP: 40 min. **COOK:** 25 min. **MAKES:** 8 servings

- ⅓ cup olive oil
- ¼ cup lemon juice
- 2 tsp. minced fresh oregano
- 2 tsp. minced fresh thyme
- 1 tsp. Dijon mustard
- 1 garlic clove, minced
- ¼ tsp. coarsely ground pepper
- ⅛ tsp. salt
- 1 can (16 oz.) kidney beans, rinsed and drained
- 1 small red onion, halved and thinly sliced
- 1 lb. small red potatoes (about 9), halved
- 1 lb. fresh asparagus, trimmed
- ½ lb. fresh green beans, trimmed
- 12 cups torn romaine (about 2 small bunches)
- 6 hard-boiled large eggs, quartered
- 1 jar (6½ oz.) marinated quartered artichoke hearts, drained
- ½ cup Nicoise or kalamata olives

1 For vinaigrette, whisk together the first 8 ingredients. In another bowl, toss the kidney beans and onion with 1 Tbsp. vinaigrette. Set aside bean mixture and remaining vinaigrette.

2 Place potatoes in a saucepan and cover with water. Bring to a boil. Reduce heat; simmer, covered, 10-15 minutes or until tender. Drain. While potatoes are warm, toss with 1 Tbsp. vinaigrette; set aside.

3 In a pot of boiling water, cook asparagus just until crisp-tender, 2-4 minutes. Remove with tongs and immediately drop into ice water. Drain and pat dry. In the same pot of boiling water, cook green beans until crisp-tender, 3-4 minutes. Remove beans; place in ice water. Drain and pat dry.

4 To serve, toss asparagus with 1 Tbsp. vinaigrette; toss green beans with 2 tsp. vinaigrette. Toss romaine with remaining vinaigrette; place on a platter. Arrange vegetables, kidney bean mixture, eggs, artichoke hearts and olives over top.

1 SERVING *329 cal., 19g fat (4g sat. fat), 140mg chol., 422mg sod., 28g carb. (6g sugars, 7g fiber), 12g pro.* ***Diabetic exchanges:*** *3 fat, 2 vegetable, 2 medium-fat meat, 1½ starch*

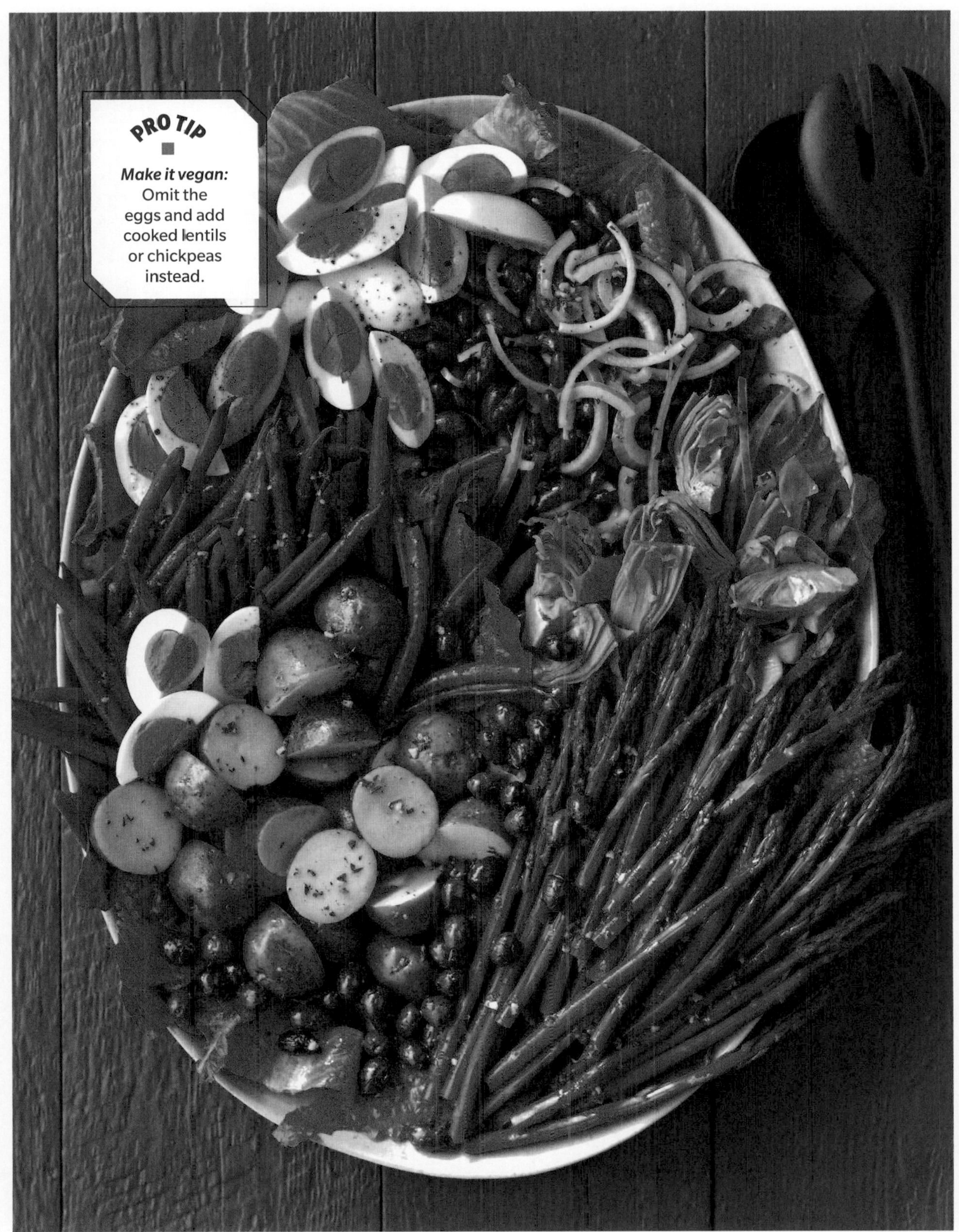
PRO TIP
Make it vegan: Omit the eggs and add cooked lentils or chickpeas instead.

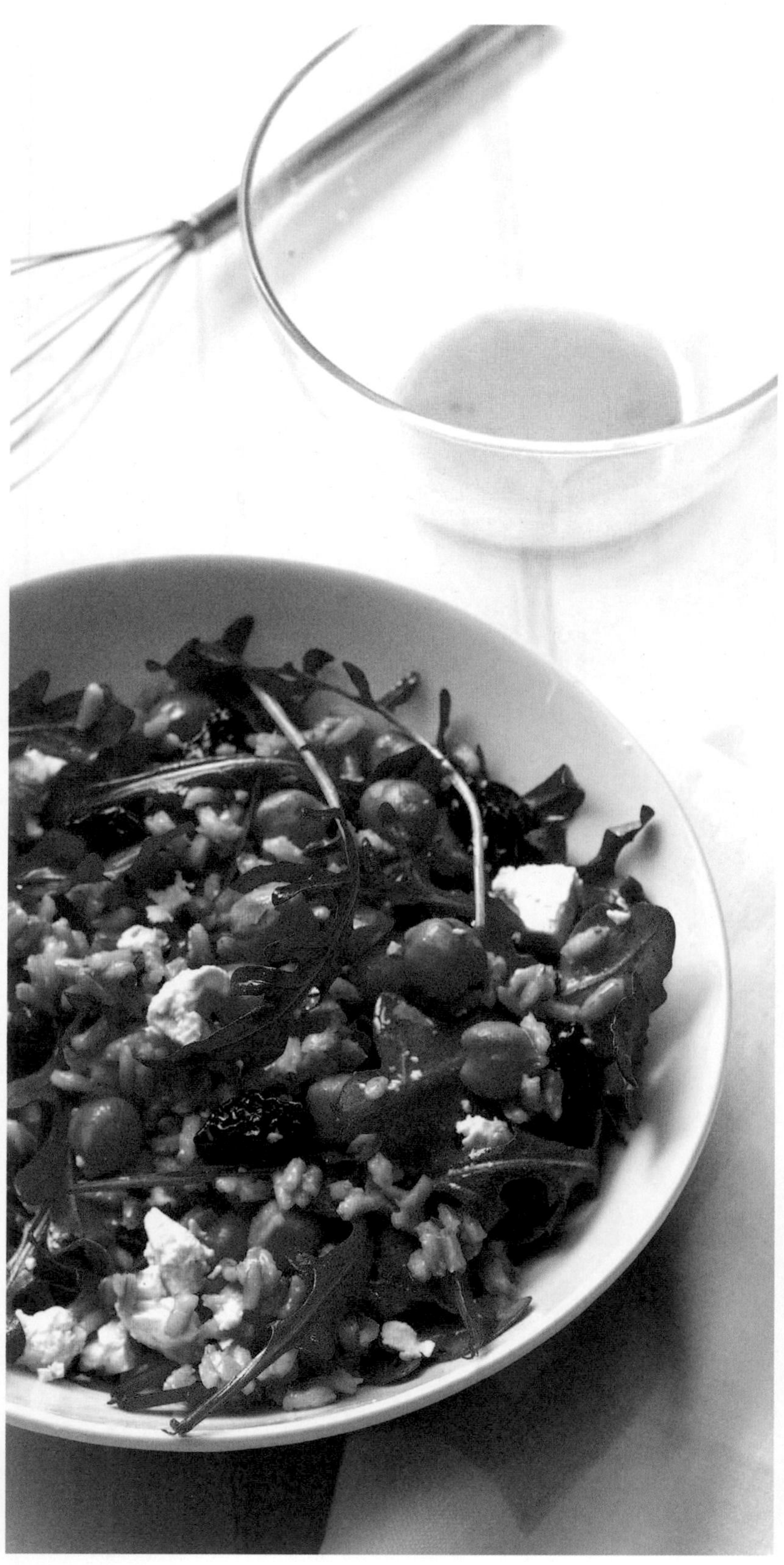

ARUGULA & BROWN RICE SALAD

TAKES: 25 min.
MAKES: 4 servings

- 1 pkg. (8.8 oz.) ready-to-serve brown rice
- 7 cups fresh arugula or baby spinach (about 5 oz.)
- 1 can (15 oz.) garbanzo beans or chickpeas, rinsed and drained
- 1 cup crumbled feta or vegan feta-style cheese
- ¾ cup loosely packed basil leaves, torn
- ½ cup dried cherries or cranberries

DRESSING

- ¼ cup olive oil
- ¼ tsp. grated lemon zest
- 2 Tbsp. lemon juice
- ¼ tsp. salt
- ⅛ tsp. pepper

1 Heat rice according to package directions. Transfer to a large bowl; cool slightly.

2 Stir arugula, beans, cheese, basil and cherries into rice. In a small bowl, whisk the dressing ingredients. Drizzle over salad; toss to coat. Serve immediately.

2 CUPS *473 cal., 22g fat (5g sat. fat), 15mg chol., 574mg sod., 53g carb. (17g sugars, 7g fiber), 13g pro.*

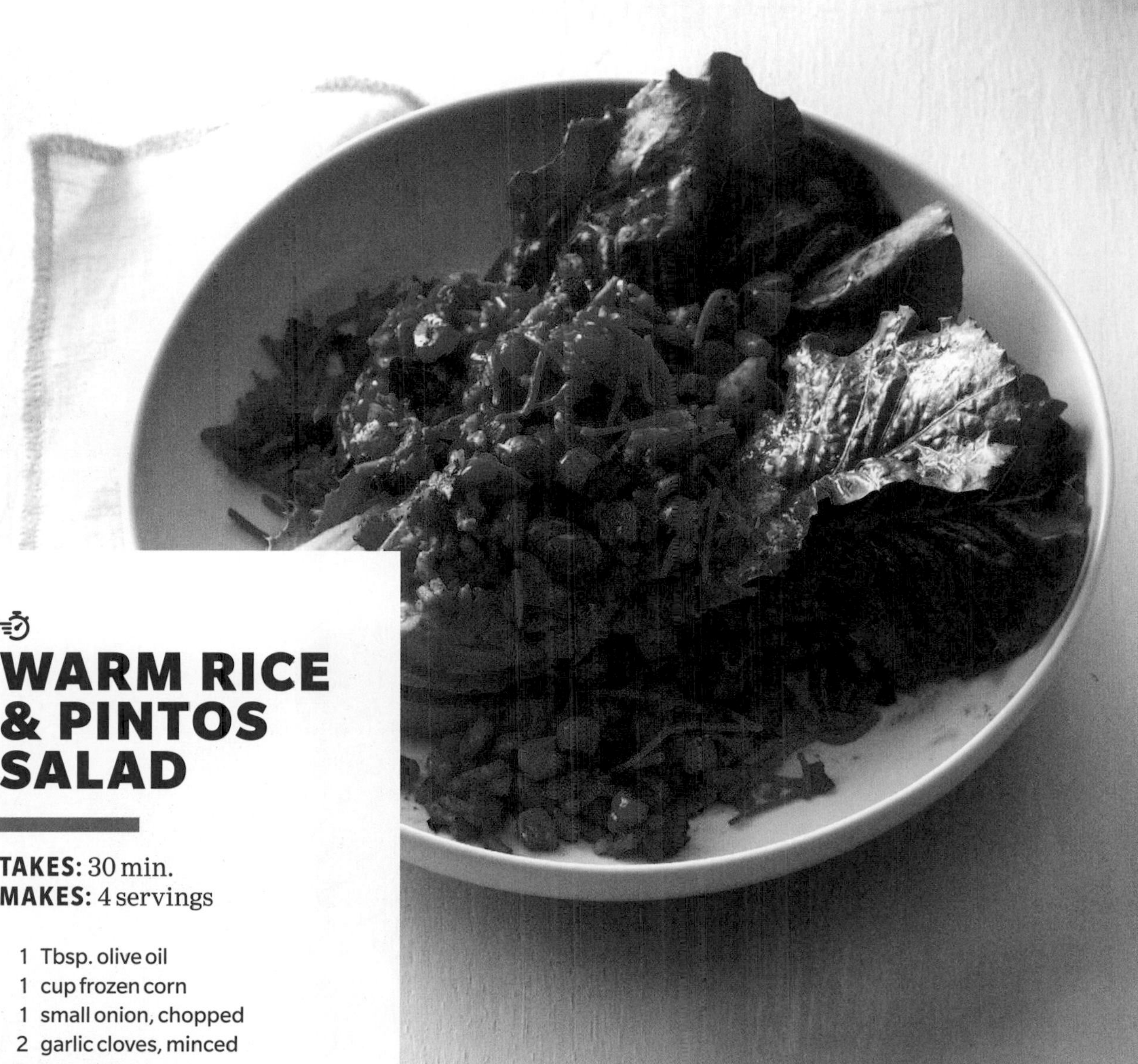

WARM RICE & PINTOS SALAD

TAKES: 30 min.
MAKES: 4 servings

- 1 Tbsp. olive oil
- 1 cup frozen corn
- 1 small onion, chopped
- 2 garlic cloves, minced
- 1½ tsp. chili powder
- 1½ tsp. ground cumin
- 1 can (15 oz.) pinto beans, rinsed and drained
- 1 pkg. (8.8 oz.) ready-to-serve brown rice
- 1 can (4 oz.) chopped green chiles
- ½ cup salsa
- ¼ cup chopped fresh cilantro
- 1 bunch romaine, quartered lengthwise through the core
- ¼ cup finely shredded cheddar or vegan cheddar-style cheese

1 In a large skillet, heat oil over medium-high heat. Add corn and onion; cook and stir 4-5 minutes or until onion is tender. Stir in garlic, chili powder and cumin; cook and stir 1 minute longer.

2 Add beans, rice, green chiles, salsa and cilantro; heat through, stirring occasionally.

3 Serve over romaine wedges. Sprinkle with cheese.

1 SERVING *331 cal., 8g fat (2g sat. fat), 7mg chol., 465mg sod., 50g carb. (5g sugars, 9g fiber), 12g pro.* ***Diabetic exchanges:*** *2½ starch, 2 vegetable, 1 lean meat, ½ fat*

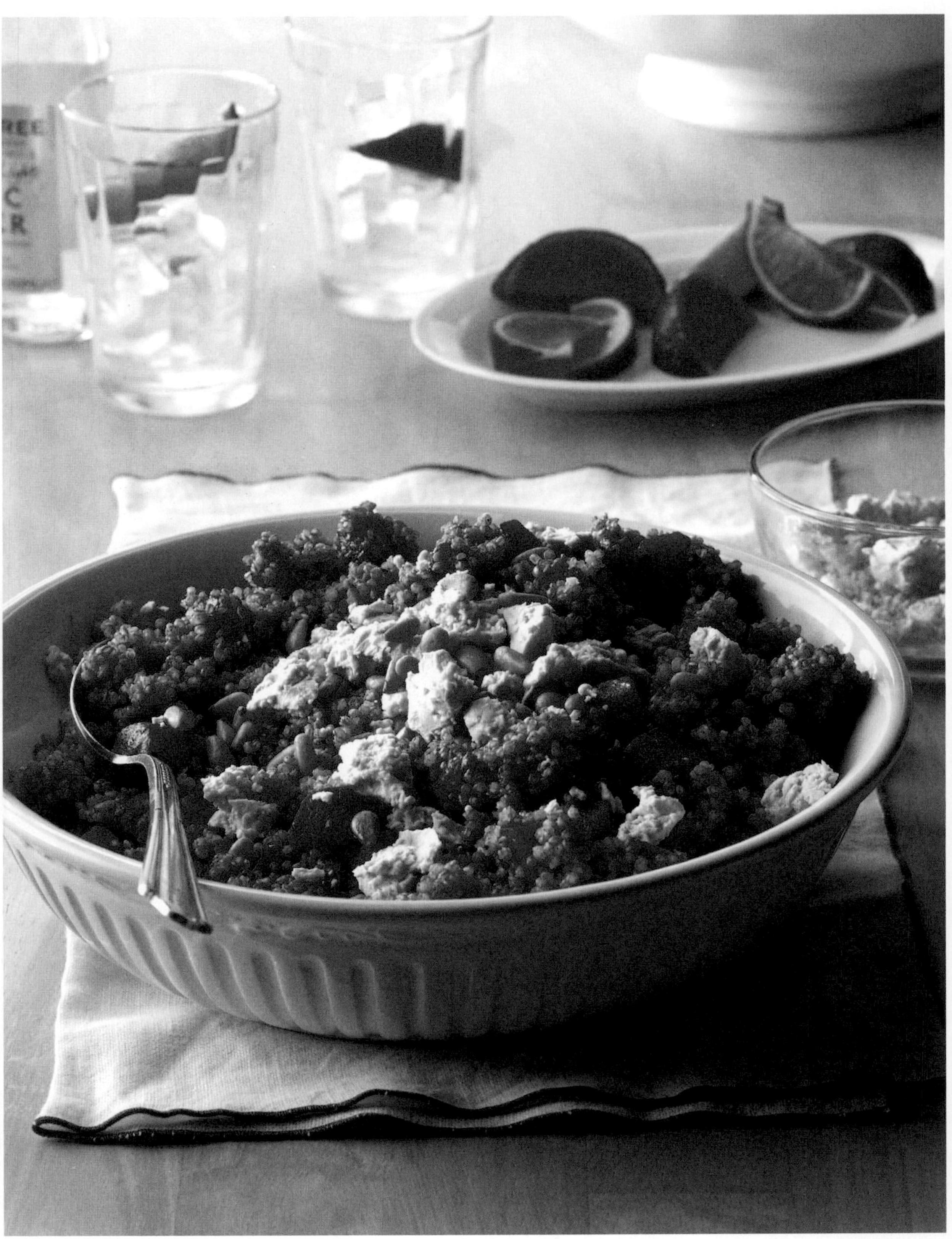

WARM SQUASH & QUINOA SALAD

TAKES: 30 min. **MAKES:** 6 servings

- 2 cups quinoa, rinsed
- 3 tsp. ground cumin
- 3 cups water
- 2 Tbsp. butter or olive oil
- 3½ cups cubed peeled butternut squash (about ½ medium)
- 1 tsp. sea salt
- ¾ tsp. Italian seasoning
- ¼ tsp. coarsely ground pepper
- ½ cup crumbled feta or vegan feta-style cheese
- Toasted pine nuts, optional

1 In a large saucepan, combine quinoa, cumin and water; bring to a boil. Reduce heat; simmer, covered, until liquid is absorbed, 10-13 minutes. Remove from heat; keep warm.

2 Meanwhile, in a large skillet, heat butter over medium-low heat 3-5 minutes or until golden brown, stirring constantly. Immediately stir in squash and seasonings; cook, covered, until tender, 10-12 minutes, stirring occasionally. Add to quinoa, stirring gently to combine. Top with feta cheese and, if desired, pine nuts.

1 CUP *314 cal., 9g fat (4g sat. fat), 15mg chol., 449mg sod., 49g carb. (2g sugars, 7g fiber), 11g pro.*

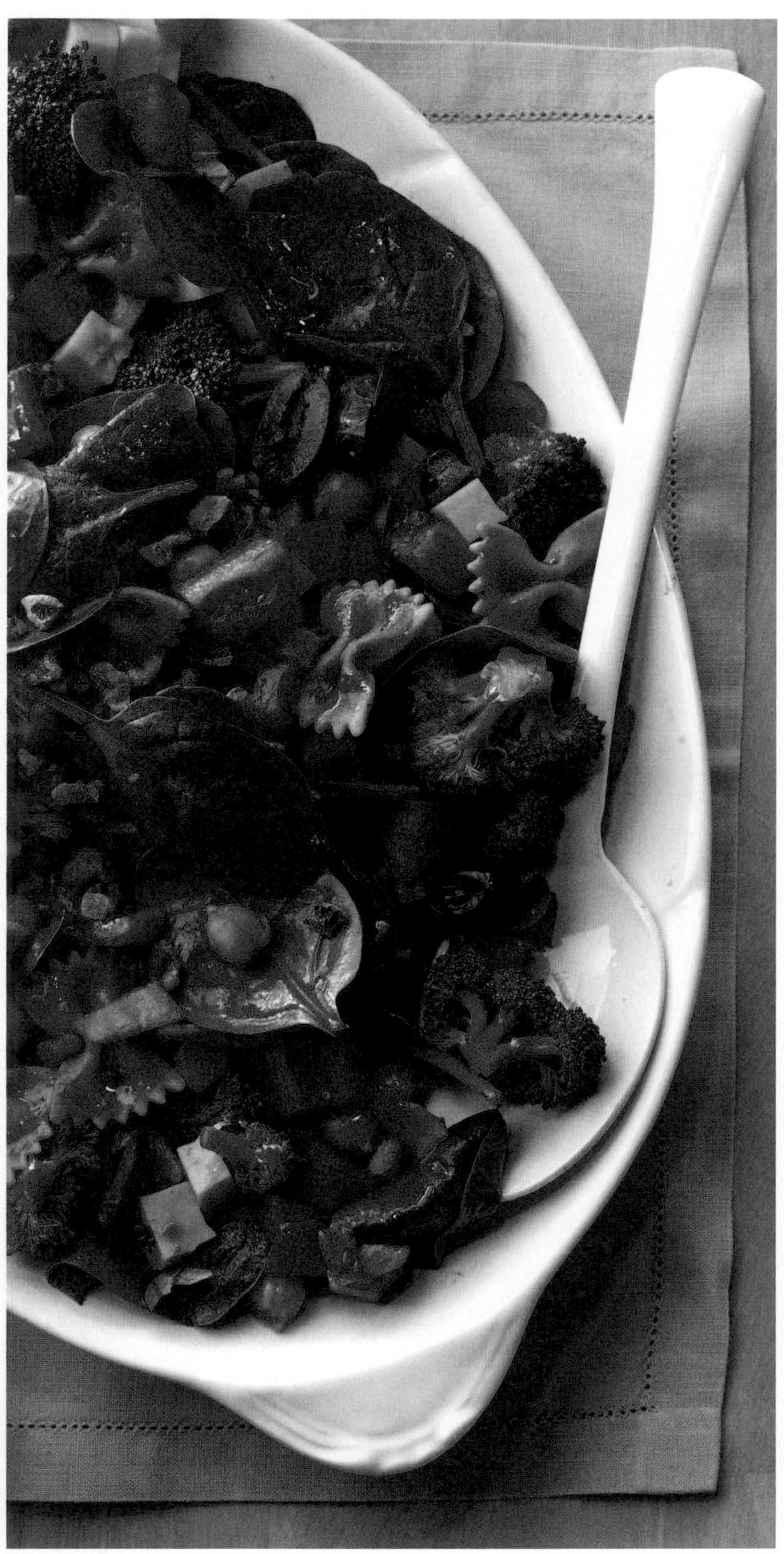

BOW TIE & SPINACH SALAD

TAKES: 30 min.
MAKES: 6 servings

- 2 cups uncooked multigrain bow tie pasta
- 1 can (15 oz.) garbanzo beans or chickpeas, rinsed and drained
- 6 cups fresh baby spinach (about 6 oz.)
- 2 cups fresh broccoli florets
- 2 plum tomatoes, chopped
- 1 medium sweet red pepper, chopped
- ½ cup cubed part-skim mozzarella or vegan mozzarella-style cheese
- ½ cup pitted Greek olives, halved
- ¼ cup minced fresh basil
- ⅓ cup red wine vinaigrette
- ¼ tsp. salt
- ¼ cup chopped walnuts, toasted

1 Cook pasta according to the package directions. Drain; transfer to a large bowl.

2 Add beans, vegetables, cheese, olives and basil to pasta. Drizzle with dressing and sprinkle with salt; toss to coat. Sprinkle with chopped walnuts.

2 CUPS *319 cal., 13g fat (2g sat. fat), 6mg chol., 730mg sod., 41g carb. (6g sugars, 7g fiber), 14g pro.* ***Diabetic exchanges:*** *2 starch, 2 fat, 1 vegetable, 1 lean meat*

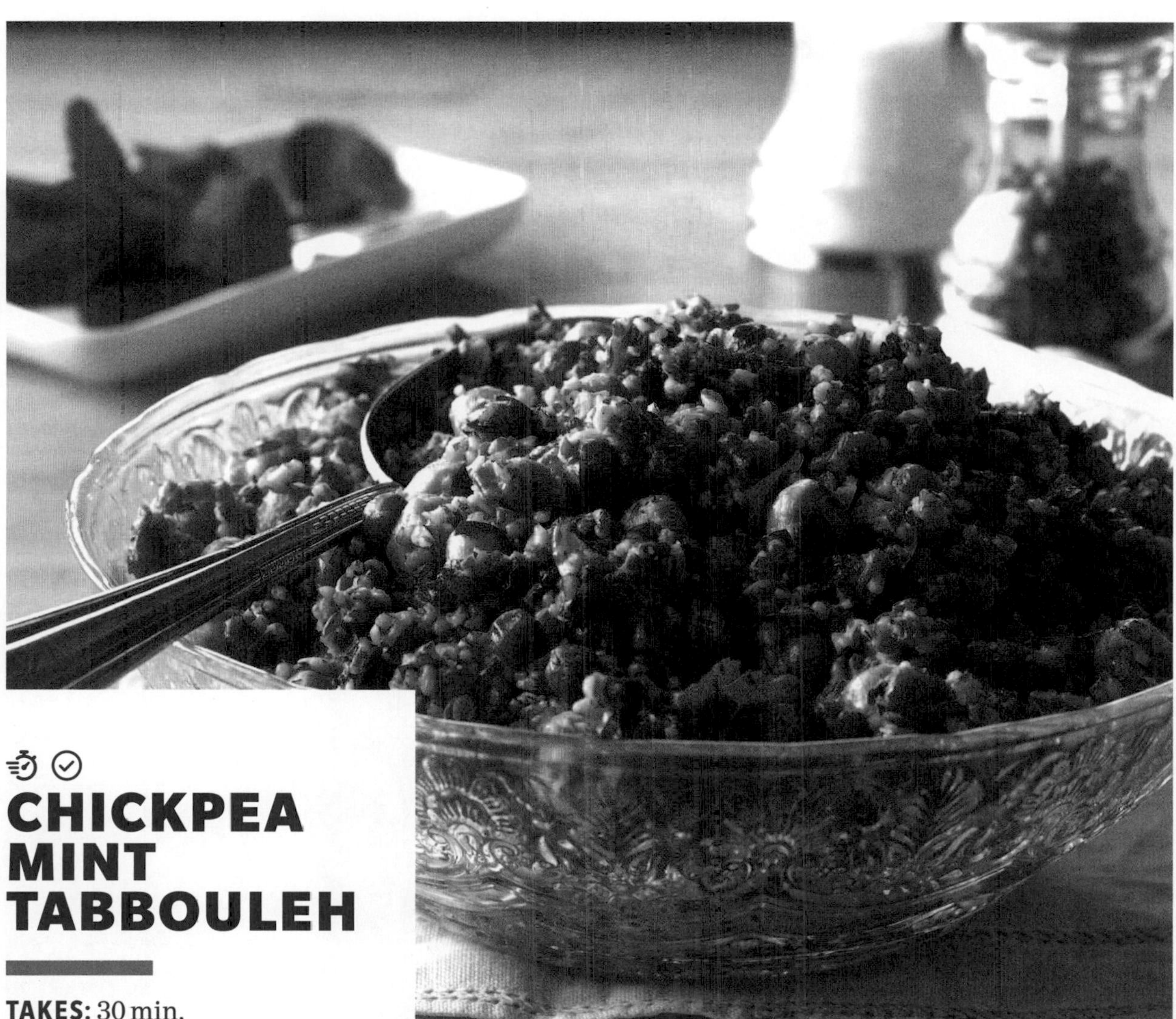

CHICKPEA MINT TABBOULEH

TAKES: 30 min.
MAKES: 4 servings

- 1 cup bulgur
- 2 cups water
- 1 cup fresh or frozen peas (about 5 oz.), thawed
- 1 can (15 oz.) chickpeas or garbanzo beans, rinsed and drained
- ½ cup minced fresh parsley
- ¼ cup minced fresh mint
- ¼ cup olive oil
- 2 Tbsp. julienned soft sun-dried tomatoes (not packed in oil)
- 2 Tbsp. lemon juice
- ½ tsp. salt
- ¼ tsp. pepper

1 In a large saucepan, combine bulgur and water; bring to a boil. Reduce heat; simmer, covered, for 10 minutes. Stir in fresh or thawed peas; cook, covered, until bulgur and peas are tender, about 5 minutes.

2 Transfer to a large bowl. Stir in the remaining ingredients. Serve warm, or refrigerate and serve cold.

1 CUP *380 cal., 16g fat (2g sat. fat), 0 chol., 450mg sod., 51g carb. (6g sugars, 11g fiber), 11g pro.* ***Diabetic exchanges:*** *3 starch, 3 fat, 1 lean meat*

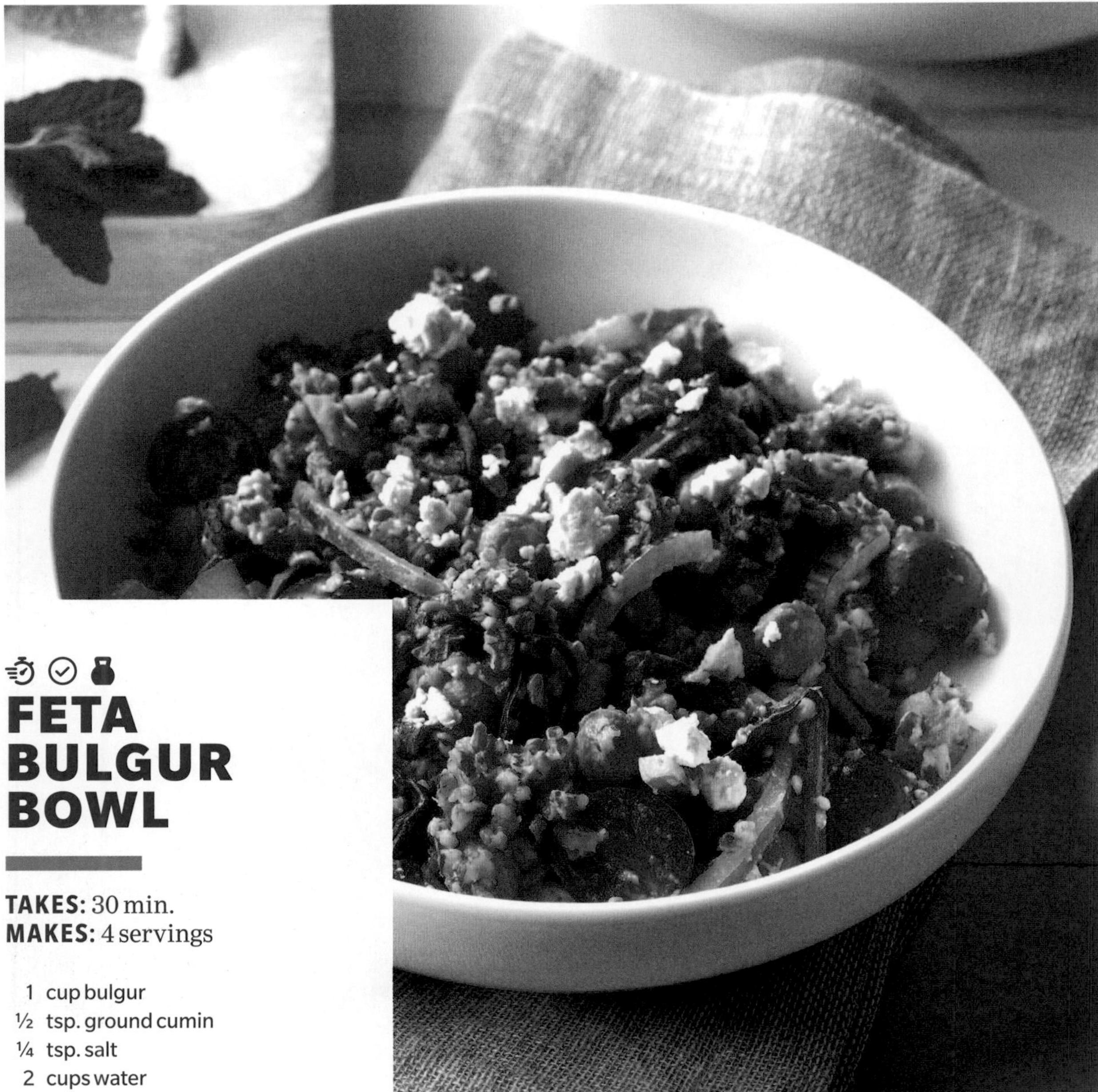

FETA BULGUR BOWL

TAKES: 30 min.
MAKES: 4 servings

- 1 cup bulgur
- ½ tsp. ground cumin
- ¼ tsp. salt
- 2 cups water
- 1 can (15 oz.) garbanzo beans or chickpeas, rinsed and drained
- 6 oz. fresh baby spinach (about 8 cups)
- 2 cups cherry tomatoes, halved
- 1 small red onion, halved and thinly sliced
- ½ cup crumbled feta or vegan feta-style cheese
- ¼ cup hummus
- 2 Tbsp. chopped fresh mint
- 2 Tbsp. lemon juice

1 In a 6-qt. stockpot, combine the first 4 ingredients; bring to a boil. Reduce heat; simmer, covered, until tender, 10-12 minutes. Stir in garbanzo beans; heat through.

2 Remove from heat; stir in the spinach. Let stand, covered, for 5 minutes or until spinach is wilted. Stir in remaining ingredients. Serve warm, or refrigerate and serve cold.

2 CUPS *311 cal., 7g fat (2g sat. fat), 8mg chol., 521mg sod., 52g carb. (6g sugars, 12g fiber), 14g pro.*

WHOLE WHEAT ORZO SALAD

TAKES: 30 min.
MAKES: 8 servings

- 2½ cups uncooked whole wheat orzo pasta (about 1 lb.)
- 1 can (15 oz.) cannellini beans, rinsed and drained
- 3 medium tomatoes, finely chopped
- 1 English cucumber, finely chopped
- 2 cups crumbled feta or vegan feta-style cheese
- 1¼ cups pitted Greek olives (about 6 oz.), chopped
- 1 medium sweet yellow pepper, finely chopped
- 1 medium green pepper, finely chopped
- 1 cup fresh mint leaves, chopped
- ½ medium red onion, finely chopped
- ¼ cup lemon juice
- 2 Tbsp. olive oil
- 1 Tbsp. grated lemon zest
- 3 garlic cloves, minced
- ½ tsp. pepper

1 Cook orzo according to package directions. Drain orzo; rinse with cold water.

2 In a large bowl, combine remaining ingredients. Stir in orzo. Refrigerate and serve cold.

1¾ CUPS *411 cal., 17g fat (4g sat. fat), 15mg chol., 740mg sod., 51g carb. (3g sugars, 13g fiber), 14g pro.*

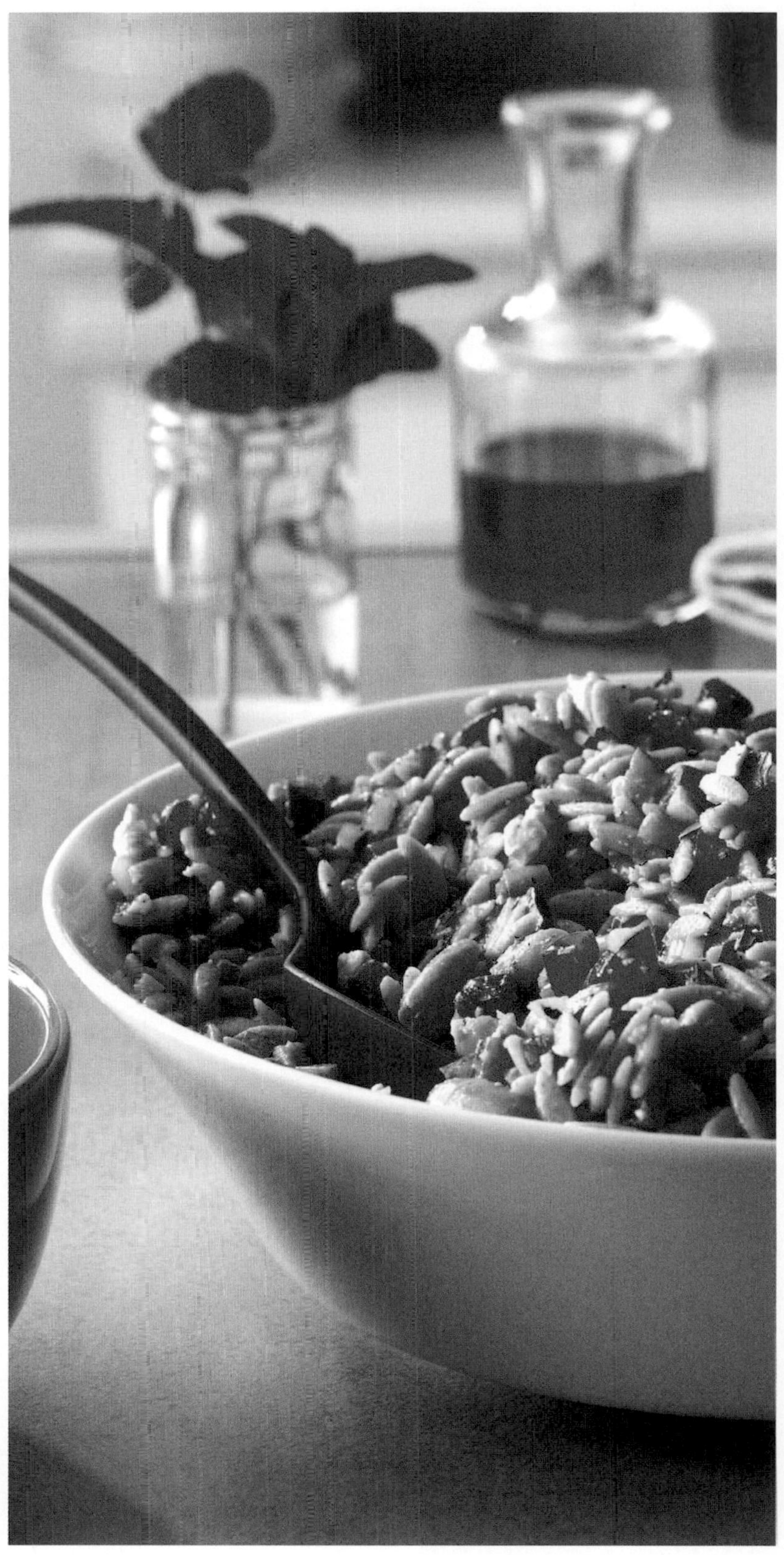

BLACK BEAN & SWEET POTATO RICE BOWLS

TAKES: 30 min. **MAKES:** 4 servings

- 3/4 cup uncooked long grain rice
- 1/4 tsp. garlic salt
- 1 1/2 cups water
- 3 Tbsp. olive oil, divided
- 1 large sweet potato, peeled and diced
- 1 medium red onion, finely chopped
- 4 cups chopped fresh kale (tough stems removed)
- 1 can (15 oz.) black beans, rinsed and drained
- 2 Tbsp. sweet chili sauce
- Lime wedges, optional
- Additional sweet chili sauce, optional

1 Place rice, garlic salt and water in a large saucepan; bring to a boil. Reduce the heat; simmer, covered, until water is absorbed and rice is tender, 15-20 minutes. Remove from heat; let stand for 5 minutes.

2 Meanwhile, in a large skillet, heat 2 Tbsp. oil over medium-high heat; saute sweet potato for 8 minutes. Add onion; cook and stir 4-6 minutes or until potato is tender. Add kale; cook and stir until tender, 3-5 minutes. Stir in beans; heat through.

3 Gently stir 2 Tbsp. chili sauce and remaining oil into rice; add to potato mixture. If desired, serve with lime wedges and additional chili sauce.

2 CUPS *435 cal., 11g fat (2g sat. fat), 0 chol., 405mg sod., 74g carb. (15g sugars, 8g fiber), 10g pro.*

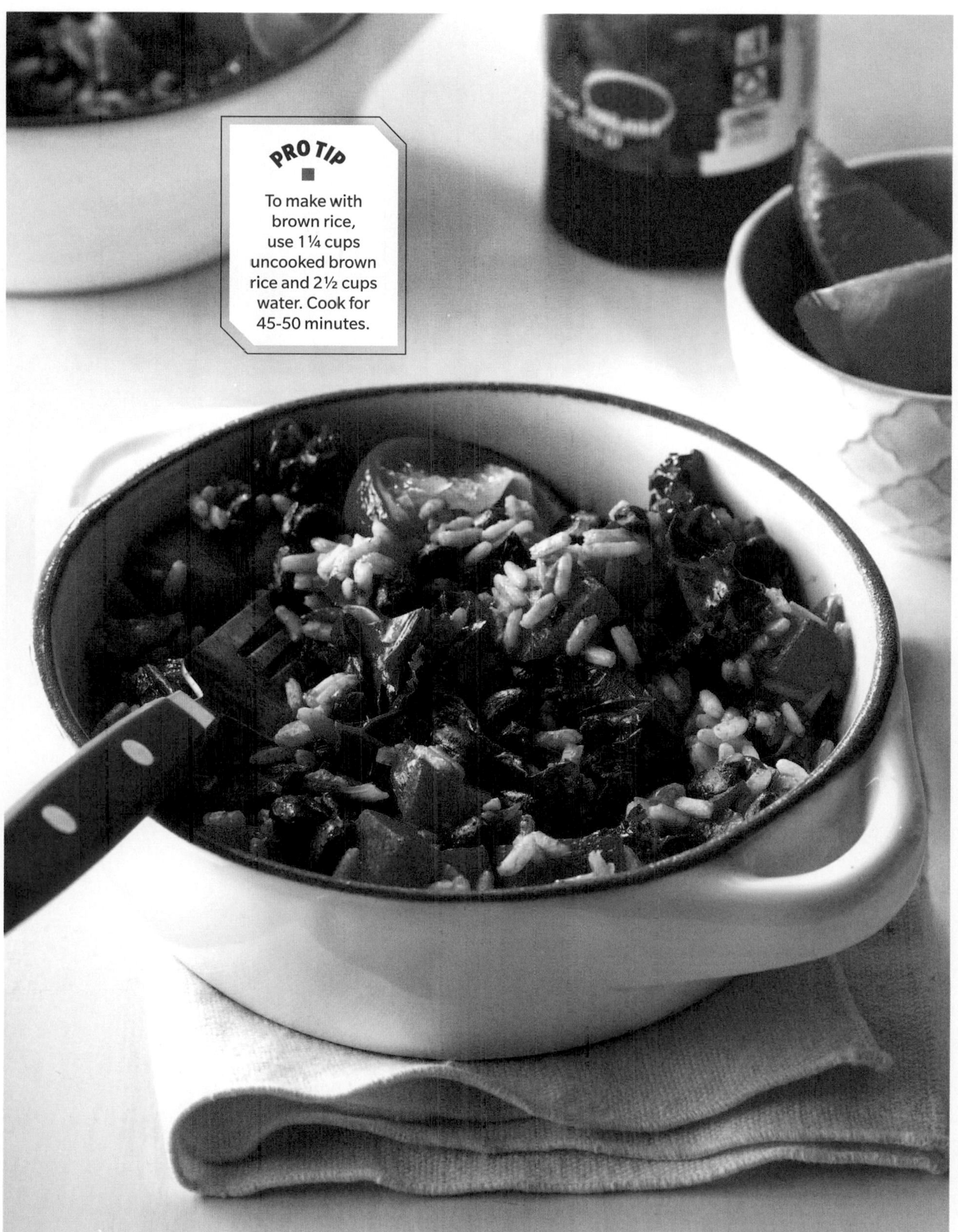
PRO TIP
To make with brown rice, use 1 ¼ cups uncooked brown rice and 2 ½ cups water. Cook for 45-50 minutes.

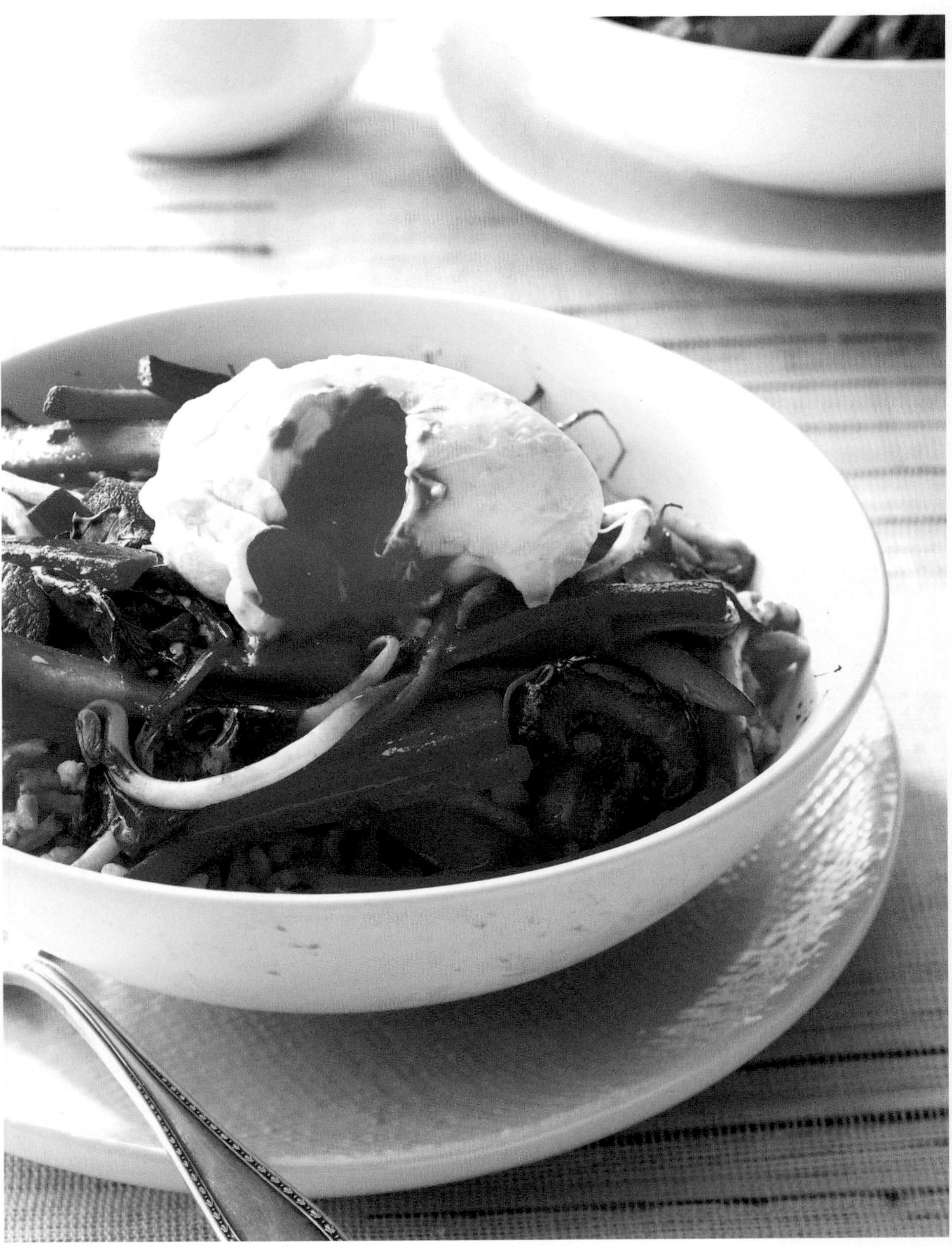

STIR-FRY RICE BOWL

TAKES: 30 min. **MAKES:** 4 servings

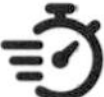

- 1 Tbsp. canola oil
- 2 medium carrots, julienned
- 1 medium zucchini, julienned
- ½ cup sliced baby portobello mushrooms
- 1 cup bean sprouts
- 1 cup fresh baby spinach
- 1 Tbsp. water
- 1 Tbsp. reduced-sodium soy sauce
- 1 Tbsp. chili garlic sauce
- 4 large eggs
- 3 cups hot cooked brown rice
- 1 tsp. sesame oil

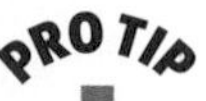

Make it vegan: Omit the eggs and stir in shelled edamame instead.

1 In a large skillet, heat oil over medium-high heat. Add the carrots, zucchini and mushrooms; cook and stir until the carrots are crisp-tender, 3-5 minutes. Add bean sprouts, spinach, water, soy sauce and chili sauce; cook and stir just until spinach is wilted. Remove from heat; keep warm.

2 Place 2-3 in. of water in a large skillet with high sides. Bring to a boil; adjust heat to maintain a gentle simmer. Break cold eggs, 1 at a time, into a small bowl; holding bowl close to surface of water, slip egg into water.

3 Cook, uncovered, 3-5 minutes or until whites are completely set and yolks begin to thicken but are not hard. Using a slotted spoon, lift eggs out of water.

4 Serve rice in bowls; top with vegetables. Drizzle with sesame oil. Top each serving with a poached egg.

1 SERVING *305 cal., 11g fat (2g sat. fat), 186mg chol., 364mg sod., 40g carb. (4g sugars, 4g fiber), 12g pro.* ***Diabetic exchanges:*** *2 starch, 1 vegetable, 1 medium-fat meat, 1 fat*

CURRY POMEGRANATE PROTEIN BOWL

PREP: 25 min. **COOK:** 25 min. **MAKES:** 6 servings

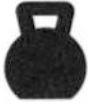

- 3 cups cubed peeled butternut squash (½-in. cubes)
- 2 Tbsp. olive oil, divided
- ½ tsp. salt, divided
- ¼ tsp. pepper
- ½ small onion, chopped
- 1 Tbsp. curry powder
- 1 Tbsp. ground cumin
- 1 garlic clove, minced
- 1 tsp. ground coriander
- 3 cups water
- 1 cup dried red lentils, rinsed
- ½ cup salted soy nuts
- ½ cup dried cranberries
- ⅓ cup thinly sliced green onions
- ⅓ cup pomegranate molasses
- ½ cup crumbled feta or vegan feta-style cheese
- ½ cup pomegranate seeds
- ¼ cup chopped fresh cilantro

1 Preheat oven to 375°. Place squash on a greased 15x10x1-in. baking pan. Drizzle with 1 Tbsp. oil; sprinkle with ¼ tsp. salt and pepper. Roast 25-30 minutes or until tender, turning once.

2 Meanwhile, in a large skillet, heat remaining 1 Tbsp. oil over medium-high heat. Add onion; cook and stir until crisp-tender, 4-6 minutes. Add curry powder, cumin, garlic, coriander and remaining ¼ tsp. salt; cook for 1 minute longer. Add water and lentils; bring to boil. Reduce heat; simmer, covered, until lentils are tender and water is absorbed, about 15 minutes.

3 Gently stir in soy nuts, cranberries, green onions and roasted squash. Divide among serving bowls. Drizzle with molasses and top with feta, pomegranate seeds and cilantro.

¾ CUP *367 cal., 9g fat (2g sat. fat), 5mg chol., 327mg sod., 60g carb. (23g sugars, 9g fiber), 14g pro.*

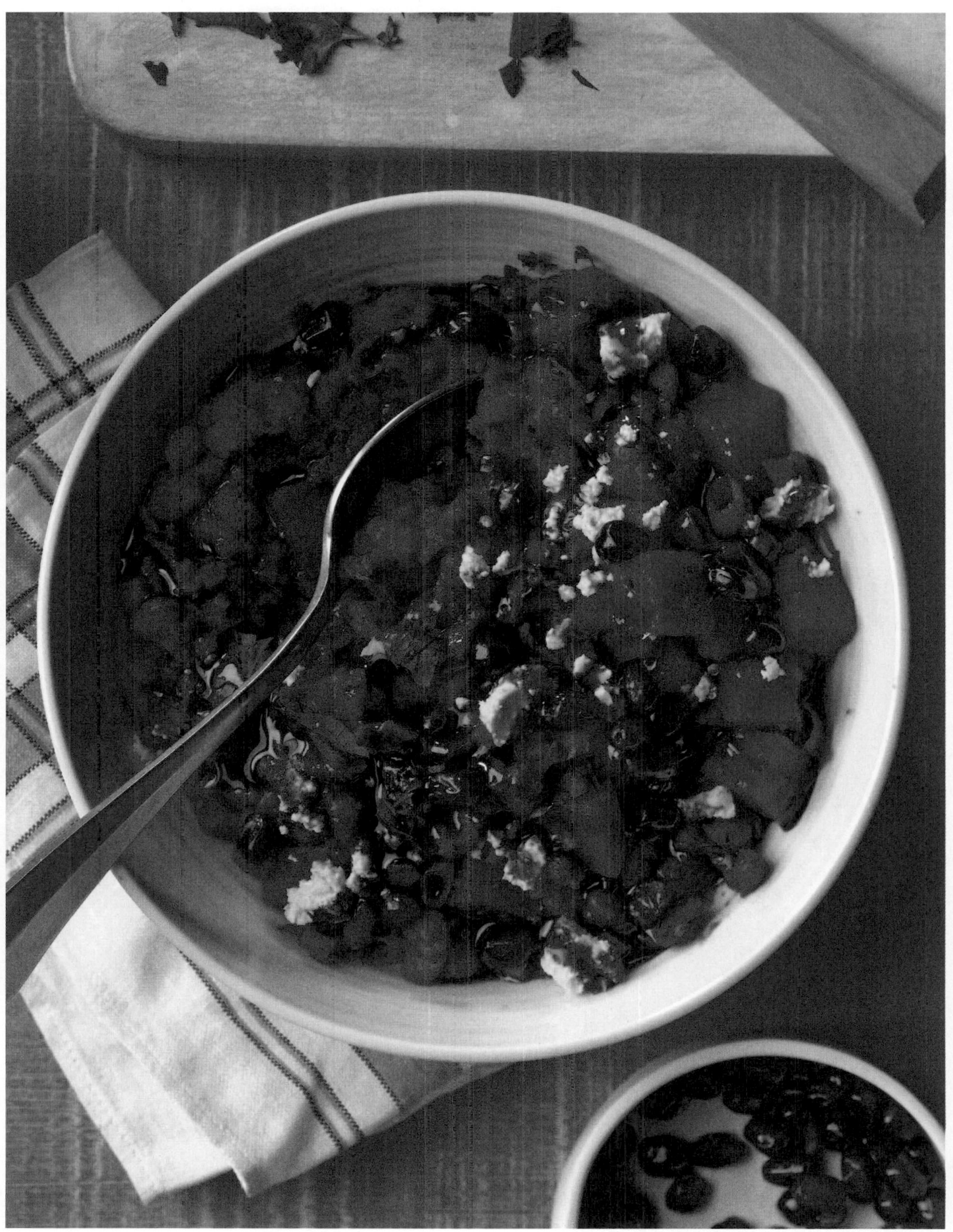

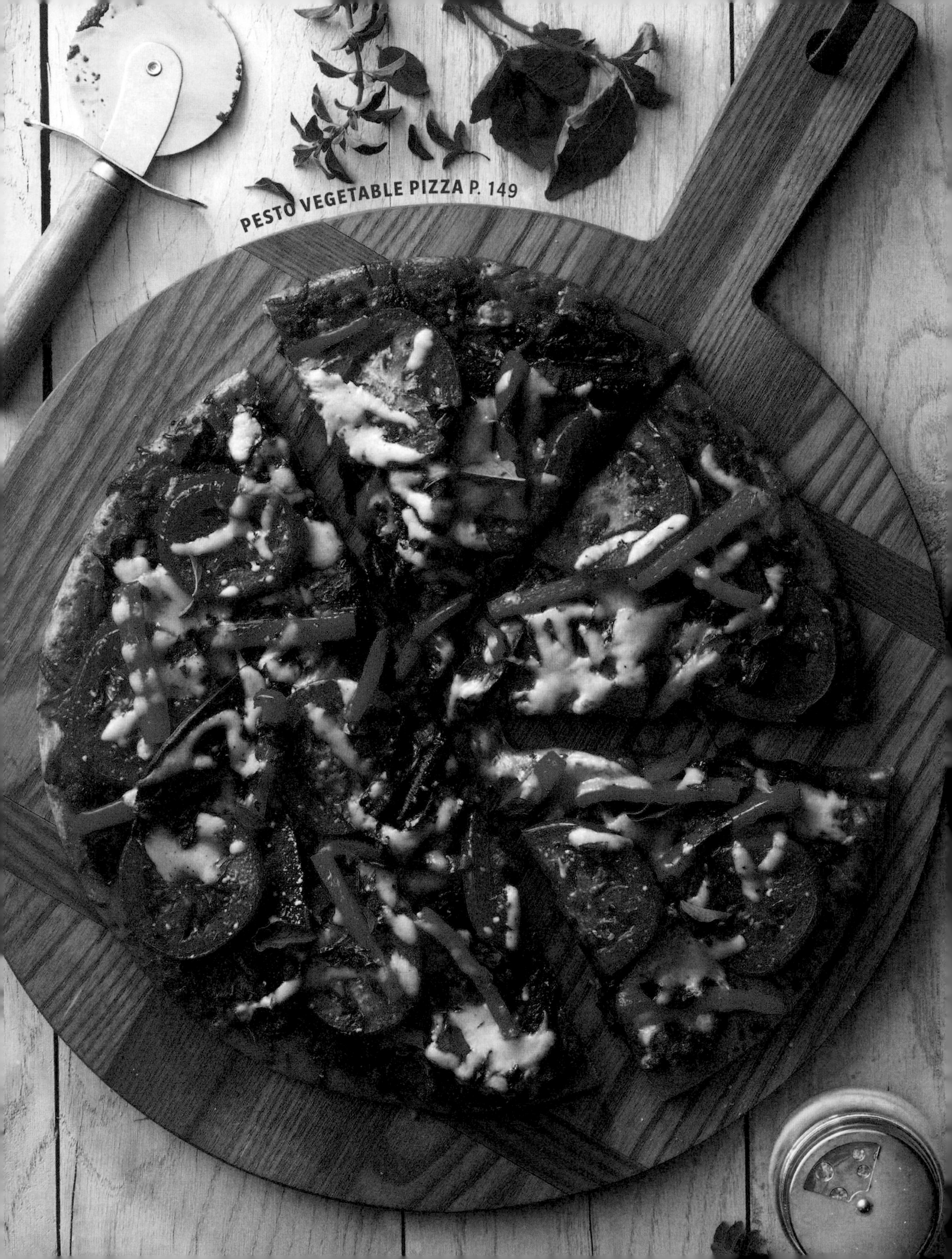

PESTO VEGETABLE PIZZA P. 149

CHAPTER 8

VEGETABLE MAINS

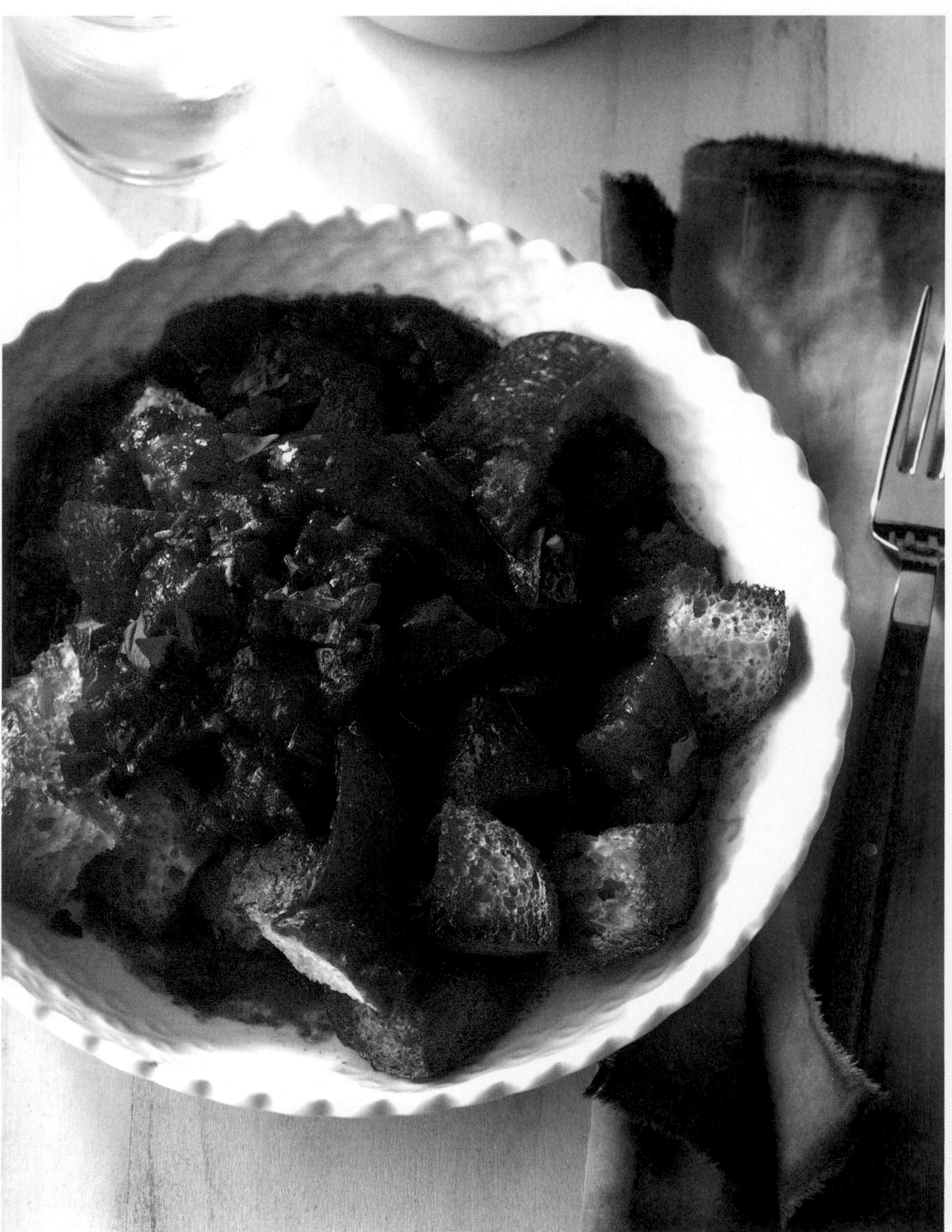

SUMMER BOUNTY RATATOUILLE

PREP: 20 min. + standing **COOK:** 1 hour **MAKES:** 12 servings

- 1 large eggplant, peeled and cut into 1-in. cubes
- 1½ tsp. kosher salt, divided
- 3 Tbsp. olive oil
- 2 medium sweet red peppers, cut into ½-in. strips
- 2 medium onions, peeled and chopped
- 4 garlic cloves, minced
- ¼ cup tomato paste
- 1 Tbsp. herbes de Provence
- ½ tsp. pepper
- 3 cans (14½ oz. each) diced tomatoes, undrained
- 1½ cups water
- 4 medium zucchini, quartered lengthwise and sliced ½-in. thick
- ¼ cup chopped fresh basil
- 2 Tbsp. minced fresh rosemary
- 2 Tbsp. minced fresh parsley
- 2 French bread baguettes (10½ oz. each), cubed and toasted

1 Place eggplant in a colander over a plate; toss with 1 tsp. kosher salt. Let stand 30 minutes. Rinse and drain well.

2 In a Dutch oven, heat oil over medium-high heat; saute peppers and onions 8-10 minutes or until tender. Add garlic; cook and stir 1 minute. Stir in tomato paste, herbs de Provence, pepper, remaining salt, tomatoes and water. Add the zucchini and eggplant; bring to a boil. Reduce the heat; simmer, uncovered, for 40-45 minutes or until flavors are blended, stirring occasionally.

3 Stir in fresh herbs. Serve over baguette cubes.

1 CUP RATATOUILLE WITH 1 CUP BREAD CUBES *205 cal., 4g fat (1g sat. fat), 0 chol., 542mg sod., 38g carb. (8g sugars, 6g fiber), 7g pro.*

JACKFRUIT CARNITAS TACOS

PREP: 20 min. **COOK:** 45 min. **MAKES:** 4 servings

- 2 medium onions, sliced
- ¼ cup olive oil, divided
- ¾ lb. portobello mushrooms, sliced
- 2 to 4 chipotle peppers in adobo sauce
- 2 Tbsp. chili powder
- 1 Tbsp. ground cumin
- 1 Tbsp. dried oregano
- 2 tsp. granulated garlic
- 1 tsp. garlic powder
- 1 to 2 tsp. kosher salt
- 4 Tbsp. water
- 2 cans (14 oz. each) jackfruit, drained and shredded
- ½ cup pumpkin seeds or pepitas, toasted
- ¼ cup nutritional yeast
- 12 corn tortillas (6 in.), warmed
- Optional: Lime wedges, sliced cabbage, salsa, cilantro leaves and avocado

1 In a large skillet, cook onions in 2 Tbsp. oil over medium-low heat until tender and lightly browned, about 10 minutes. Add portobello mushrooms; cook until liquid evaporates and mushrooms are tender, 8-10 minutes.

2 Meanwhile, in a blender, process chipotle peppers and seasonings with water until smooth. Add jackfruit and sauce to onion mixture; cook, stirring occasionally, until sauce darkens in color and starts to caramelize onto jackfruit, about 15 minutes. Reduce heat to low; stir in the toasted pumpkin seeds and nutritional yeast. Cook for 10 minutes. Serve the jackfruit mixture in tortillas; add optional toppings as desired.

2 TACOS *325 cal., 10g fat (2g sat. fat), 0 chol., 1249mg sod., 51g carb. (1g sugars, 17g fiber), 14g pro.*

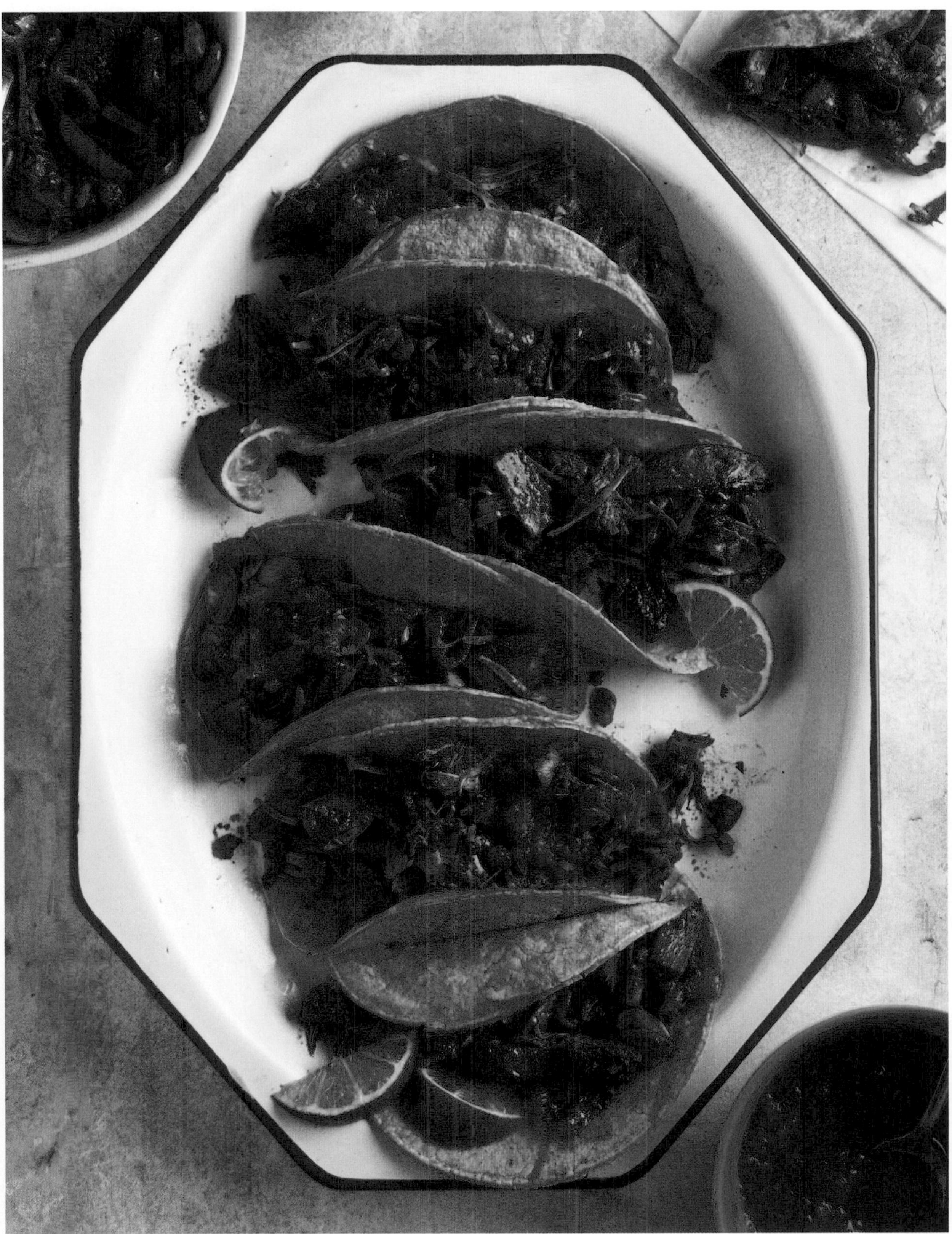

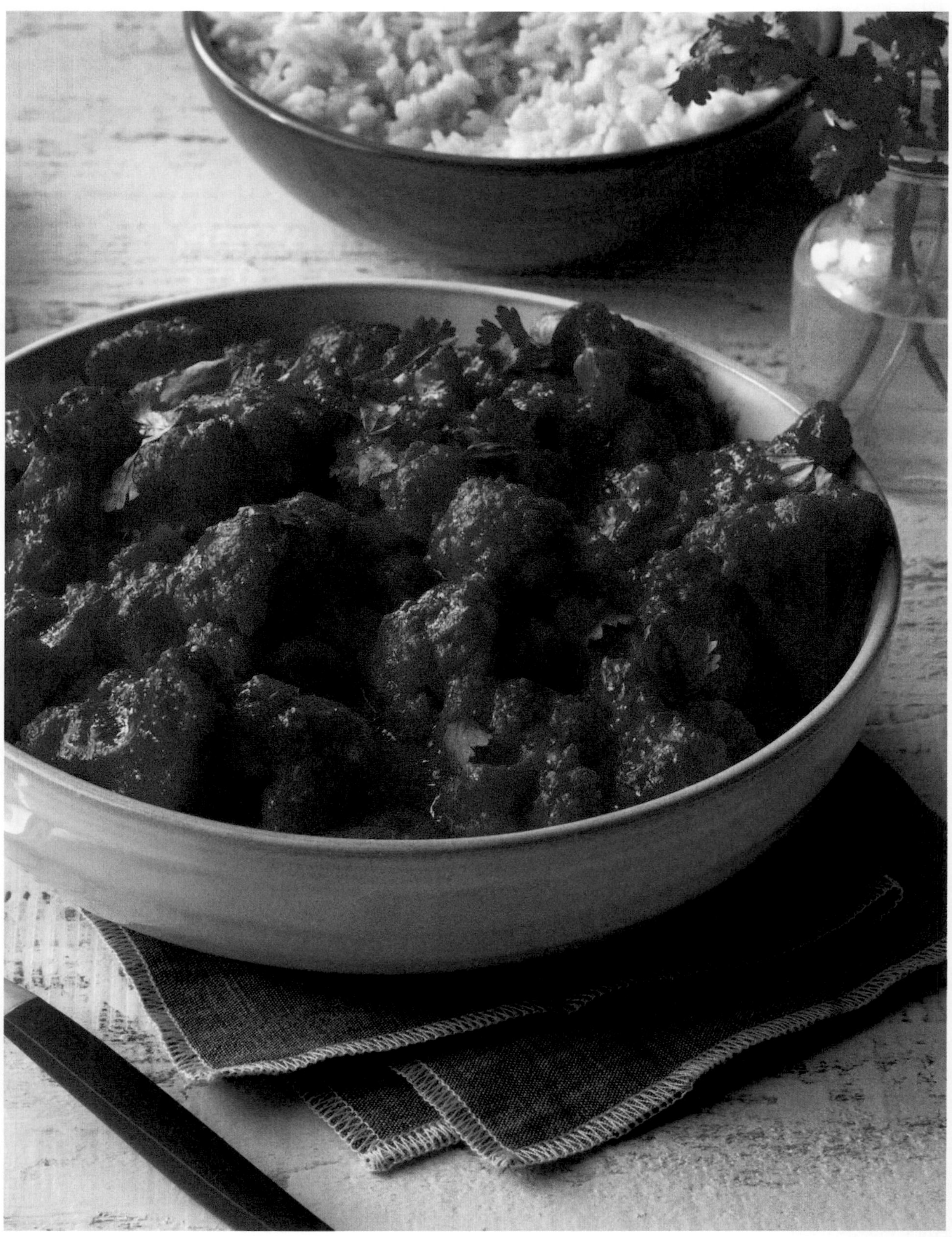

CAULIFLOWER TIKKA MASALA

PREP: 45 min. **COOK:** 15 min. **MAKES:** 4 servings

- 2 Tbsp. canola oil
- 1 large head cauliflower, cut into florets
- 1 tsp. ground mustard
- ½ tsp. paprika
- ½ tsp. ground turmeric
- ½ tsp. garam masala

MASALA

- 2 Tbsp. canola oil
- 1 small onion, chopped
- ¼ cup salted cashews
- 4 cardamom pods
- 2 whole cloves
- 1 can (14½ oz.) diced tomatoes, undrained
- ½ cup water
- 1½ tsp. minced garlic
- 1½ tsp. minced fresh gingerroot
- ¼ cup water
- 2 Tbsp. almond flour
- 1 Tbsp. ground fenugreek
- 1 Tbsp. maple syrup
- ½ tsp. salt
- ½ tsp. garam masala
- ¼ to ½ tsp. cayenne pepper
- 2 Tbsp. plain dairy or vegan yogurt
- Fresh cilantro leaves

1 Select saute setting on a 6-qt. electric pressure cooker. Adjust for medium heat; add canola oil. When oil is hot, cook and stir the cauliflower, mustard, paprika, turmeric and garam masala until crisp-tender, 6-8 minutes. Remove and keep warm.

2 For masala, add oil to pressure cooker. When hot, add onion, cashews, cardamom and cloves. Cook and stir until onion is tender, 4-5 minutes. Add the tomatoes and ½ cup water. Press cancel. Lock lid; close pressure-release valve. Adjust to pressure-cook on high for 5 minutes. Let pressure release naturally for 5 minutes; quick-release any remaining pressure. Discard cardamom and cloves. Cool the sauce slightly; transfer to a food processor. Process until smooth. Return to pressure cooker.

3 Select saute setting and adjust for low heat. Add garlic and ginger; cook and stir 1 minute. Add water, almond flour, fenugreek, maple syrup, salt, garam masala and cayenne; simmer, uncovered, until mixture is slightly thickened, 10-12 minutes, stirring occasionally. Press cancel. Stir in yogurt and cauliflower; heat through. Sprinkle with cilantro.

1¼ CUPS *312 cal., 22g fat (3g sat. fat), 0 chol., 573mg sod., 26g carb. (13g sugars, 7g fiber), 8g pro.*

EGGPLANT ROLL-UPS

PREP: 50 min. **BAKE:** 20 min. **MAKES:** 6 servings

- 2 medium eggplants (about 2½ lbs.)
- Cooking spray
- ½ tsp. salt
- 3 cups fresh spinach leaves

SAUCE

- 1 Tbsp. olive oil
- 2 garlic cloves, minced
- 1 can (14½ oz.) diced tomatoes
- 1 can (15 oz.) tomato puree
- 3 Tbsp. minced fresh basil or 3 tsp. dried basil
- 2 tsp. sugar
- 1 tsp. dried oregano
- ¼ tsp. salt
- ¼ tsp. pepper

FILLING

- 1 carton (15 oz.) reduced-fat ricotta or vegan ricotta-style cheese
- ¼ cup grated Parmesan or vegan Parmesan-style cheese
- ½ tsp. dried oregano
- ¼ tsp. pepper
- Dash ground nutmeg

TOPPING

- ¼ cup grated Parmesan or vegan Parmesan-style cheese
- 3 Tbsp. panko bread crumbs
- Minced fresh parsley, optional

1 Preheat oven to 400°. Cut eggplants lengthwise into eighteen ¼-in.-thick slices; reserve leftover pieces. Line 2 baking sheets with foil. Coat both sides of eggplant slices with cooking spray; place in a single layer on prepared pans. Sprinkle eggplant with ½ tsp. salt. Bake until slices are just pliable (do not soften completely), 10-12 minutes; cool slightly.

2 Meanwhile, in a large saucepan, bring ½ in. of water to a boil. Add spinach; cover and boil 2-3 minutes or until wilted. Drain spinach and squeeze dry. Chop spinach and set aside.

3 Finely chop leftover eggplant to measure 1 cup (discard remaining or save for another use). In a large saucepan, heat oil over medium heat. Add chopped eggplant; cook and stir until tender. Add garlic; cook 1 minute longer. Stir in tomatoes, puree, basil, sugar, oregano, salt and pepper. Bring to a boil. Reduce heat; simmer, uncovered, 8-10 minutes or until flavors are blended.

4 Spread 1 cup sauce into a 13x9-in. baking dish coated with cooking spray. In a small bowl, combine the filling ingredients and spinach. Place a rounded

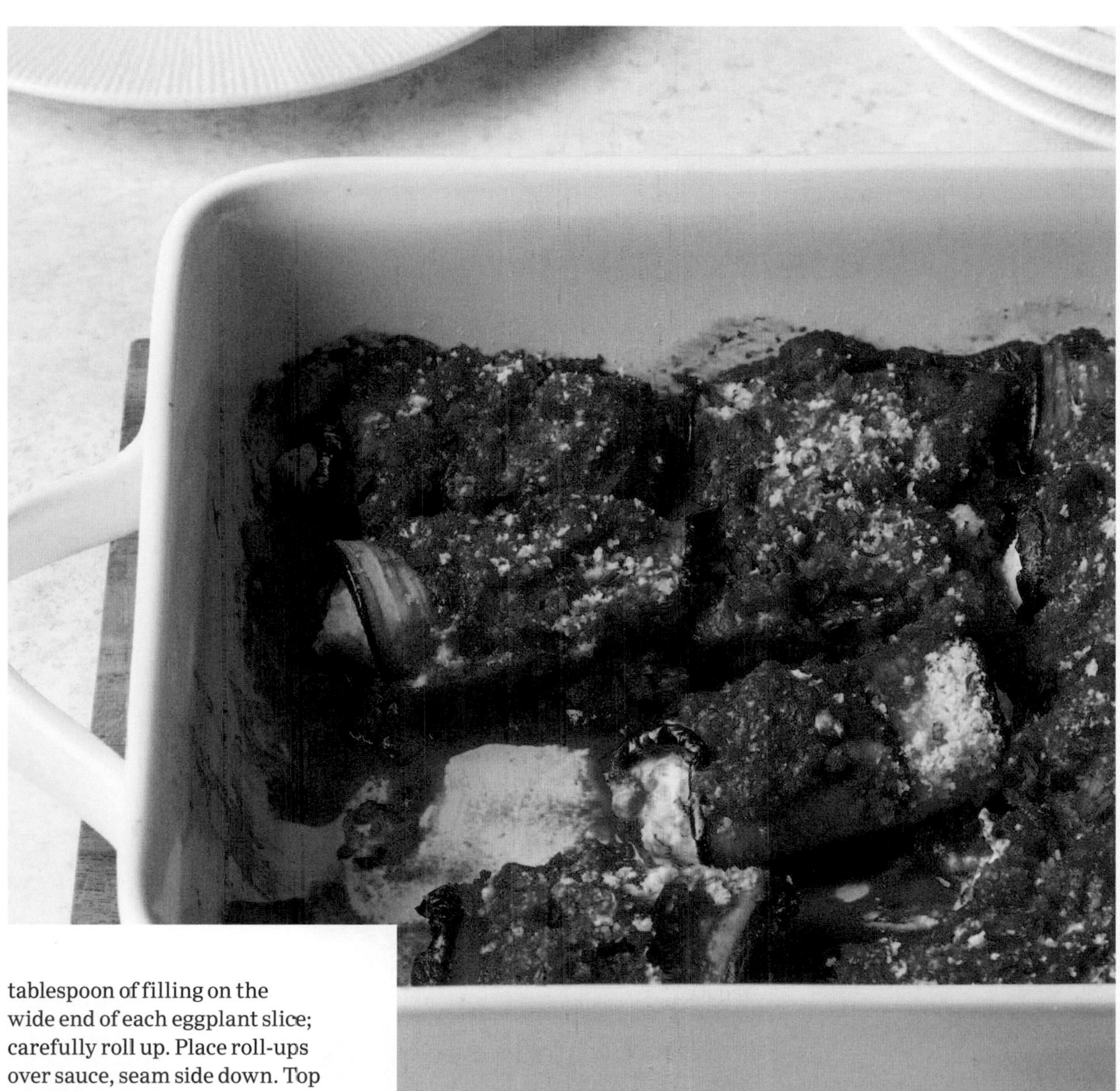

tablespoon of filling on the wide end of each eggplant slice; carefully roll up. Place roll-ups over sauce, seam side down. Top with 1½ cups sauce. In a small bowl, mix Parmesan cheese and bread crumbs; sprinkle over top. Bake until heated through and bubbly, 20-25 minutes. Serve with remaining sauce and, if desired, sprinkle with parsley.

3 ROLL-UPS *257 cal., 10g fat (3g sat. fat), 23mg chol., 652mg sod., 28g carb. (14g sugars, 8g fiber), 12g pro.* ***Diabetic exchanges:*** *2 starch, 2 medium-fat meat, ½ fat*

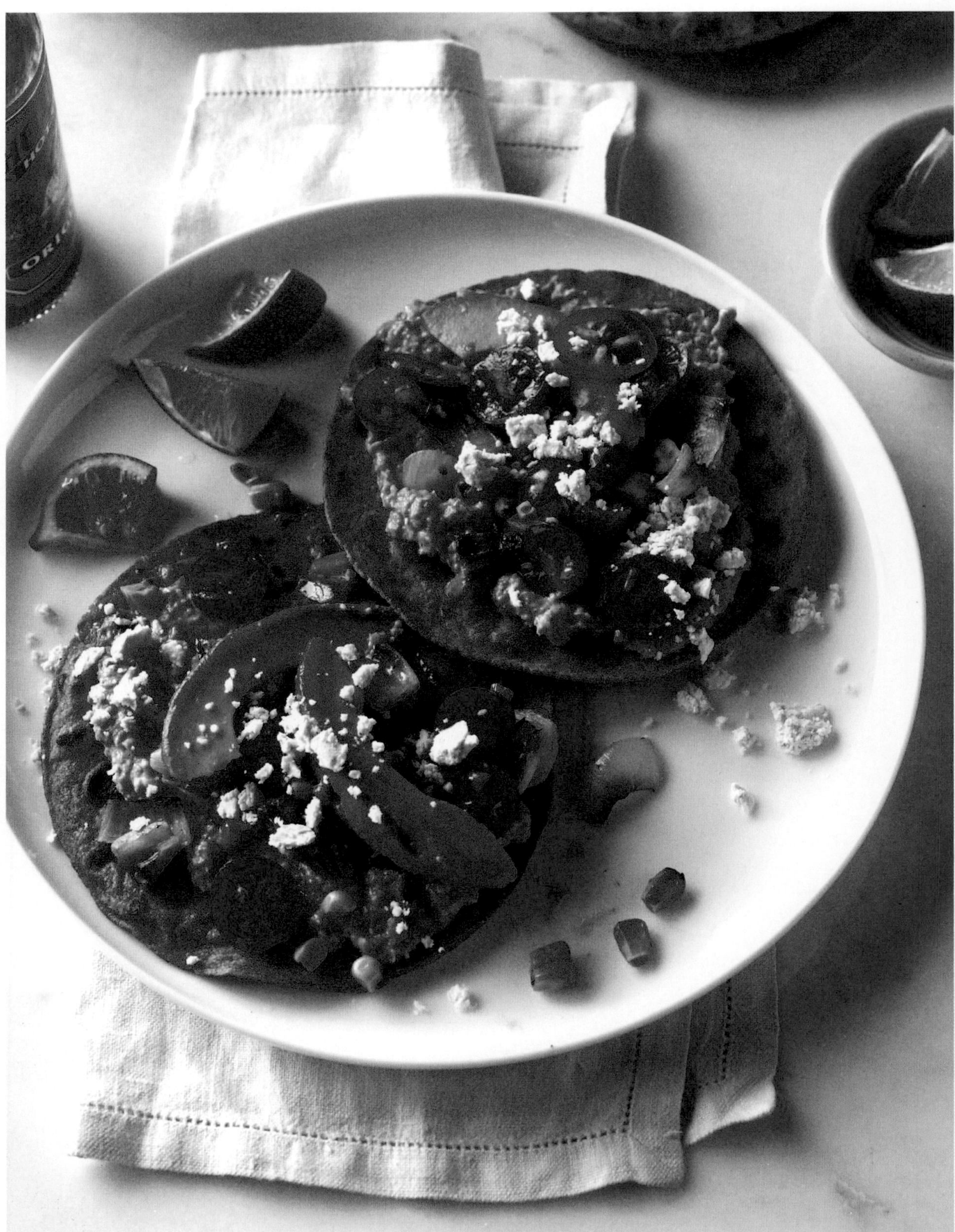

GRILLED CORN HUMMUS TOSTADAS

TAKES: 30 min. **MAKES:** 4 servings

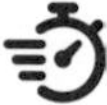

- 4 medium ears sweet corn, husks removed
- 1 small red onion, cut crosswise into ½-in. slices
- 2 Tbsp. olive oil, divided
- 8 corn tortillas (6 in.)
- 1 container (8 oz.) hummus
- ¼ tsp. ground chipotle pepper
- 1 cup cherry tomatoes, halved
- ½ tsp. salt
- 1 medium ripe avocado, peeled and sliced
- ½ cup crumbled feta or vegan feta-style cheese
- 1 jalapeno pepper, thinly sliced
- Optional: Lime wedges, fresh cilantro leaves and Mexican hot pepper sauce

1 Brush corn and onion with 1 Tbsp. oil. Grill the corn and onion, covered, over medium-high heat until tender and lightly charred, 5-7 minutes, turning occasionally. Cool slightly.

2 Meanwhile, brush tortillas with the remaining oil. Grill, covered, until crisp and lightly browned, 2-3 minutes per side.

3 Cut corn from cobs. Process hummus, chipotle pepper and 2 cups of the cut corn in a food processor until almost smooth. Coarsely chop grilled onion; toss with cherry tomatoes, salt and any remaining corn.

4 Spread hummus mixture over tortillas; top with onion mixture, avocado, cheese and jalapeno. If desired, serve with lime wedges, cilantro and pepper sauce.

2 TOSTADAS *453 cal., 23g fat (5g sat. fat), 8mg chol., 692mg sod., 55g carb. (9g sugars, 12g fiber), 14g pro.*

MUSHROOM & SWEET POTATO POTPIE

PREP: 45 min. **BAKE:** 30 min. **MAKES:** 8 servings

- 1/3 cup olive oil, divided
- 1 lb. sliced fresh shiitake mushrooms
- 1 lb. sliced baby portobello mushrooms
- 2 large onions, chopped
- 2 garlic cloves, minced
- 1 tsp. minced fresh rosemary, plus more for topping
- 1 bottle (12 oz.) porter or stout beer
- 1½ cups mushroom broth or vegetable broth, divided
- 2 bay leaves
- 1 Tbsp. balsamic vinegar
- 2 Tbsp. reduced-sodium soy sauce
- 1/4 cup cornstarch
- 3 to 4 small sweet potatoes, peeled and thinly sliced
- 3/4 tsp. coarsely ground pepper
- 1/2 tsp. salt

1 Preheat oven to 400°. In a Dutch oven, heat 1 Tbsp. oil over medium heat. Add shiitake mushrooms and cook in batches 8-10 minutes or until dark golden brown; remove with a slotted spoon. Repeat with 1 Tbsp. oil and the portobello mushrooms.

2 In same pan, heat 1 Tbsp. oil over medium heat. Add onions; cook and stir 8-10 minutes or until tender. Add garlic and 1 tsp. rosemary; cook for 30 seconds longer. Stir in beer, 1 cup broth, bay leaves, vinegar, soy sauce and sauteed mushrooms.

3 Bring to a boil. Reduce heat; simmer, uncovered, 10 minutes. In a small bowl, mix cornstarch and the remaining broth until smooth; stir into the mushroom mixture. Return to a boil, stirring constantly; cook and stir until thickened, 1-2 minutes. Remove and discard bay leaves; transfer mushroom mixture to 8 greased 8-oz. ramekins. Place on a rimmed baking sheet.

4 Layer sweet potatoes in a circular pattern on top of each ramekin; brush with remaining oil and sprinkle with pepper, salt and additional rosemary. Bake, covered, until the potatoes are tender, 20-25 minutes. Remove cover and bake until potatoes are lightly browned, 8-10 minutes. Let potpies stand for 5 minutes before serving.

1 SERVING *211 cal., 10g fat (1g sat. fat), 0 chol., 407mg sod., 26g carb. (10g sugars, 4g fiber), 5g pro.*

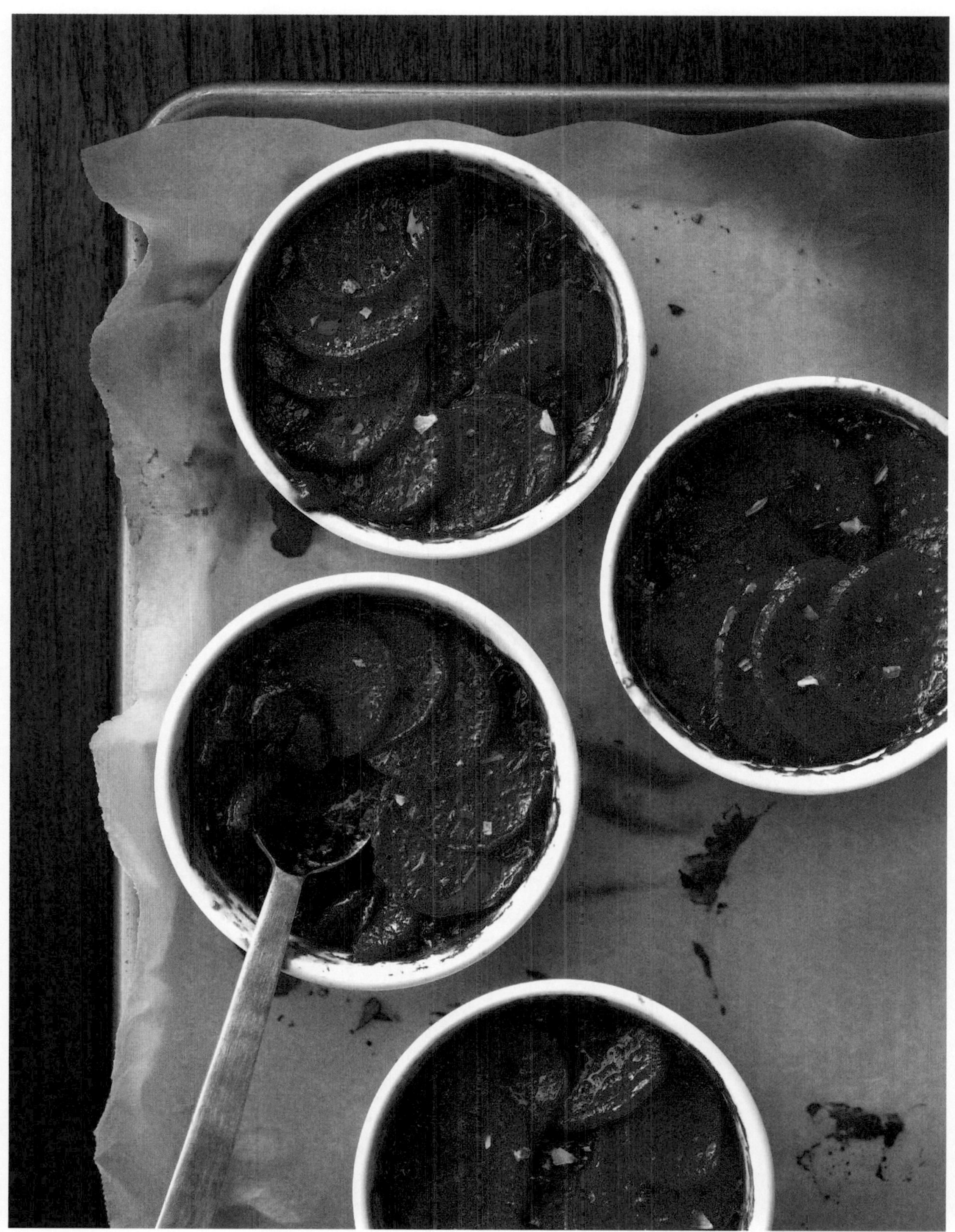

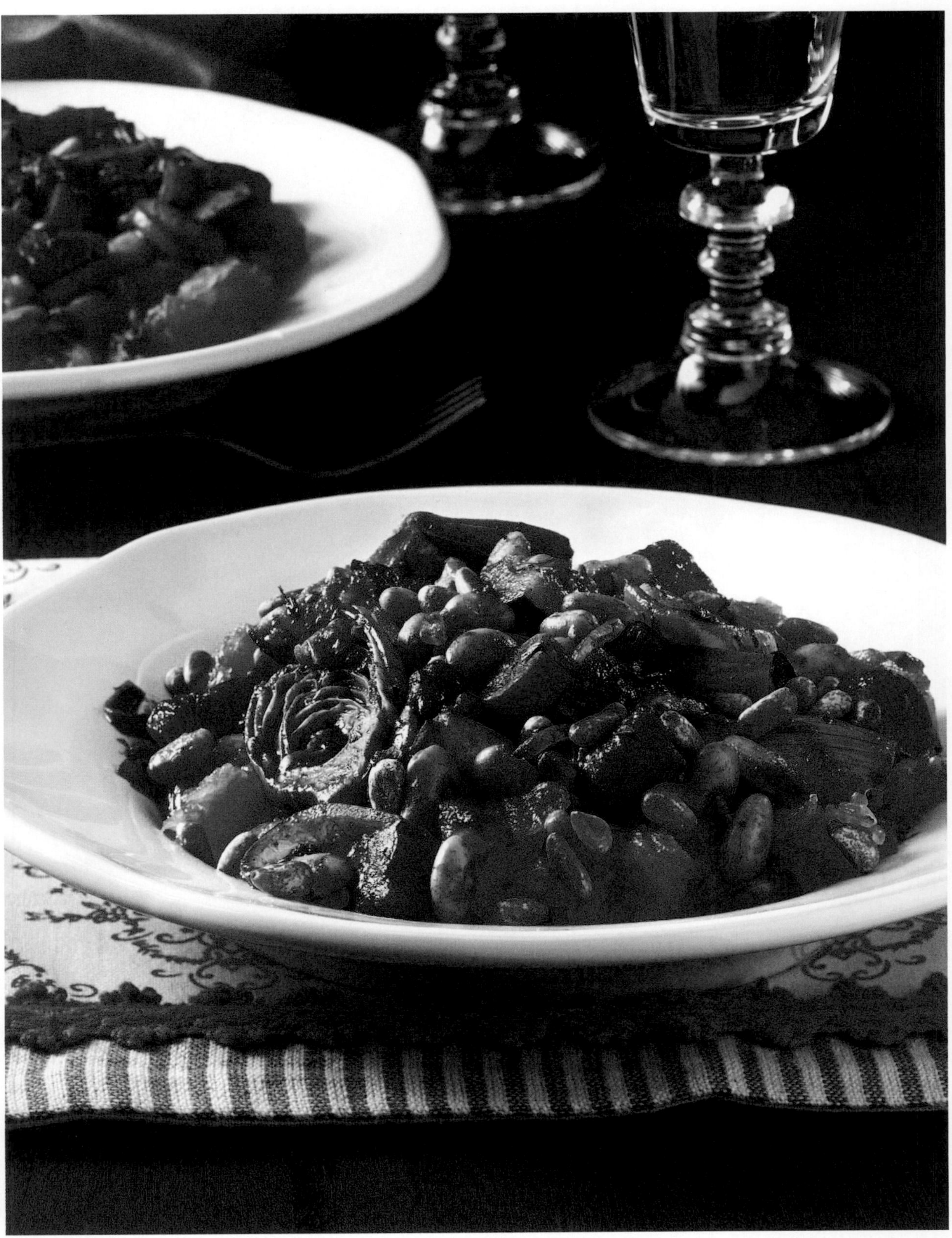

SPAGHETTI SQUASH & BALSAMIC VEGETABLES

PREP: 20 min. **COOK:** 15 min. **MAKES:** 6 servings

- 1 medium spaghetti squash (about 4 lbs.)
- 1 cup chopped carrots
- 1 small red onion, halved and sliced
- 1 Tbsp. olive oil
- 4 garlic cloves, minced
- 1 can (15½ oz.) great northern beans, rinsed and drained
- 1 can (14½ oz.) diced tomatoes, drained
- 1 can (14 oz.) water-packed artichoke hearts, rinsed, drained and halved
- 1 medium zucchini, chopped
- 3 Tbsp. balsamic vinegar
- 2 tsp. minced fresh thyme or ½ tsp. dried thyme
- ¼ tsp. salt
- ¼ tsp. pepper
- ½ cup pine nuts, toasted

1 Cut squash in half lengthwise; discard seeds. Place squash cut side down on a microwave-safe plate. Microwave, uncovered, on high until tender, 15-18 minutes.

2 Meanwhile, in a large nonstick skillet, saute carrots and onion in oil until tender. Add garlic; cook 1 minute. Stir in beans, tomatoes, artichokes, zucchini, vinegar, thyme, salt and pepper. Cook and stir over medium heat until heated through, 8-10 minutes.

3 When squash is cool enough to handle, use a fork to separate strands. Serve with the bean mixture. Sprinkle with nuts.

¾ CUP BEAN MIXTURE WITH ⅔ CUP SQUASH AND 4 TSP. NUTS *275 cal., 10g fat (1g sat. fat), 0 chol., 510mg sod., 41g carb. (6g sugars, 10g fiber), 11g pro.* ***Diabetic exchanges:*** *2½ starch, 1½ fat, 1 lean meat*

MUSHROOM BROCCOLI PIZZA

PREP: 30 min. + rising **BAKE:** 15 min. **MAKES:** 6 servings

- 1 pkg. (¼ oz.) active dry yeast
- ¾ cup warm water (110° to 115°)
- 1 tsp. olive oil
- ½ tsp. sugar
- ½ cup whole wheat flour
- ½ tsp. salt
- 1½ cups all-purpose flour

TOPPINGS

- 1 Tbsp. olive oil
- 1 cup sliced fresh mushrooms
- ¼ cup chopped onion
- 4 garlic cloves, minced
- 3 cups broccoli florets
- 2 Tbsp. water
- ½ cup pizza sauce
- 4 plum tomatoes, sliced
- ¼ cup chopped fresh basil
- 1½ cups shredded part-skim mozzarella or vegan mozzarella-style cheese
- ⅓ cup shredded Parmesan or vegan Parmesan-style cheese

1 In a bowl, dissolve yeast in warm water. Add oil and sugar; mix well. Combine whole wheat flour and salt; stir into yeast mixture until smooth. Stir in enough all-purpose flour to form a soft dough.

2 Turn onto a floured surface; knead until smooth and elastic, about 6-8 minutes. Place in a bowl coated with cooking spray, turning once to coat top. Cover and let rise in a warm place until doubled, about 1½ hours. Preheat oven to 425°.

3 Punch down dough; press onto a 12-in. pizza pan coated with cooking spray. Prick dough several times with a fork. Bake until edges are light golden brown, 10-12 minutes.

4 In a nonstick skillet, heat oil over medium-high heat; saute mushrooms, onion and garlic until tender. Place broccoli and water in a microwave-safe bowl; microwave, covered, on high until broccoli is crisp-tender, about 2 minutes. Drain well.

5 Spread pizza sauce over crust. Top with mushroom mixture, tomatoes, broccoli, basil and cheeses. Bake until crust is golden brown and cheese is melted, 12-14 minutes.

1 PIECE *317 cal., 11g fat (5g sat. fat), 21mg chol., 558mg sod., 40g carb. (4g sugars, 4g fiber), 16g pro.* ***Diabetic exchanges:*** *2 starch, 2 medium-fat meat, 1 vegetable, ½ fat*

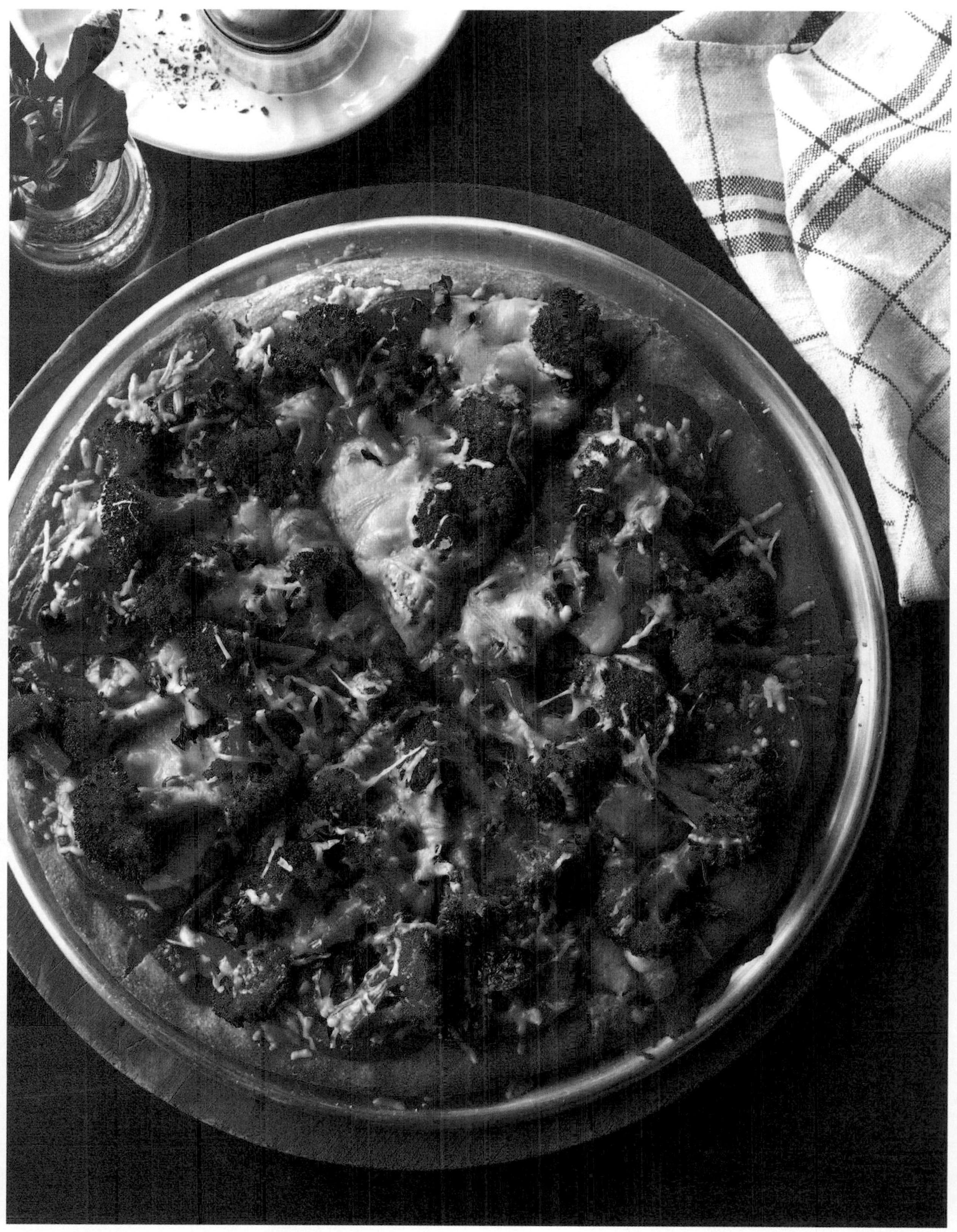

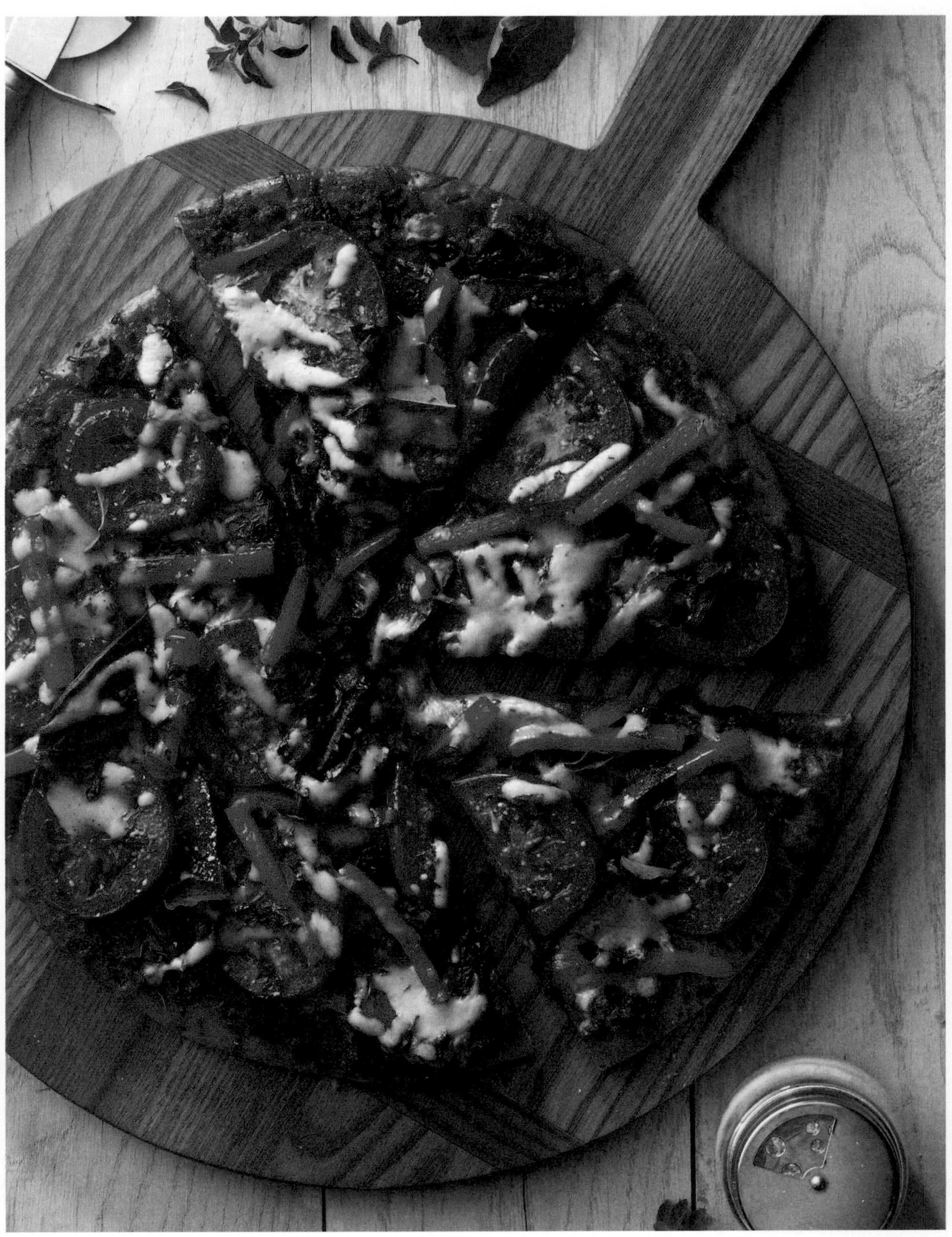

PESTO VEGETABLE PIZZA

TAKES: 30 min. **MAKES:** 6 servings

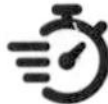

- 1 prebaked 12-in. thin pizza crust
- 2 garlic cloves, halved
- ½ cup pesto sauce
- ¾ cup packed fresh spinach, chopped
- 2 large portobello mushrooms, thinly sliced
- 1 medium sweet yellow pepper, julienned
- 2 plum tomatoes, seeded and sliced
- ⅓ cup packed fresh basil, chopped
- 1 cup shredded vegan mozzarella-style cheese
- ¼ cup grated vegan Parmesan-style cheese
- ½ tsp. fresh or dried oregano

1 Preheat oven to 450°. Place crust on an ungreased 12-in. pizza pan. Rub cut side of garlic cloves over crust; discard garlic. Spread pesto sauce over crust. Top with spinach, mushrooms, yellow pepper, tomatoes and basil. Sprinkle with cheeses and oregano.

2 Bake until pizza is heated through and cheese is melted, 10-15 minutes.

1 PIECE *350 cal., 18g fat (6g sat. fat), 0 chol., 860mg sod., 38g carb. (3g sugars, 4g fiber), 7g pro.*

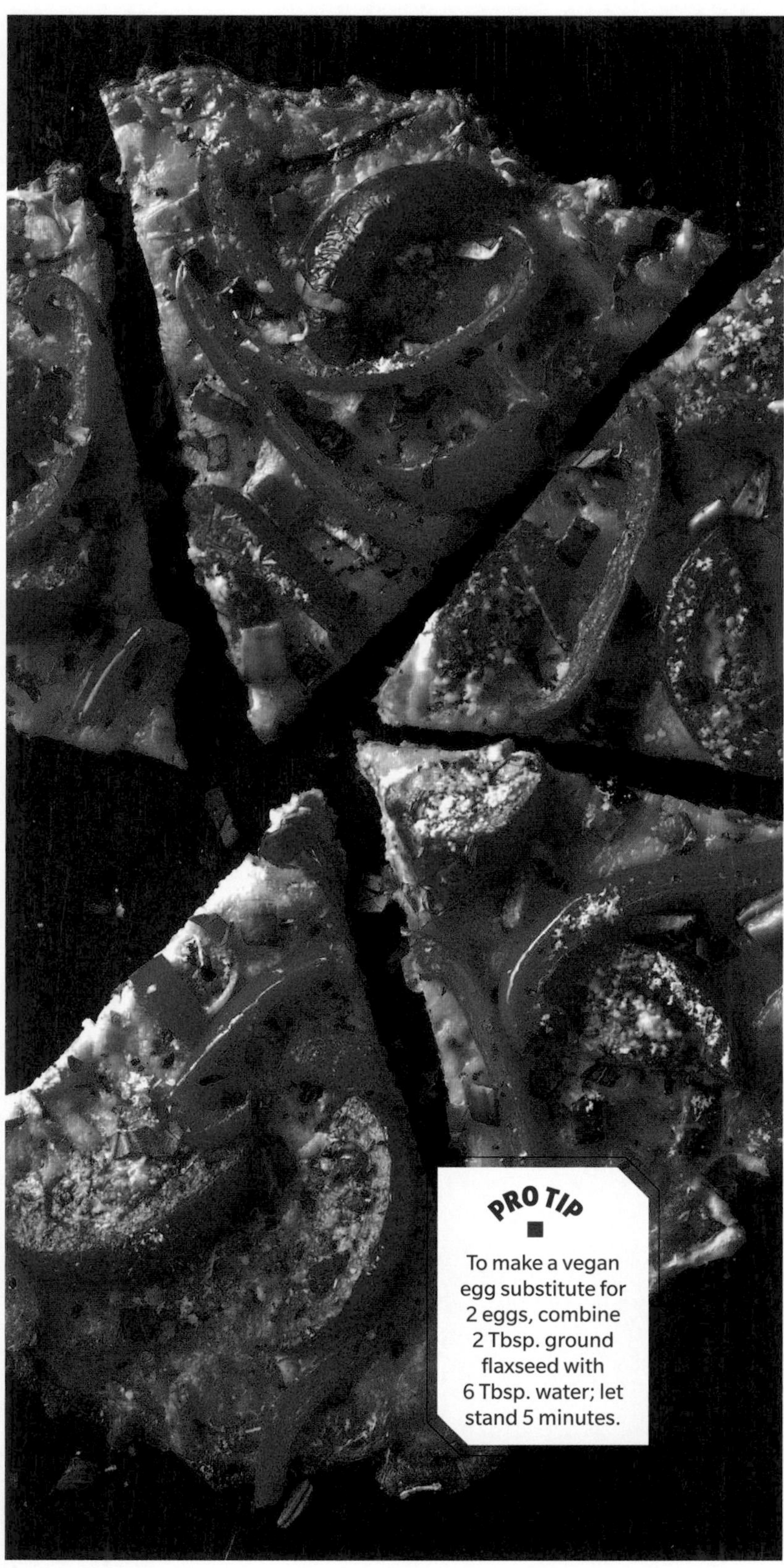

PRO TIP

To make a vegan egg substitute for 2 eggs, combine 2 Tbsp. ground flaxseed with 6 Tbsp. water; let stand 5 minutes.

ZUCCHINI CRUST PIZZA

PREP: 20 min. **BAKE:** 25 min.
MAKES: 6 servings

- 2 cups shredded zucchini (1 to 1½ medium), squeezed dry
- 2 large eggs, lightly beaten or vegan egg substitute
- ¼ cup all-purpose flour
- ¼ tsp. salt
- 2 cups shredded part-skim mozzarella or vegan mozzarella-style cheese, divided
- ½ cup grated Parmesan or vegan Parmesan-style cheese, divided
- 2 small tomatoes, halved and sliced
- ½ cup chopped red onion
- ½ cup julienned bell pepper
- 1 tsp. dried oregano
- ½ tsp. dried basil

1 Preheat oven to 450°. In a large bowl, combine first 4 ingredients; stir in ½ cup mozzarella cheese and ¼ cup Parmesan cheese. Transfer to a 12-in. pizza pan coated generously with cooking spray; spread to an 11-in. circle.

2 Bake 13-16 minutes or until golden brown. Reduce the oven setting to 400°. Sprinkle with remaining mozzarella; top with tomatoes, onion, pepper, herbs and remaining Parmesan cheese. Bake until edge is golden brown and cheese is melted, 10-15 minutes.

1 PIECE *200 cal., 11g fat (6g sat. fat), 90mg chol., 500mg sod., 11g carb. (3g sugars, 1g fiber), 14g pro.* ***Diabetic exchanges:*** *2 vegetable, 2 lean meat, ½ fat*

PRO TIP
Make it vegan: Omit the halibut and top the veggie mixture with cubes of lightly browned tofu.

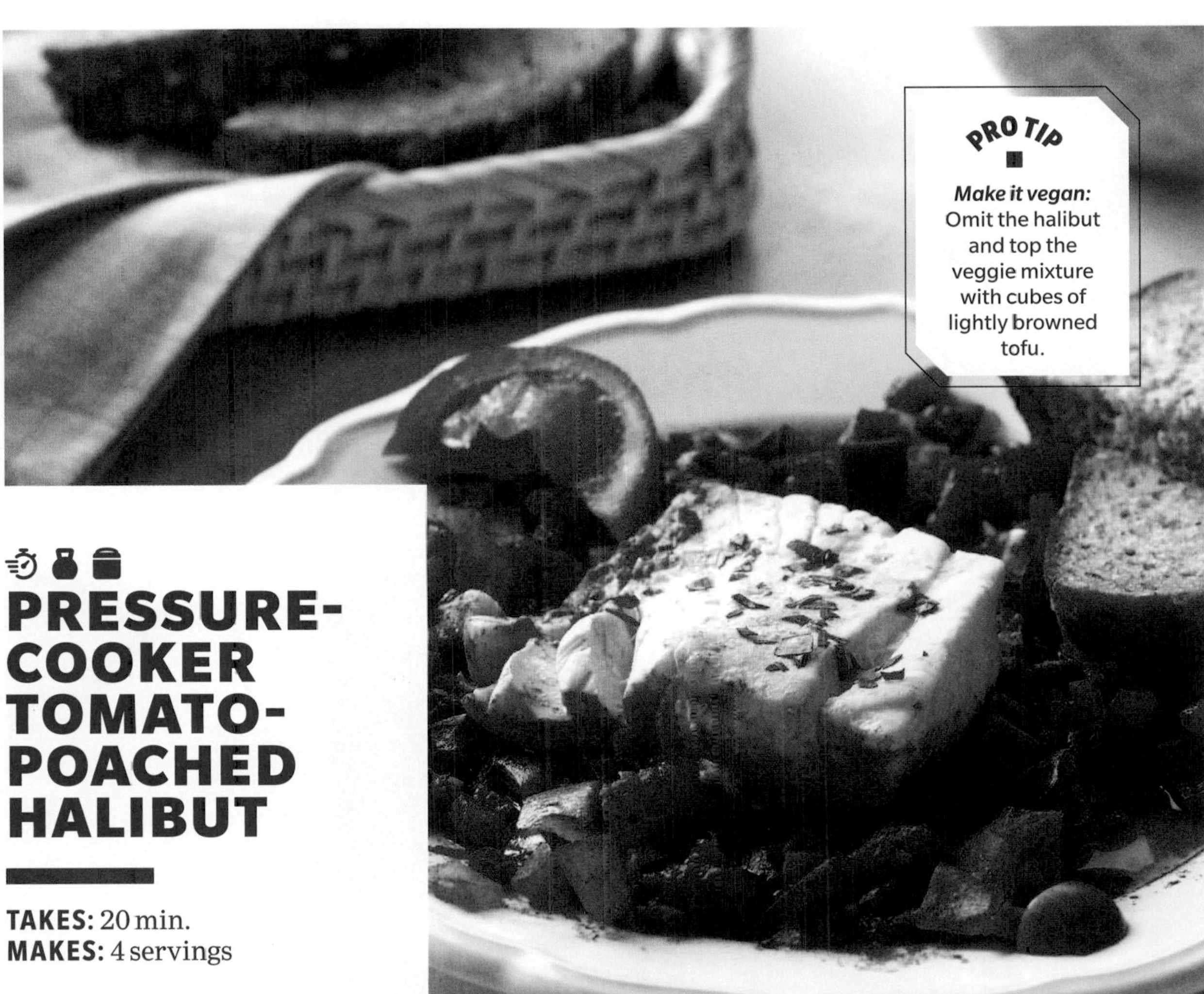

PRESSURE-COOKER TOMATO-POACHED HALIBUT

TAKES: 20 min.
MAKES: 4 servings

- 1 Tbsp. olive oil
- 2 poblano peppers, finely chopped
- 1 small onion, finely chopped
- 1 can (14½ oz.) fire-roasted diced tomatoes, undrained
- 1 can (14½ oz.) no-salt-added diced tomatoes, undrained
- ½ cup water
- ¼ cup chopped pitted green olives
- 3 garlic cloves, minced
- ¼ tsp. pepper
- ⅛ tsp. salt
- 4 halibut fillets (4 oz. each)
- ⅓ cup chopped fresh cilantro
- 4 lemon wedges
- Crusty whole grain bread, optional

1 Select saute setting on a 6-qt. electric pressure cooker. Adjust for medium heat; add oil. When oil is hot, cook and stir poblano peppers and onion until crisp-tender, 2-3 minutes. Press cancel. Stir in tomatoes, water, olives, garlic, pepper and salt. Top with halibut fillets.

2 Lock lid; close pressure-release valve. Adjust to pressure-cook on high for 3 minutes. Quick-release pressure. A thermometer inserted in fish should read at least 145°.

3 Sprinkle with fresh cilantro. Serve with lemon wedges and, if desired, bread.

1 FILLET WITH 1 CUP SAUCE *215 cal., 7g fat (1g sat. fat), 56mg chol., 614mg sod., 16g carb. (7g sugars, 3g fiber), 23g pro.* ***Diabetic exchanges:*** *3 lean meat, 1 starch, ½ fat*

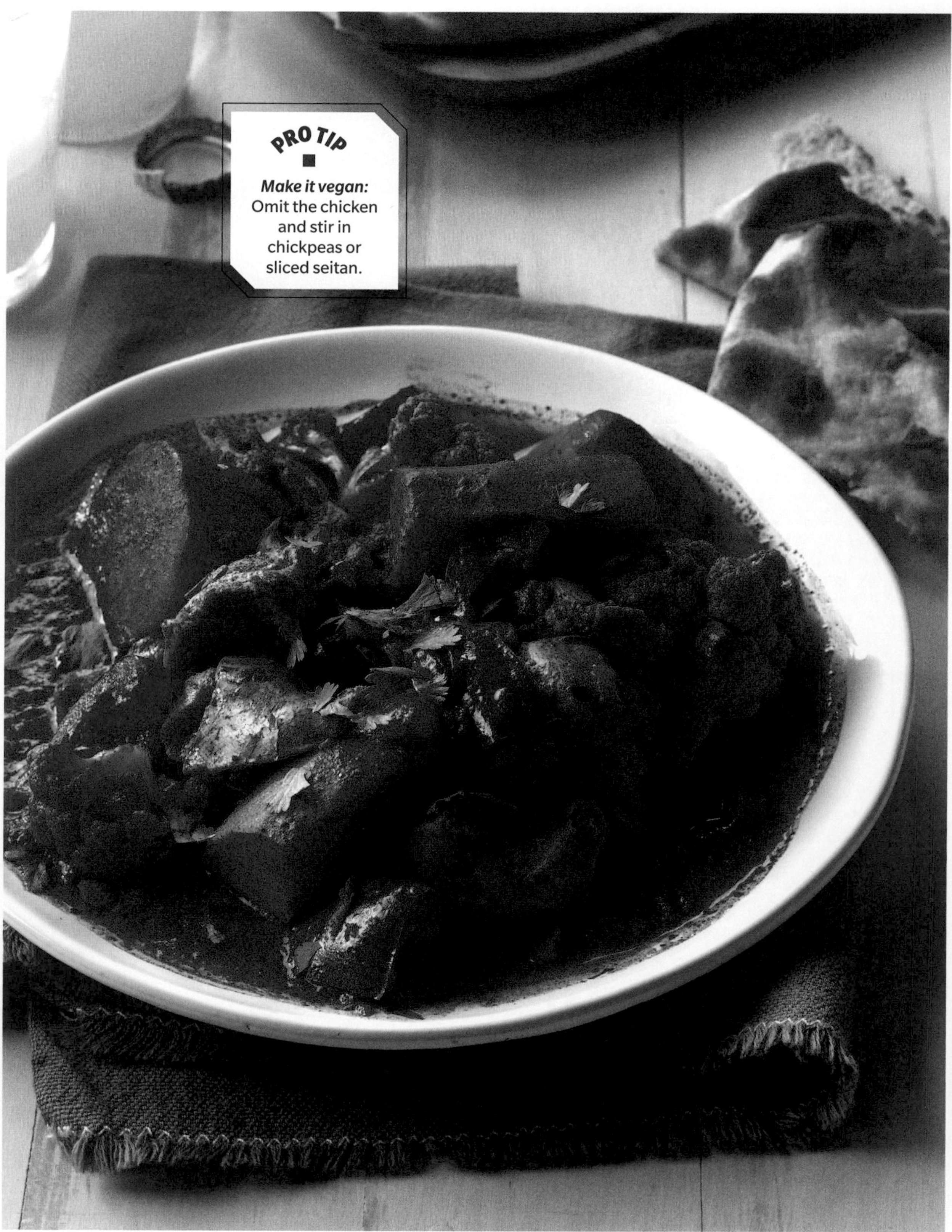
PRO TIP
Make it vegan:
Omit the chicken and stir in chickpeas or sliced seitan.

PRESSURE-COOKER INDIAN-STYLE CHICKEN

TAKES: 20 min. **MAKES:** 8 servings

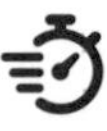

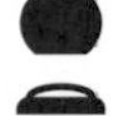

- 2 lbs. boneless skinless chicken thighs, cubed
- 2 medium sweet potatoes, peeled and cut into 1½-in. pieces
- 2 medium sweet red peppers, cut into 1-in. pieces
- 3 cups fresh cauliflowerets
- 2 jars (15 oz. each) tikka masala curry sauce
- ½ cup water
- ¾ tsp. salt
- Minced fresh cilantro, optional
- Naan flatbreads, warmed

In a 6-qt. electric pressure cooker, combine chicken and vegetables; add sauce, water and salt. Lock lid; close pressure-release valve. Adjust to pressure-cook on high for 3 minutes. Quick-release pressure. A thermometer inserted in chicken should read at least 170°. If desired, top with cilantro; serve with warmed naan flatbreads.

TO FREEZE Omitting cilantro and naan, freeze the cooled chicken and vegetable mixture in freezer containers. To use, partially thaw in the refrigerator overnight. Microwave, covered, on high in a microwave-safe dish until heated through, stirring gently; add water if necessary. If desired, sprinkle with cilantro. Serve with warmed naan.

1¼ CUPS *334 cal., 15g fat (4g sat. fat), 80mg chol., 686mg sod., 25g carb. (12g sugars, 5g fiber), 25g pro.* ***Diabetic exchanges:*** *3 lean meat, 2 fat, 1½ starch*

BEEF DAUBE PROVENCAL

PREP: 30 min. **COOK:** 5 hours **MAKES:** 8 servings

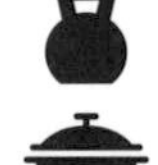

- 2 tsp. olive oil
- 1 boneless beef chuck roast or venison roast (about 2 lbs.), cut into 1-in. cubes
- 1½ tsp. salt, divided
- ½ tsp. coarsely ground pepper, divided
- 2 cups chopped carrots
- 1½ cups chopped onion
- 12 garlic cloves, crushed
- 1 Tbsp. tomato paste
- 1 cup dry red wine
- 1 can (14½ oz.) diced tomatoes
- ½ cup beef broth
- 1 tsp. chopped fresh rosemary
- 1 tsp. chopped fresh thyme
- 1 bay leaf
- Dash ground cloves
- Hot cooked pasta or mashed potatoes
- Fresh thyme leaves, optional

1 In a large skillet, heat oil over medium-high heat. Sprinkle meat with ½ tsp. salt and ¼ tsp. pepper; brown meat in batches. Transfer beef to 4-qt. slow cooker.

2 Add carrot, onion, garlic and remaining salt and pepper to skillet; cook and stir until golden brown, 4-6 minutes. Add the tomato paste; cook and stir until fragrant, about 1 minute. Add wine, stirring to loosen browned bits from pan; bring to a boil.

3 Transfer the meat mixture, tomatoes, broth and seasonings to slow cooker. Cook, covered, on low 5-7 hours or until tender. Discard bay leaf. Serve with hot cooked pasta or mashed potatoes. If desired, sprinkle with fresh thyme leaves.

1 CUP BEEF MIXTURE *237 cal., 12g fat (4g sat. fat), 74mg chol., 651mg sod., 8g carb. (3g sugars, 2g fiber), 23g pro.* ***Diabetic exchanges:*** *3 lean meat, 1 vegetable*

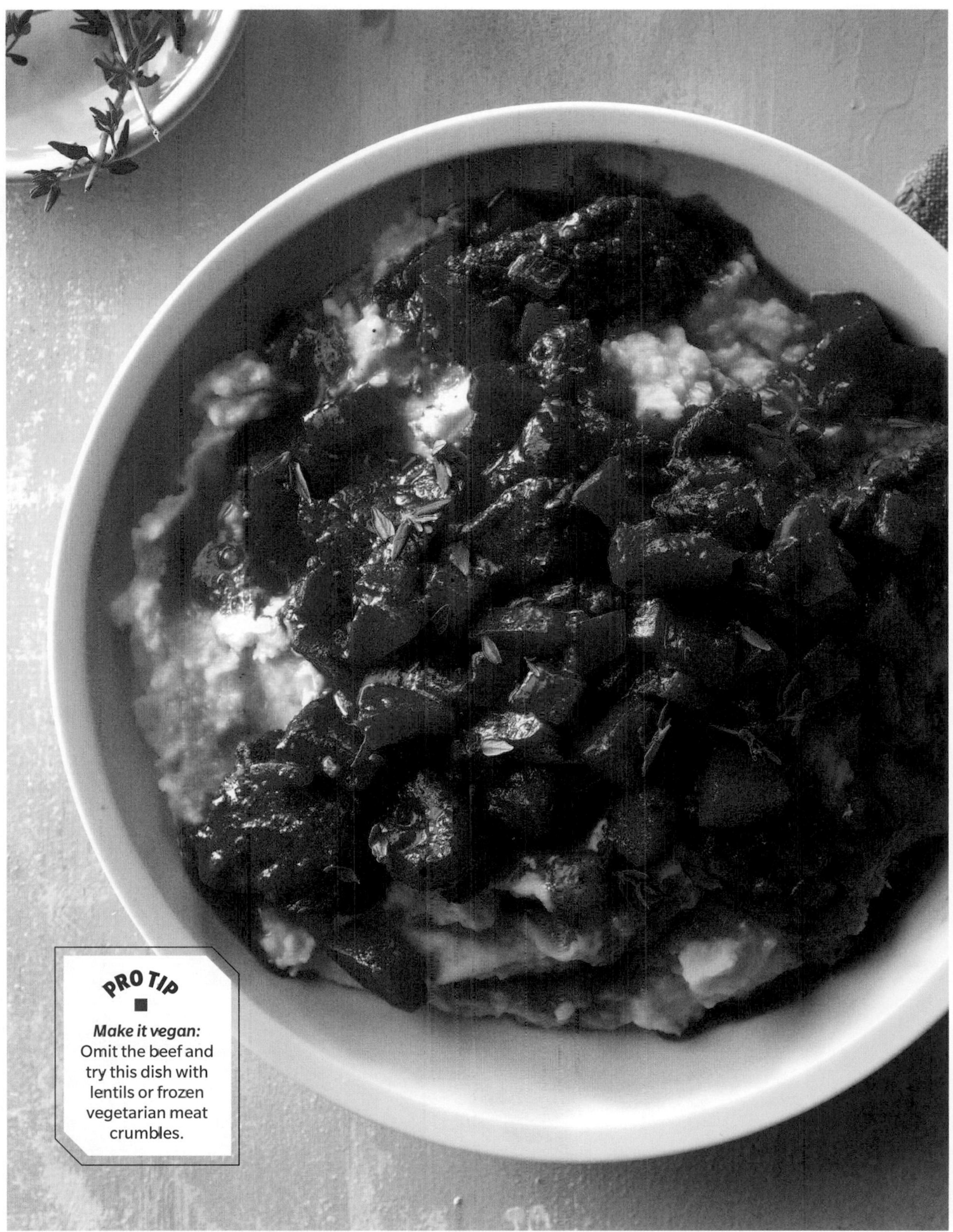
PRO TIP
Make it vegan: Omit the beef and try this dish with lentils or frozen vegetarian meat crumbles.

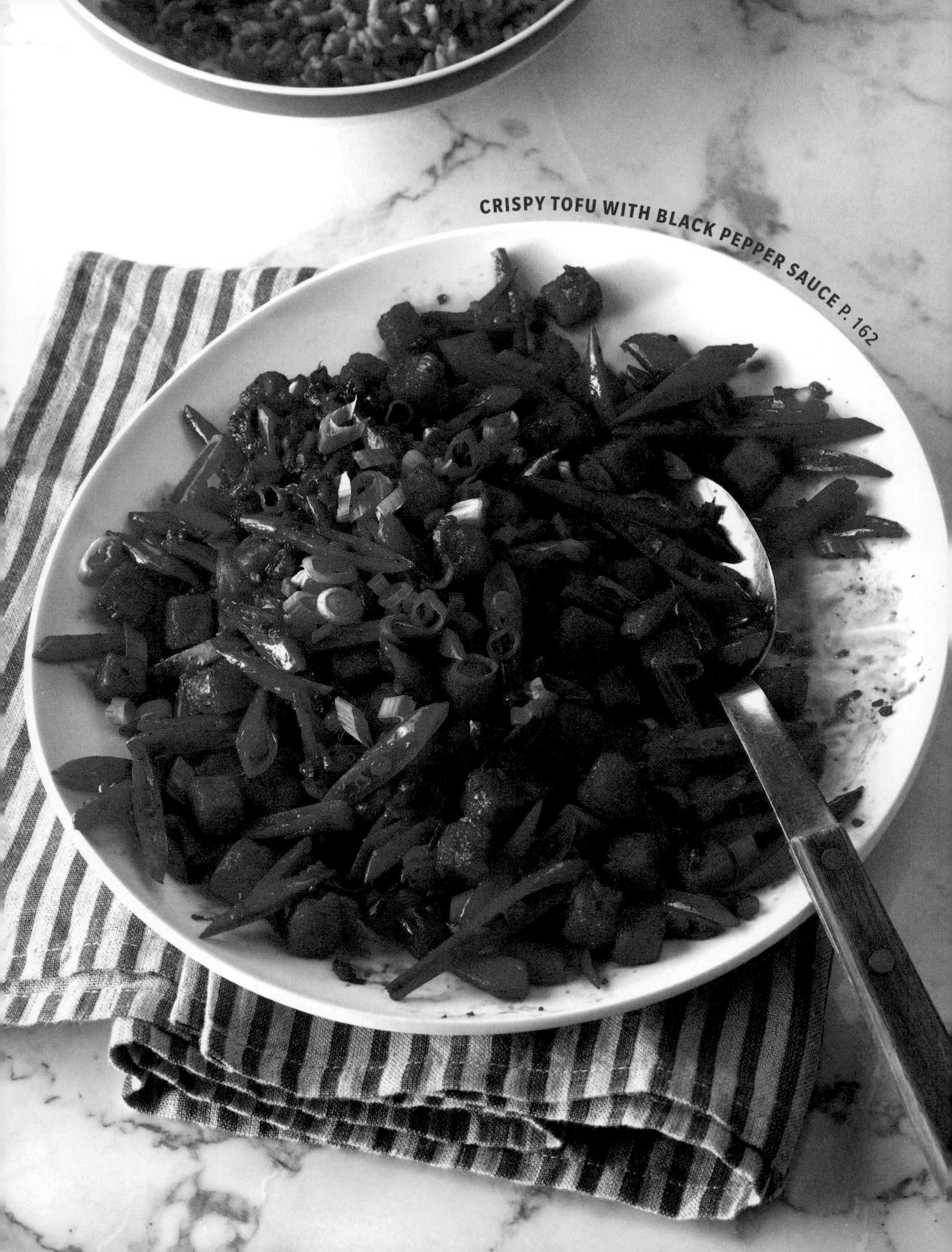
CRISPY TOFU WITH BLACK PEPPER SAUCE P. 162

CHAPTER 9

BEANS & LEGUMES

ASPARAGUS TOFU STIR-FRY

PREP: 15 min. **COOK:** 20 min. **MAKES:** 4 servings

- 1 Tbsp. cornstarch
- ½ tsp. sugar
- 1¼ cups vegetable broth
- 4 tsp. reduced-sodium soy sauce
- 2 tsp. minced fresh gingerroot, divided
- 3 tsp. canola oil, divided
- 1 lb. fresh asparagus, trimmed and cut into 1-in. pieces
- 1 medium yellow summer squash, halved and sliced
- 2 green onions, thinly sliced
- 1 pkg. (14 oz.) extra-firm tofu, drained and cut into ½-in. cubes
- ¼ tsp. salt
- ¼ tsp. pepper
- 2 cups hot cooked brown rice
- 2 Tbsp. sliced almonds, toasted

1 In a small bowl, combine the cornstarch, sugar, broth and soy sauce until smooth; set aside.

2 In a large nonstick skillet or wok, stir-fry 1 tsp. ginger in 1 tsp. oil for 1 minute. Add asparagus; stir-fry for 2 minutes. Add the squash; stir-fry 2 minutes longer. Add onions; stir-fry 1 minute longer or until vegetables are crisp-tender. Remove mixture and keep warm.

3 In the same pan, stir-fry tofu, salt, pepper and remaining ginger in remaining oil until lightly browned, 7-9 minutes. Remove and keep warm.

4 Stir cornstarch mixture and add to the pan. Bring to a boil; cook and stir for 2 minutes or until thickened. Add asparagus mixture and tofu; heat through. Serve with rice; sprinkle with almonds.

1 CUP *278 cal., 11g fat (1g sat. fat), 0 chol., 682mg sod., 34g carb. (4g sugars, 4g fiber), 14g pro.* ***Diabetic exchanges:*** *2 starch, 1 vegetable, 1 lean meat, 1 fat*

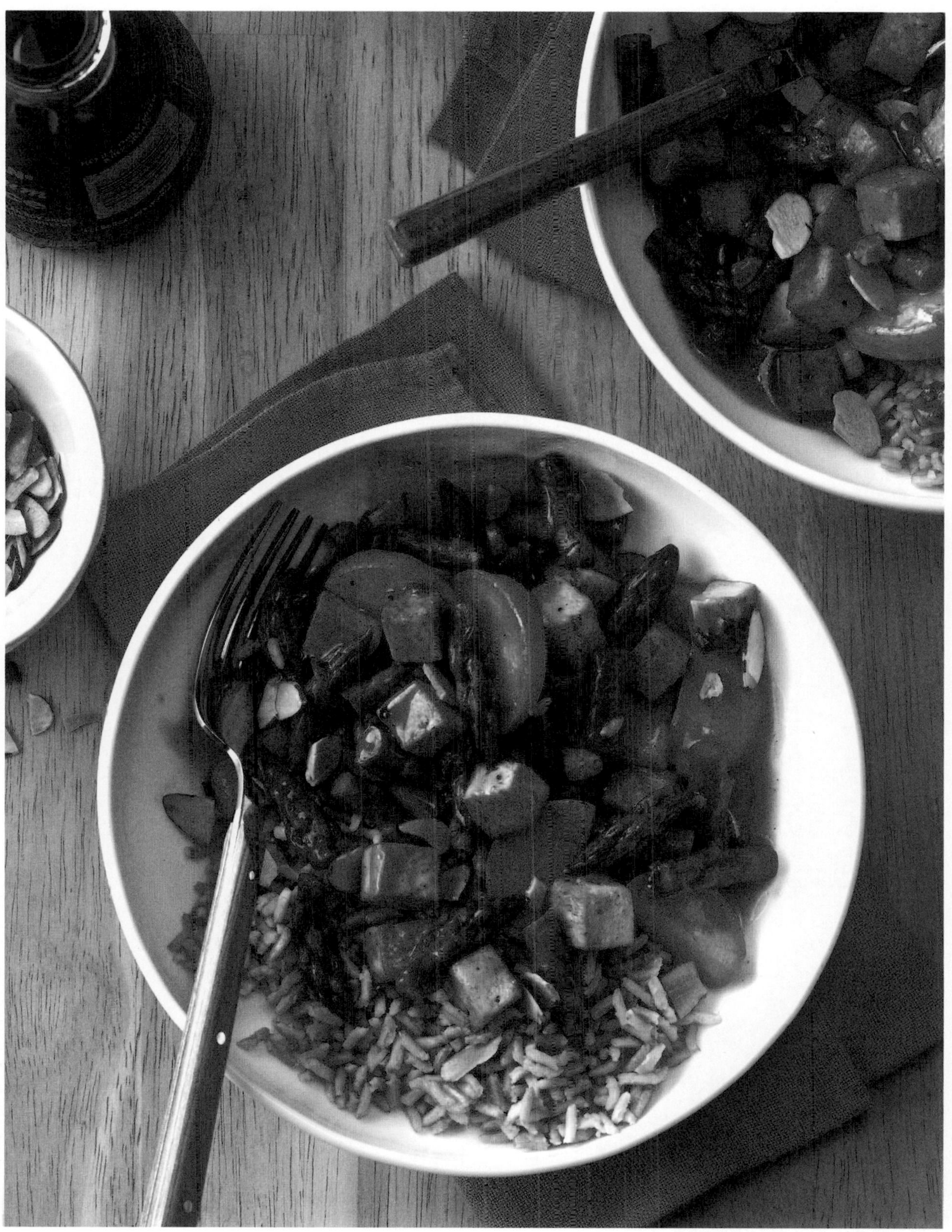

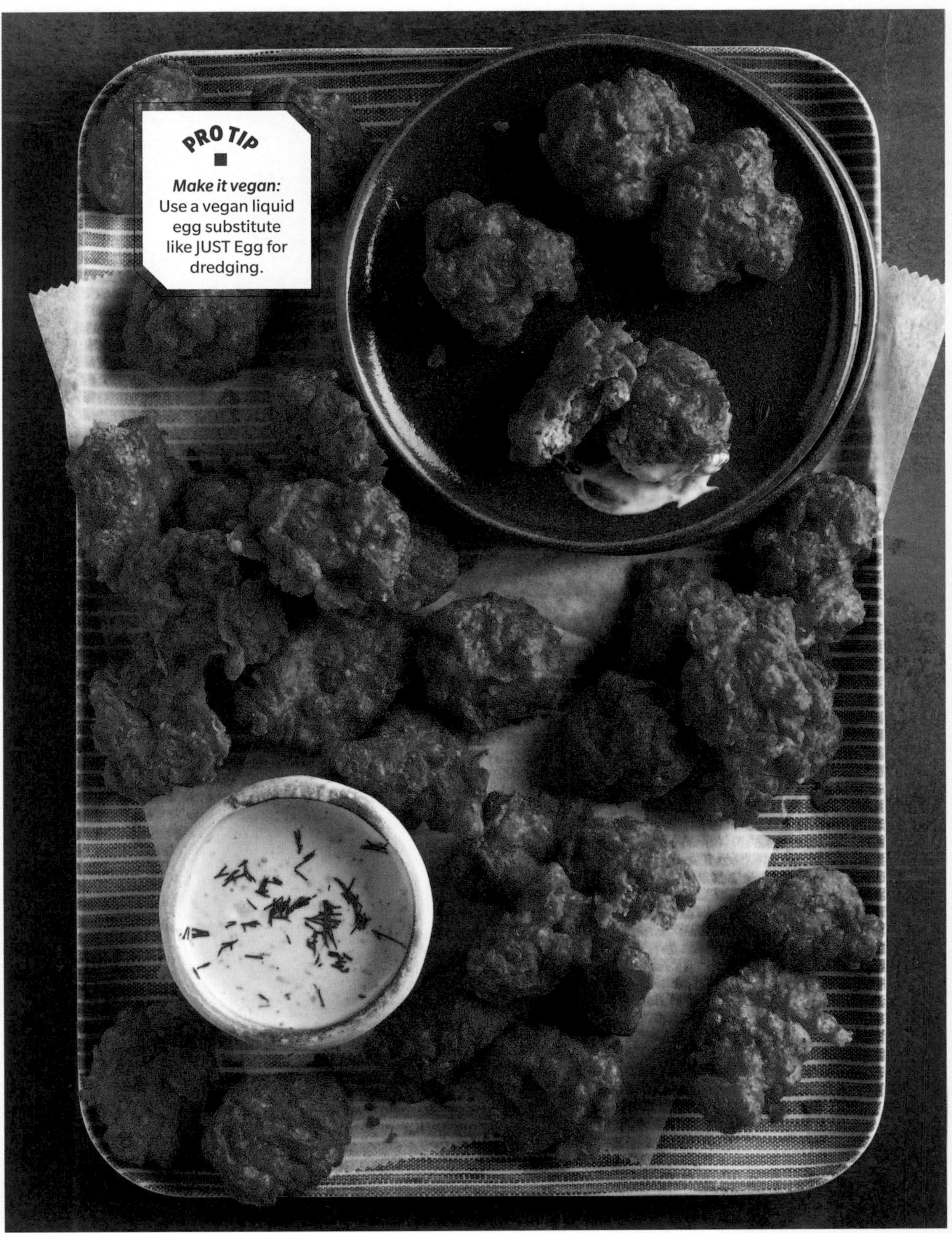

PRO TIP

Make it vegan: Use a vegan liquid egg substitute like JUST Egg for dredging.

TOFU CHICKEN NUGGETS

PREP: 15 min. **COOK:** 40 min. **MAKES:** 10 servings

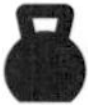

- 1 pkg. (14 oz.) soft tofu, patted dry
- 2¾ cups vital wheat gluten, divided
- 1½ tsp. poultry seasoning
- ½ tsp. salt
- ½ tsp. garlic powder
- ½ tsp. white pepper
- 1¼ cups water, divided
- ¼ cup vegan egg substitute (powdered)
- Oil for frying

1 Combine tofu, 1½ cups vital wheat gluten, poultry seasoning, salt, garlic powder and pepper in large bowl just until combined. Add ¼ cup water, a little at a time, until dough forms a ball. On a surface lightly dusted with vital wheat gluten, roll the dough into a circle about ½ in. thick. Gently cut or tear dough into 50 pieces.

2 In a large saucepan, place a steamer basket over 1 in. of water. In batches, place pieces in basket. Bring remaining water to a boil. Reduce heat to maintain a low boil; steam, covered, until pieces look puffed and firm, 10-15 minutes. Remove; keep warm.

3 Place remaining 1¼ cups vital wheat gluten in a shallow bowl. In a separate shallow bowl, mix egg substitute with 1 cup water, let stand 5 minutes to thicken. Dip pieces in egg mix, then vital wheat gluten. In a Dutch oven, heat oil to 375°. Fry in batches for 2-3 minutes on each side or until golden brown. Drain on paper towels. Serve immediately.

5 PIECES *268 cal., 11g fat (1g sat. fat), 0 chol., 56mg sod., 14g carb. (0 sugars, 0 fiber), 26g pro.*

CRISPY TOFU WITH BLACK PEPPER SAUCE

TAKES: 30 min. **MAKES:** 4 servings

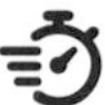

- 2 Tbsp. reduced-sodium soy sauce
- 2 Tbsp. chili garlic sauce
- 1 Tbsp. packed brown sugar
- 1 Tbsp. rice vinegar
- 4 green onions
- 8 oz. extra-firm tofu, drained
- 3 Tbsp. cornstarch
- 6 Tbsp. canola oil, divided
- 8 oz. fresh sugar snap peas (about 2 cups), trimmed and thinly sliced
- 1 tsp. freshly ground pepper
- 3 garlic cloves, minced
- 2 tsp. grated fresh gingerroot

1 Mix the first 4 ingredients. Mince white parts of green onions; thinly slice green parts.

2 Cut tofu into ½-in. cubes; pat dry with paper towels. Toss the tofu with cornstarch. In a large skillet, heat 4 Tbsp. oil over medium-high heat. Add tofu; cook until crisp and golden brown, 5-7 minutes, stirring occasionally. Remove from pan; drain on paper towels.

3 In same pan, heat 1 Tbsp. oil over medium-high heat. Add peas; stir-fry until crisp-tender, 2-3 minutes. Remove from pan.

4 In same pan, heat remaining oil over medium-high heat. Add pepper; cook 30 seconds. Add garlic, ginger and minced green onions; stir-fry 30-45 seconds. Stir in soy sauce mixture; cook and stir until slightly thickened. Remove from heat; stir in tofu and peas. Sprinkle with sliced green onions.

1 CUP *316 cal., 24g fat (2g sat. fat), 0 chol., 583mg sod., 20g carb. (8g sugars, 2g fiber), 7g pro.*

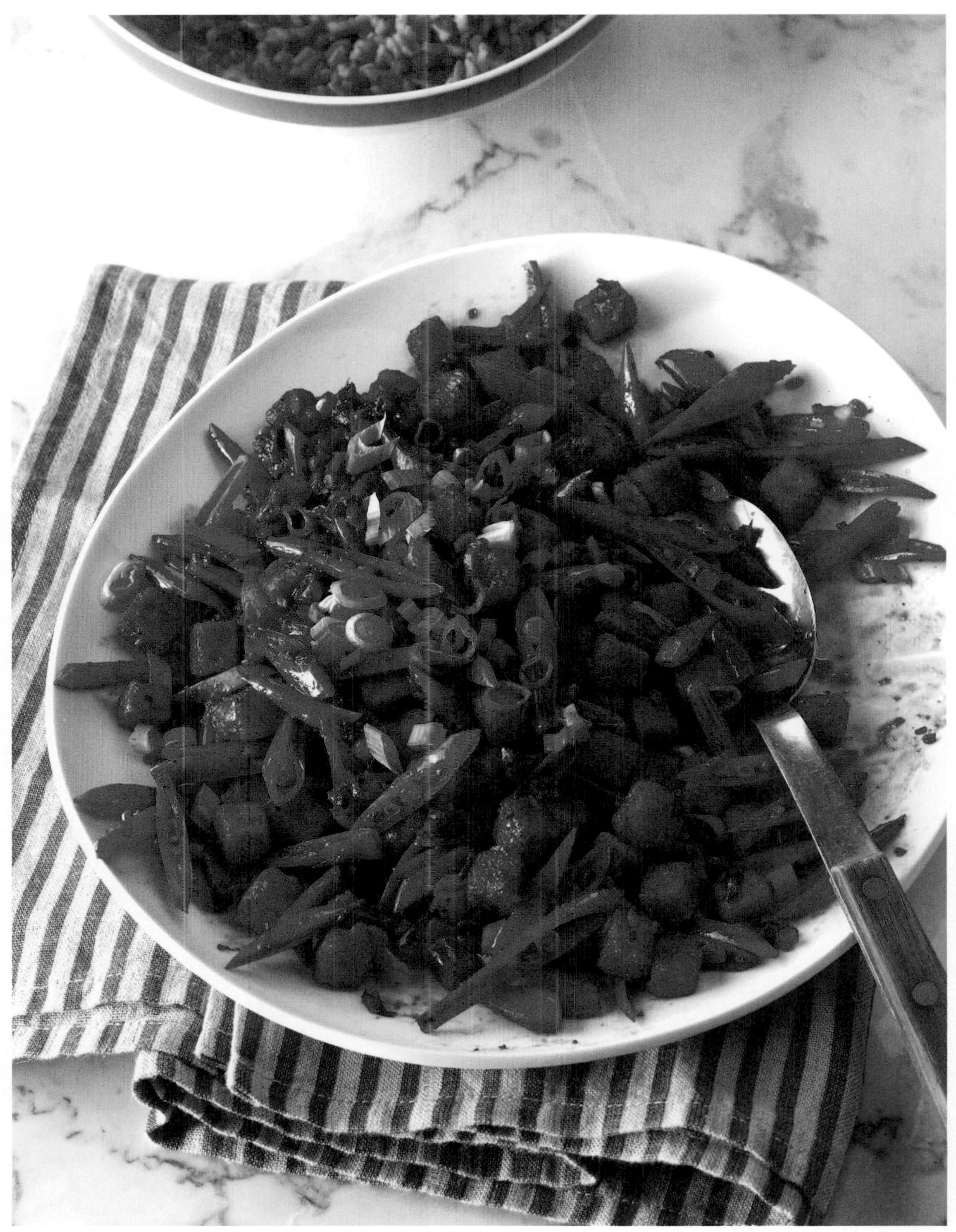

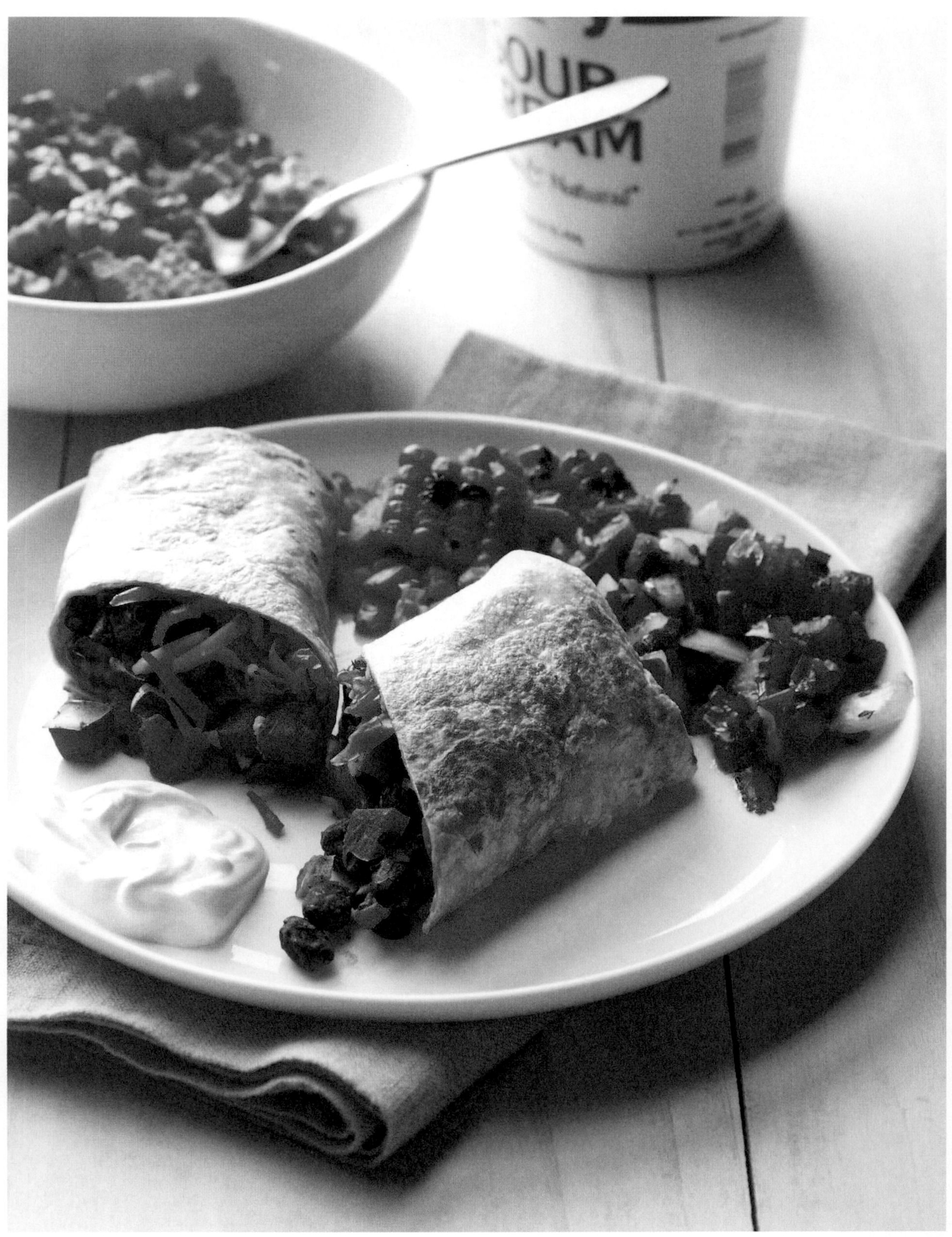

BLACK BEAN BURRITOS

TAKES: 10 min. **MAKES:** 4 servings

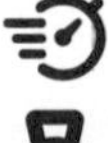

- 1 Tbsp. canola oil
- 3 Tbsp. chopped onion
- 3 Tbsp. chopped green pepper
- 1 can (15 oz.) black beans, rinsed and drained
- 4 flour tortillas (8 in.), warmed
- 1 cup shredded Mexican or vegan Mexican-style cheese blend
- 1 medium tomato, chopped
- 1 cup shredded lettuce
- Optional toppings: Salsa, dairy or vegan sour cream, minced fresh cilantro and cubed avocado

1 In a nonstick skillet, heat oil over medium heat; saute onion and green pepper until tender. Stir in beans; heat through.

2 Spoon about ½ cup of the vegetable mixture off-center on each tortilla. Sprinkle with the cheese, tomato and lettuce. Fold sides and ends over filling and roll up. Serve with optional toppings as desired.

1 BURRITO *395 cal., 16g fat (6g sat. fat), 25mg chol., 610mg sod., 46g carb. (2g sugars, 7g fiber), 16g pro.* ***Diabetic exchanges:*** *2½ starch, 1 vegetable, 1 lean meat, 1 fat*

CORNBREAD-TOPPED FRIJOLES

PREP: 20 min. **COOK:** 3 hours **MAKES:** 8 servings

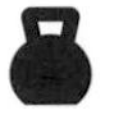
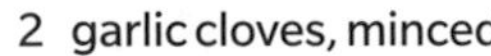

- 1 medium onion, chopped
- 1 medium green pepper, chopped
- 1 Tbsp. canola oil
- 2 garlic cloves, minced
- 1 can (16 oz.) kidney beans, rinsed and drained
- 1 can (15 oz.) pinto beans, rinsed and drained
- 1 can (14½ oz.) diced tomatoes, undrained
- 1 can (8 oz.) tomato sauce
- 1 tsp. chili powder
- ½ tsp. pepper
- ⅛ tsp. hot pepper sauce

CORNBREAD TOPPING

- 1 cup all-purpose flour
- 1 cup yellow cornmeal
- 1 Tbsp. sugar
- 1½ tsp. baking powder
- ½ tsp. salt
- 2 large eggs, room temperature, lightly beaten or vegan egg substitute
- 1¼ cups fat-free milk or milk alternative
- 1 can (8¼ oz.) cream-style corn
- 3 Tbsp. canola oil

1 In a large skillet, saute onion and green pepper in oil until tender. Add garlic; cook 1 minute longer. Transfer to a greased 5-qt. slow cooker.

2 Stir in the beans, tomatoes, tomato sauce, chili powder, pepper and pepper sauce. Cover and cook on high for 1 hour.

3 In a large bowl, combine the flour, cornmeal, sugar, baking powder and salt. Combine the eggs, milk, corn and oil; add to dry ingredients and mix well. Spoon evenly over bean mixture.

4 Cover and cook on high for 2½-3 hours or until a toothpick inserted in center of cornbread comes out clean.

1 SERVING *367 cal., 9g fat (1g sat. fat), 54mg chol., 708mg sod., 59g carb. (10g sugars, 9g fiber), 14g pro.*

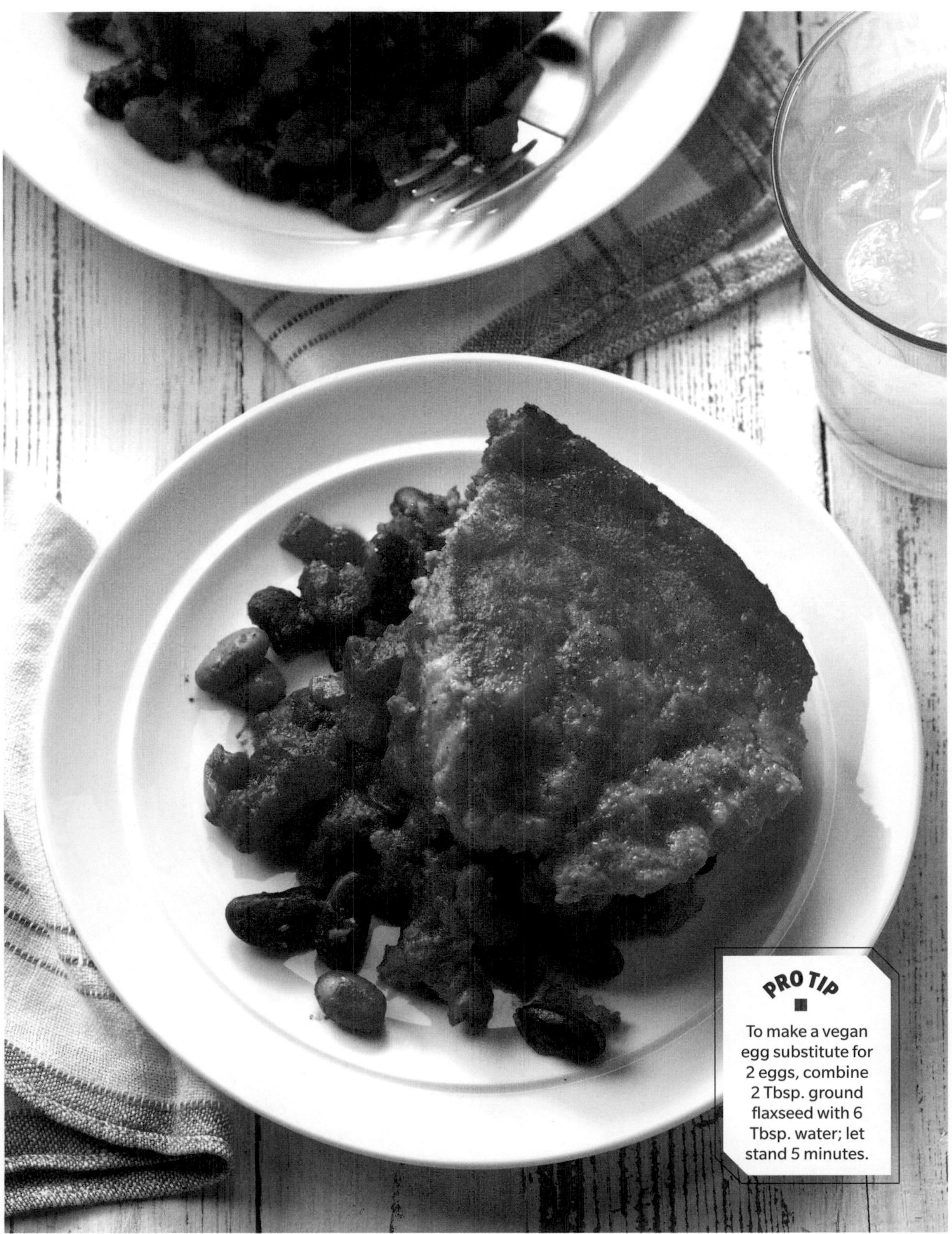

PRO TIP

To make a vegan egg substitute for 2 eggs, combine 2 Tbsp. ground flaxseed with 6 Tbsp. water; let stand 5 minutes.

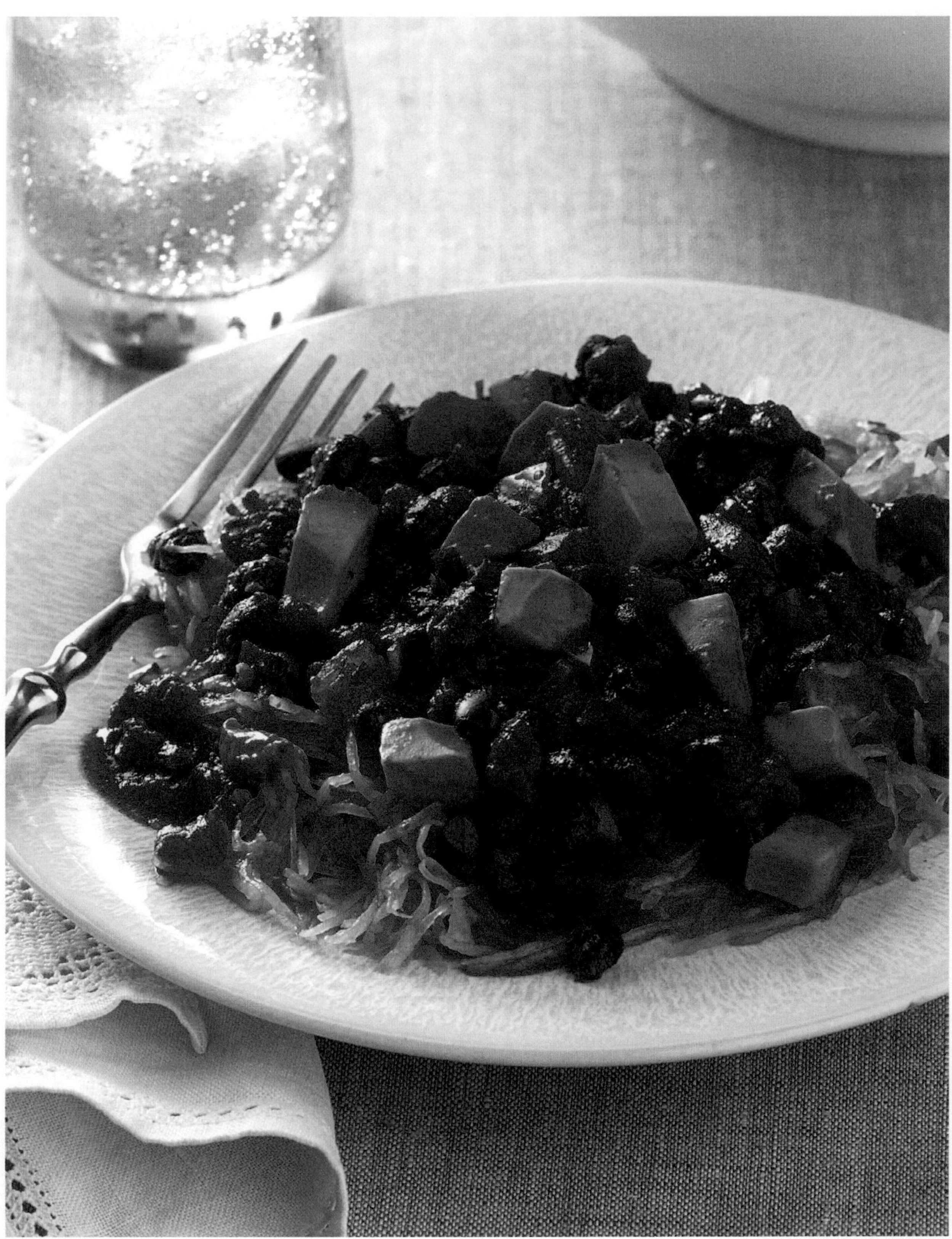

SALSA SPAGHETTI SQUASH

TAKES: 30 min. **MAKES:** 4 servings

- 1 medium spaghetti squash
- 1 medium onion, chopped
- 2 cups salsa
- 1 can (15 oz.) black beans, rinsed and drained
- 3 Tbsp. minced fresh cilantro
- 1 medium ripe avocado, peeled and cubed

1 Cut squash lengthwise in half; discard seeds. Place squash on a microwave-safe plate, cut side down. Microwave, uncovered, on high for 15-18 minutes or until tender.

2 Meanwhile, in a lightly oiled nonstick skillet, cook and stir onion over medium heat until tender. Stir in salsa, beans and fresh cilantro; heat through. Gently stir in avocado; cook for 1 minute longer.

3 When squash is cool enough to handle, use a fork to separate strands. Serve squash topped with salsa mixture.

1 CUP *308 cal., 9g fat (2g sat. fat), 0 chol., 822mg sod., 46g carb. (6g sugars, 16g fiber), 8g pro.*

CREAMY LENTILS WITH KALE ARTICHOKE SAUTE

TAKES: 30 min. **MAKES:** 4 servings

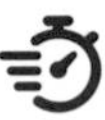

- ½ cup dried red lentils, rinsed and sorted
- ¼ tsp. dried oregano
- ⅛ tsp. pepper
- 1¼ cups vegetable broth
- ¼ tsp. sea salt, divided
- 1 Tbsp. olive oil or grapeseed oil
- 16 cups chopped fresh kale (about 12 oz.)
- 1 can (14 oz.) water-packed artichoke hearts, drained and chopped
- 3 garlic cloves, minced
- ½ tsp. Italian seasoning
- 2 Tbsp. grated Romano or vegan Romano-style cheese
- 2 cups hot cooked brown or basmati rice

1 Place first 4 ingredients and ⅛ tsp. salt in a small saucepan; bring to a boil. Reduce heat; simmer, covered, until lentils are tender and liquid is almost absorbed, 12-15 minutes. Remove from heat.

2 In a 6-qt. stockpot, heat oil over medium heat. Add the kale and remaining salt; cook, covered, until kale is wilted, 4-5 minutes, stirring occasionally. Add the artichoke hearts, garlic and Italian seasoning; cook and stir 3 minutes. Remove from heat; stir in cheese.

3 Serve lentils and kale mixture over rice.

1 SERVING *321 cal., 6g fat (2g sat. fat), 1mg chol., 661mg sod., 53g carb. (1g sugars, 5g fiber), 15g pro.*

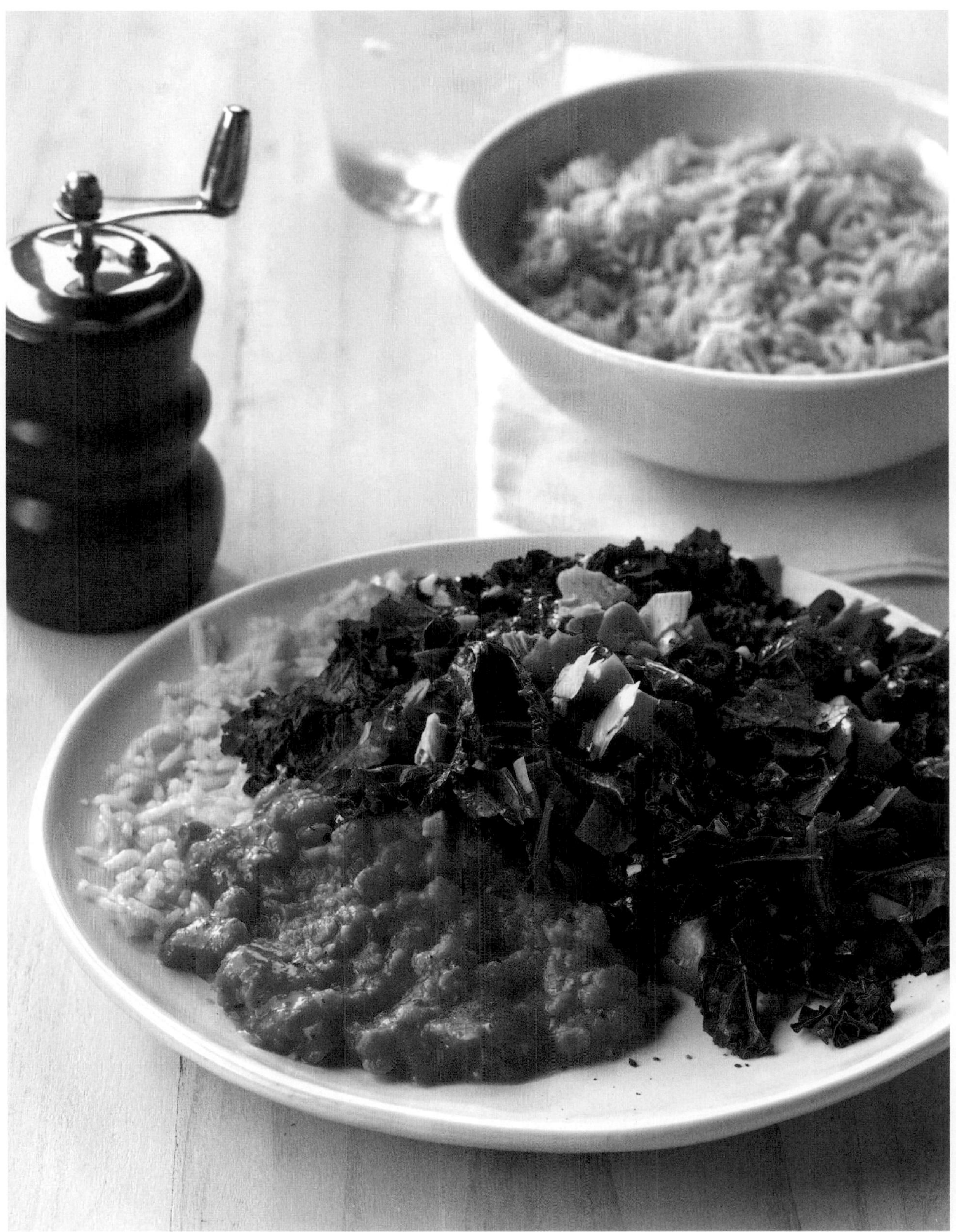

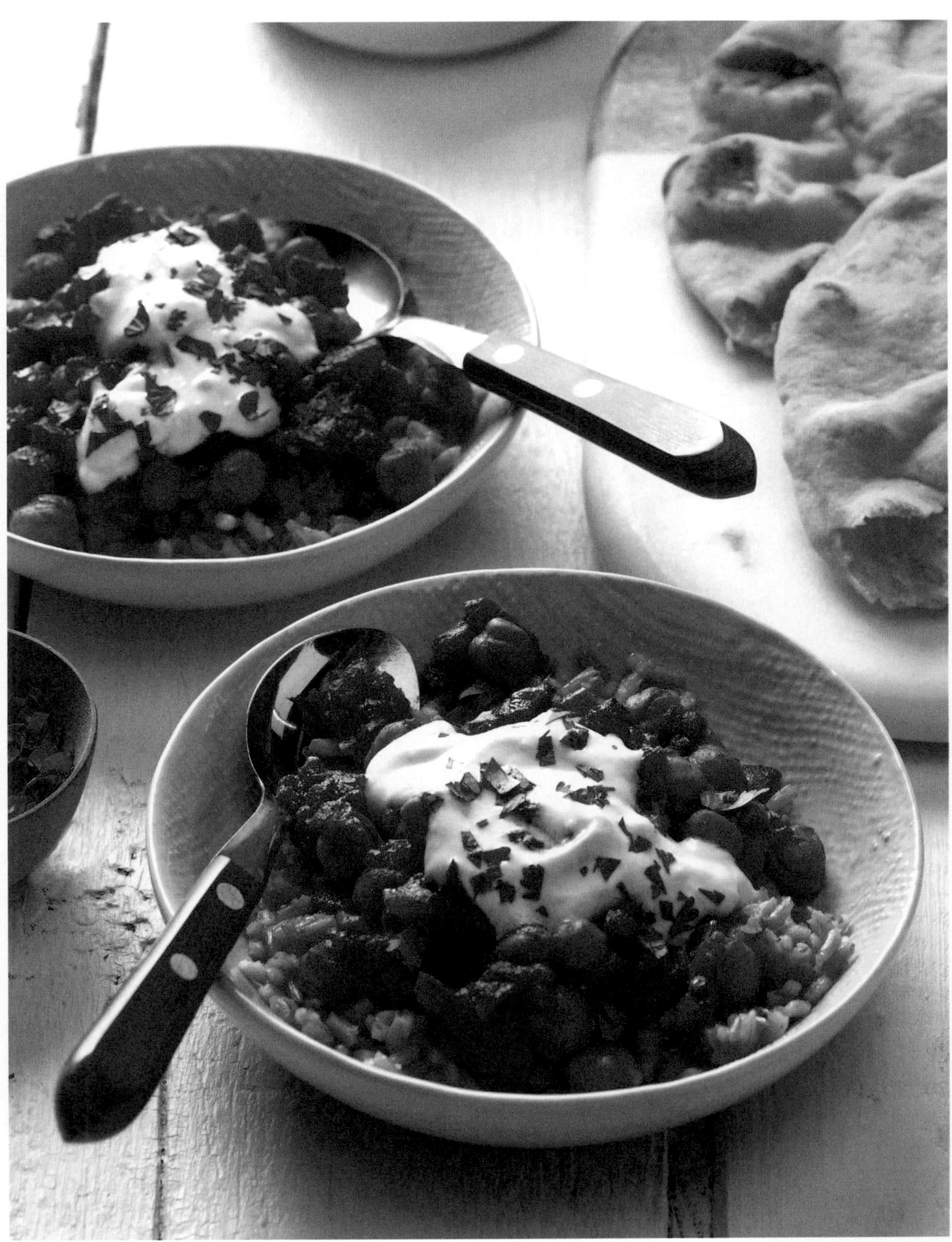

EASY CHANA MASALA

TAKES: 30 min. **MAKES:** 4 servings

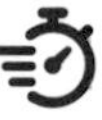

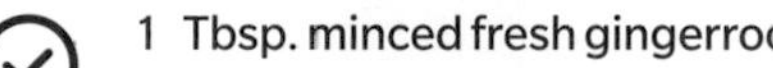

- 1 Tbsp. canola oil
- ½ cup finely chopped onion
- 1 Tbsp. minced fresh gingerroot
- 2 garlic cloves, minced
- 1 jalapeno pepper, seeded and finely chopped, optional
- ½ tsp. salt
- 1 tsp. garam masala
- ½ tsp. ground coriander
- ½ tsp. ground cumin
- 1 can (15 oz.) diced tomatoes, undrained
- 1 can (15 oz.) garbanzo beans or chickpeas, rinsed and drained
- 3 cups hot cooked brown rice
- ¼ cup plain vegan yogurt
- Minced fresh cilantro

1 In a large skillet, heat oil over medium heat. Add onion, ginger, garlic and, if desired, jalapeno; cook and stir until the onion is softened and lightly browned, 4-5 minutes. Add seasonings; cook and stir 1 minute.

2 Stir in the tomatoes and garbanzo beans; bring to a boil. Reduce heat; simmer, covered, 12-15 minutes or until the flavors are blended, stirring occasionally. Serve with rice. Top with yogurt and cilantro.

TO FREEZE Freeze the cooled garbanzo bean mixture in freezer containers. To use, partially thaw in refrigerator overnight. Heat through in a saucepan, stirring occasionally; add water if necessary.

¾ CUP CHICKPEA MIXTURE WITH ¾ CUP RICE *359 cal., 8g fat (1g sat. fat), 0 chol., 610mg sod., 63g carb. (7g sugars, 9g fiber), 10g pro.*

FIERY STUFFED POBLANOS

PREP: 50 min. + standing **BAKE:** 20 min. **MAKES:** 8 servings

- 8 poblano peppers
- 1 can (15 oz.) black beans, rinsed and drained
- 1 medium zucchini, chopped
- 1 small red onion, chopped
- 4 garlic cloves, minced
- 1 can (15¼ oz.) whole kernel corn, drained
- 1 can (14½ oz.) fire-roasted diced tomatoes, undrained
- 1 cup cooked brown rice
- 1 Tbsp. ground cumin
- 1 to 1½ tsp. ground ancho chile pepper
- ¼ tsp. salt
- ¼ tsp. pepper
- 1 cup shredded reduced-fat Mexican or vegan Mexican-style cheese blend, divided
- 3 green onions, chopped
- ½ cup reduced-fat dairy or vegan sour cream

1 Broil peppers 3 in. from heat until the skins blister, about 5 minutes. With tongs, rotate peppers a quarter turn. Broil and rotate until all sides are blistered and blackened. Immediately place the peppers in a large bowl; cover and let stand for 20 minutes.

2 Meanwhile, in a small bowl, coarsely mash beans; set aside. In a large nonstick skillet, cook and stir zucchini and onion until tender. Add garlic; cook 1 minute longer. Add corn, tomatoes, rice, seasonings and beans. Remove from heat; stir in ½ cup cheese. Set aside.

3 Preheat oven to 375°. Peel the charred skins from poblanos and discard. Cut a lengthwise slit through each pepper, leaving stem intact; discard membranes and seeds. Spoon ⅔ cup filling into each pepper.

4 Place peppers in a 13x9-in. baking dish coated with cooking spray. Bake until heated through, 18-22 minutes, sprinkling with green onions and remaining cheese during last 5 minutes of baking. Serve with sour cream.

1 STUFFED PEPPER *223 cal., 5g fat (2g sat. fat), 15mg chol., 579mg sod., 32g carb. (9g sugars, 7g fiber), 11g pro.* ***Diabetic exchanges:*** *2 vegetable, 1 starch, 1 lean meat, 1 fat*

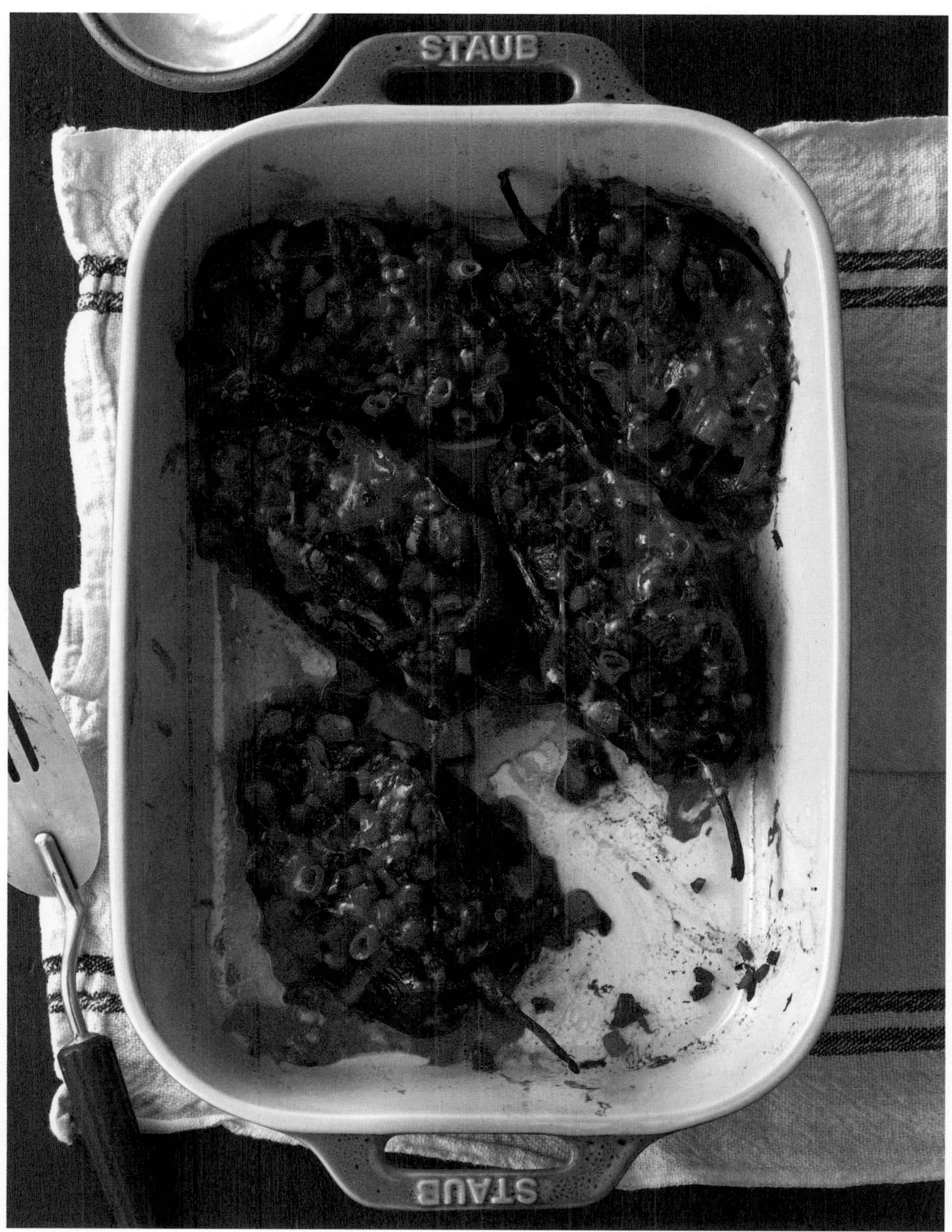
STAUB
STAUB

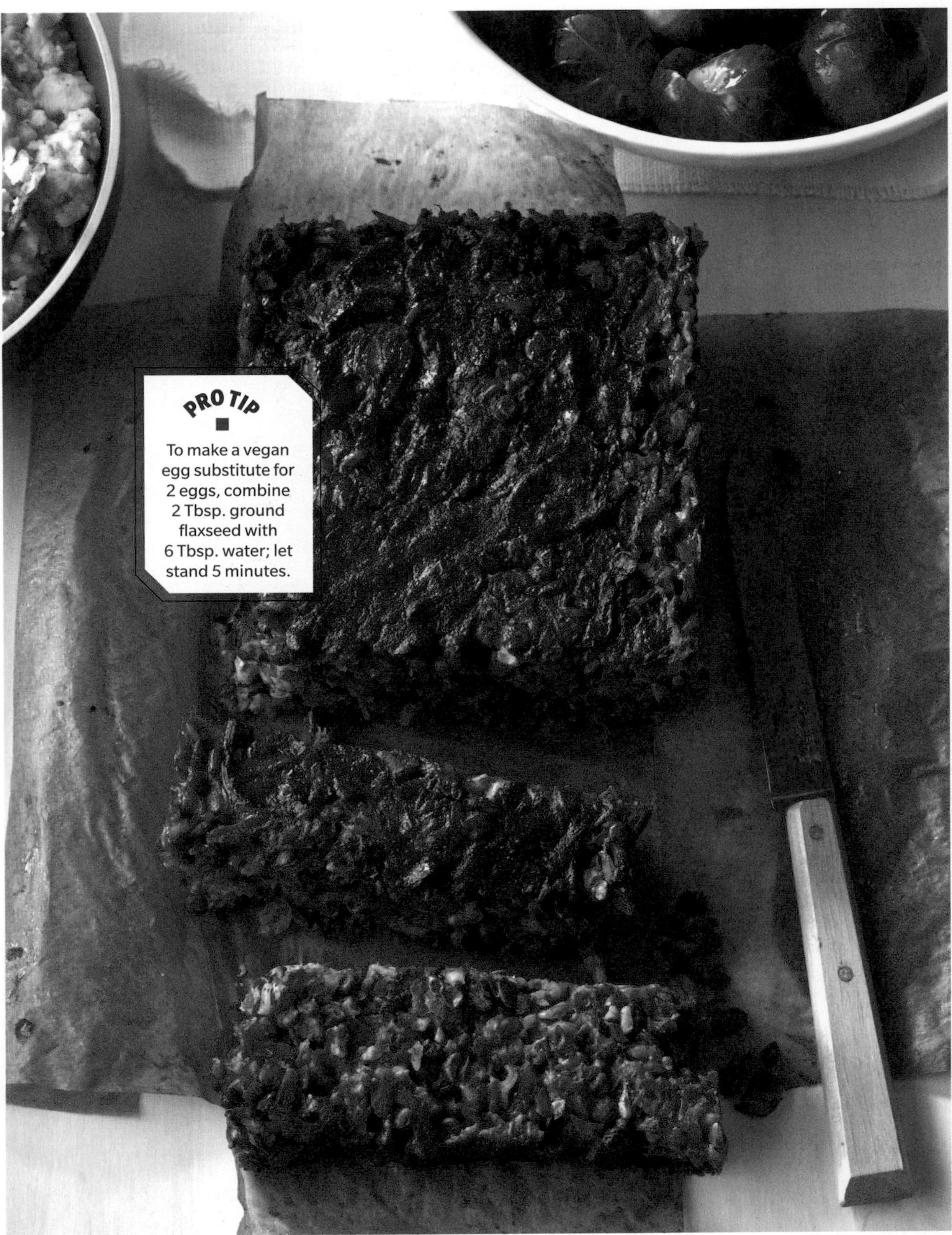

PRO TIP

To make a vegan egg substitute for 2 eggs, combine 2 Tbsp. ground flaxseed with 6 Tbsp. water; let stand 5 minutes.

LENTIL LOAF

PREP: 35 min. **BAKE:** 45 min. + standing **MAKES:** 6 servings

¾ cup brown lentils, rinsed
1 can (14½ oz.) vegetable broth
1 Tbsp. olive oil
1¾ cups shredded carrots
1 cup finely chopped onion
1 cup chopped fresh mushrooms
2 Tbsp. minced fresh basil or 2 tsp. dried basil
1 Tbsp. minced fresh parsley
1 cup shredded part-skim mozzarella or vegan mozzarella-style cheese
½ cup cooked brown rice
1 large egg or vegan egg substitute
1 large egg white or vegan egg substitute
½ tsp. salt
½ tsp. garlic powder
¼ tsp. pepper
2 Tbsp. tomato paste
2 Tbsp. water

1 Place lentils and broth in a small saucepan; bring to a boil. Reduce heat; simmer, covered, until tender, about 30 minutes.

2 Preheat oven to 350°. Line a 9x5-in. loaf pan with parchment, letting ends extend up sides. Coat paper with cooking spray.

3 In a large skillet, heat oil over medium heat; saute carrots, onion and mushrooms until tender, about 10 minutes. Stir in herbs. Transfer to a large bowl; cool slightly.

4 Add cheese, rice, egg, egg white, seasonings and lentils to the vegetables; mix well. Transfer to prepared loaf pan. Mix tomato paste and water; spread over loaf.

5 Bake until a thermometer inserted into the center reads 160°, 45-50 minutes. Let stand 10 minutes before slicing.

1 PIECE *213 cal., 5g fat (3g sat. fat), 43mg chol., 580mg sod., 29g carb. (5g sugars, 5g fiber), 14g pro.* ***Diabetic exchanges:*** *2 lean meat, 1½ starch, 1 vegetable, ½ fat*

MUSHROOM-BEAN BOURGUIGNON

PREP: 15 min. **COOK:** 1¼ hours **MAKES:** 10 servings (2½ qt.)

- 4 Tbsp. olive oil, divided
- 5 medium carrots, cut into 1-in. pieces
- 2 medium onions, halved and sliced
- 2 garlic cloves, minced
- 8 large portobello mushrooms, cut into 1-in. pieces
- 1 Tbsp. tomato paste
- 1 bottle (750 ml) dry red wine
- 2 cups mushroom broth or vegetable broth, divided
- 1 tsp. salt
- 1 tsp. minced fresh thyme or ½ tsp. dried thyme
- ½ tsp. pepper
- 2 cans (15½ oz. each) navy beans, rinsed and drained
- 1 pkg. (14.4 oz.) frozen pearl onions
- 3 Tbsp. all-purpose flour

1 In a Dutch oven, heat 2 Tbsp. oil over medium-high heat. Add carrots and onions; cook and stir 8-10 minutes or until onions are tender. Add garlic; cook 1 minute longer. Remove from pan.

2 In same pan, heat 1 Tbsp. oil over medium-high heat. Add half the mushrooms; cook and stir until lightly browned. Remove from pan; repeat with remaining 1 Tbsp. oil and mushrooms.

3 Return all mushrooms to pan. Add tomato paste; cook and stir 1 minute. Stir in wine, 1½ cups broth, salt, thyme, pepper and carrot mixture; bring to a boil. Reduce heat; simmer, covered, 25 minutes.

4 Add beans and pearl onions; cook 30 minutes longer. In a small bowl, whisk flour and remaining broth until smooth; stir into pan. Bring to a boil; cook and stir until the mixture is slightly thickened, about 2 minutes.

1 CUP *234 cal., 6g fat (1g sat. fat), 0 chol., 613mg sod., 33g carb. (6g sugars, 7g fiber), 9g pro.* ***Diabetic exchanges:*** *2 starch, 2 vegetable, 1 lean meat, 1 fat*

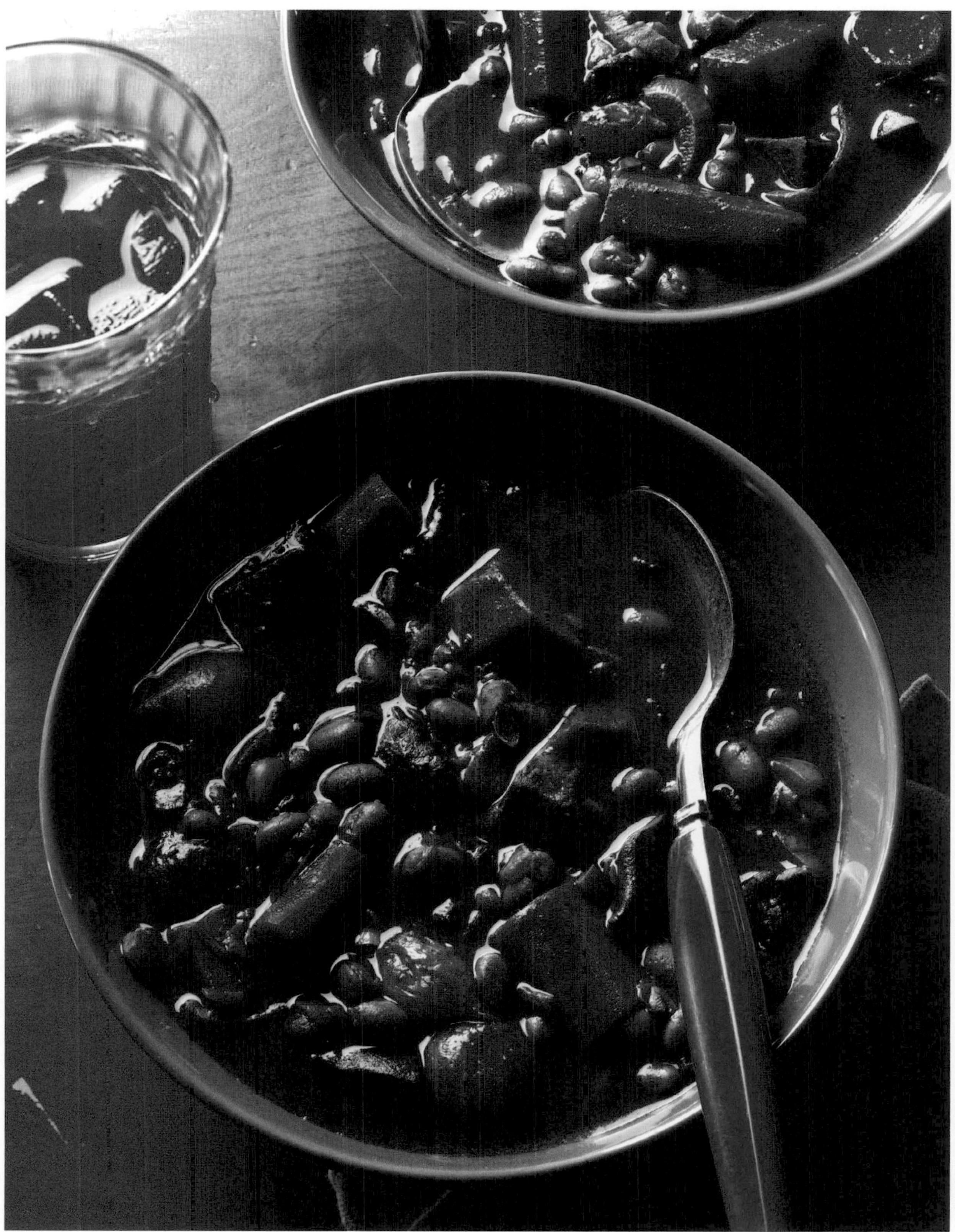

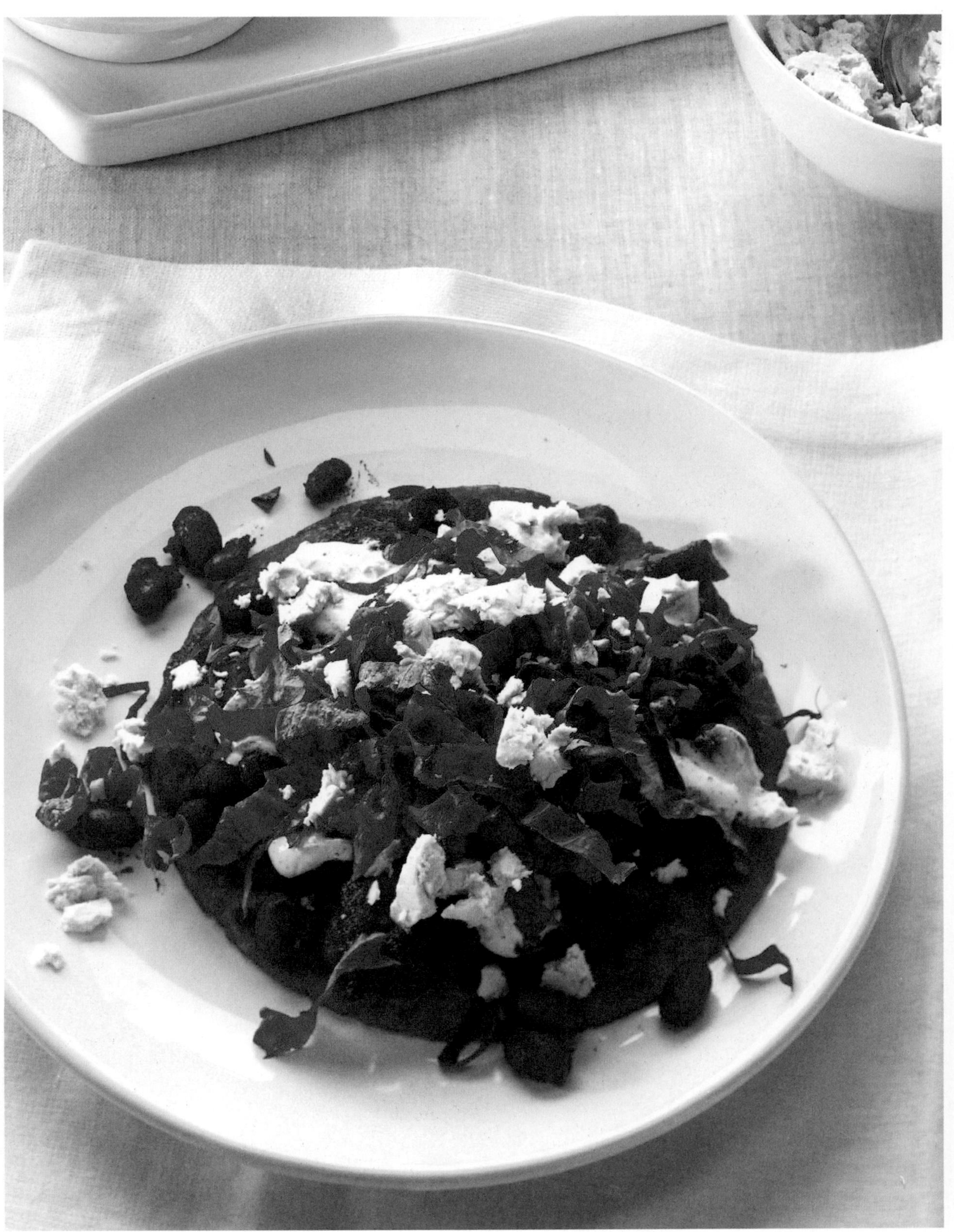

PINTO BEAN TOSTADAS

TAKES: 30 min. **MAKES:** 6 servings

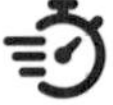

- ¼ cup dairy or vegan sour cream
- ¾ tsp. grated lime zest
- ¼ tsp. ground cumin
- ½ tsp. salt, divided
- 2 Tbsp. canola oil, divided
- 2 garlic cloves, minced
- 2 cans (15 oz. each) pinto beans, rinsed and drained
- 1 to 2 tsp. hot pepper sauce
- 1 tsp. chili powder
- 6 corn tortillas (6 in.)
- 2 cups shredded lettuce
- ½ cup salsa
- ¾ cup crumbled feta or vegan feta-style cheese
- Lime wedges

1 In a small bowl, mix sour cream, lime zest, cumin and ¼ tsp. salt. In a large saucepan, heat 1 Tbsp. oil over medium heat. Add garlic; cook and stir just until fragrant, about 45 seconds. Stir in beans, pepper sauce, chili powder and remaining salt; heat through, stirring occasionally. Keep warm.

2 Brush both sides of tortillas with remaining oil. Place a large skillet over medium-high heat. Add tortillas in 2 batches; cook until lightly browned and crisp, 2-3 minutes on each side.

3 To serve, arrange beans and lettuce over tostada shells; top with salsa, sour cream mixture and cheese. Serve tostadas with lime wedges.

1 TOSTADA *291 cal., 10g fat (3g sat. fat), 14mg chol., 658mg sod., 38g carb. (4g sugars, 8g fiber), 11g pro.* ***Diabetic exchanges:*** *2½ starch, 1 lean meat, 1 fat*

PORTOBELLO & CHICKPEA SHEET-PAN SUPPER

PREP: 15 min. **BAKE:** 35 min. **MAKES:** 4 servings

- ¼ cup olive oil
- 2 Tbsp. balsamic vinegar
- 1 Tbsp. minced fresh oregano
- ¾ tsp. garlic powder
- ½ tsp. salt
- ¼ tsp. pepper
- 1 can (15 oz.) chickpeas or garbanzo beans, rinsed and drained
- 4 large portobello mushrooms (4 to 4½ in.), stems removed
- 1 lb. fresh asparagus, trimmed and cut into 2-in. pieces
- 8 oz. cherry tomatoes

1 Preheat oven to 400°. In a small bowl, combine first 6 ingredients. Toss chickpeas with 2 Tbsp. oil mixture. Transfer chickpeas to a 15x10x1-in. baking pan. Bake 20 minutes.

2 Brush mushrooms with 1 Tbsp. oil mixture; add to pan. Toss asparagus and tomatoes with remaining oil mixture; arrange around the mushrooms. Bake until the vegetables are tender, 15-20 minutes longer.

1 MUSHROOM WITH 1 CUP VEGETABLES
279 cal., 16g fat (2g sat. fat), 0 chol., 448mg sod., 28g carb. (8g sugars, 7g fiber), 8g pro. ***Diabetic exchanges:*** *3 fat, 2 starch*

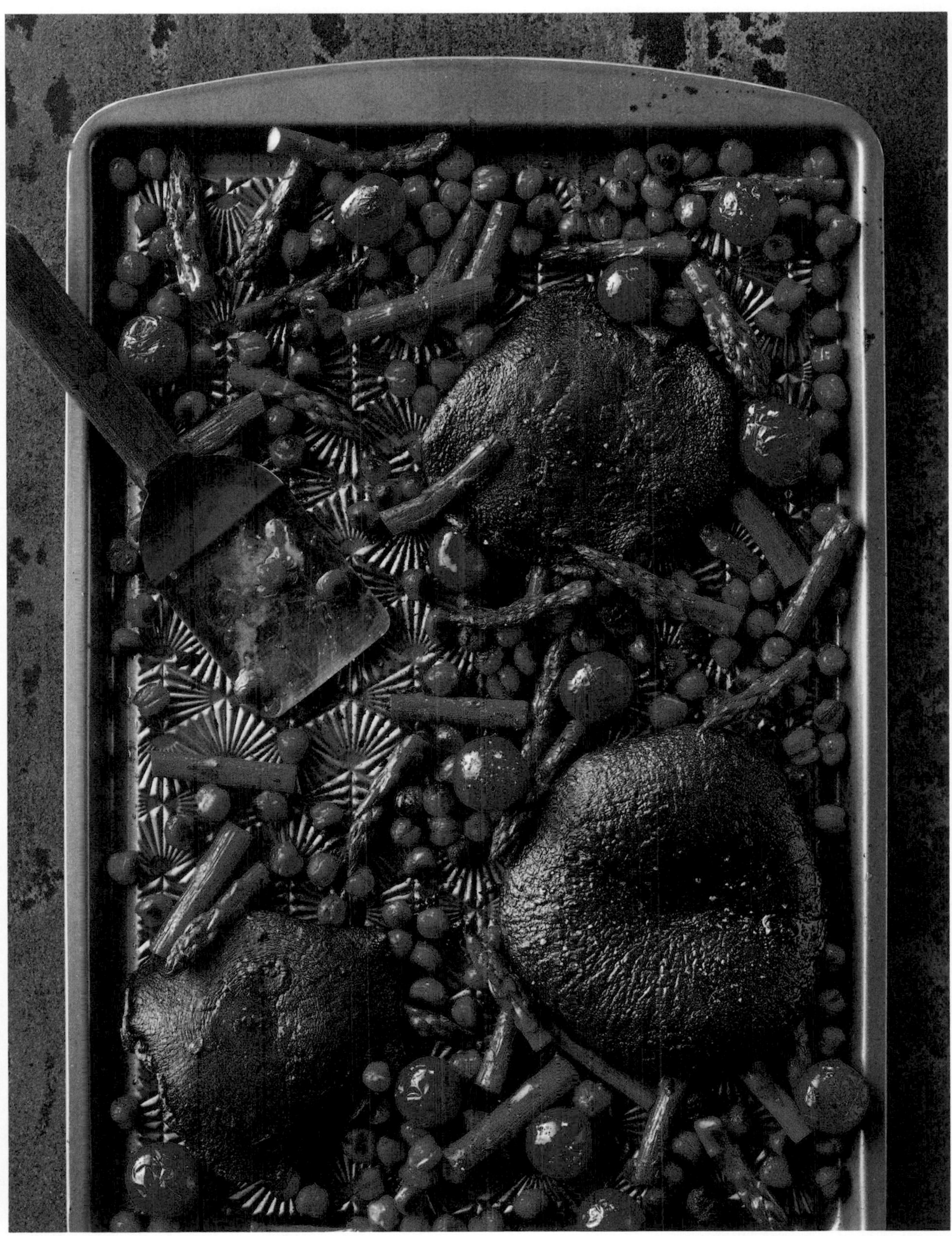

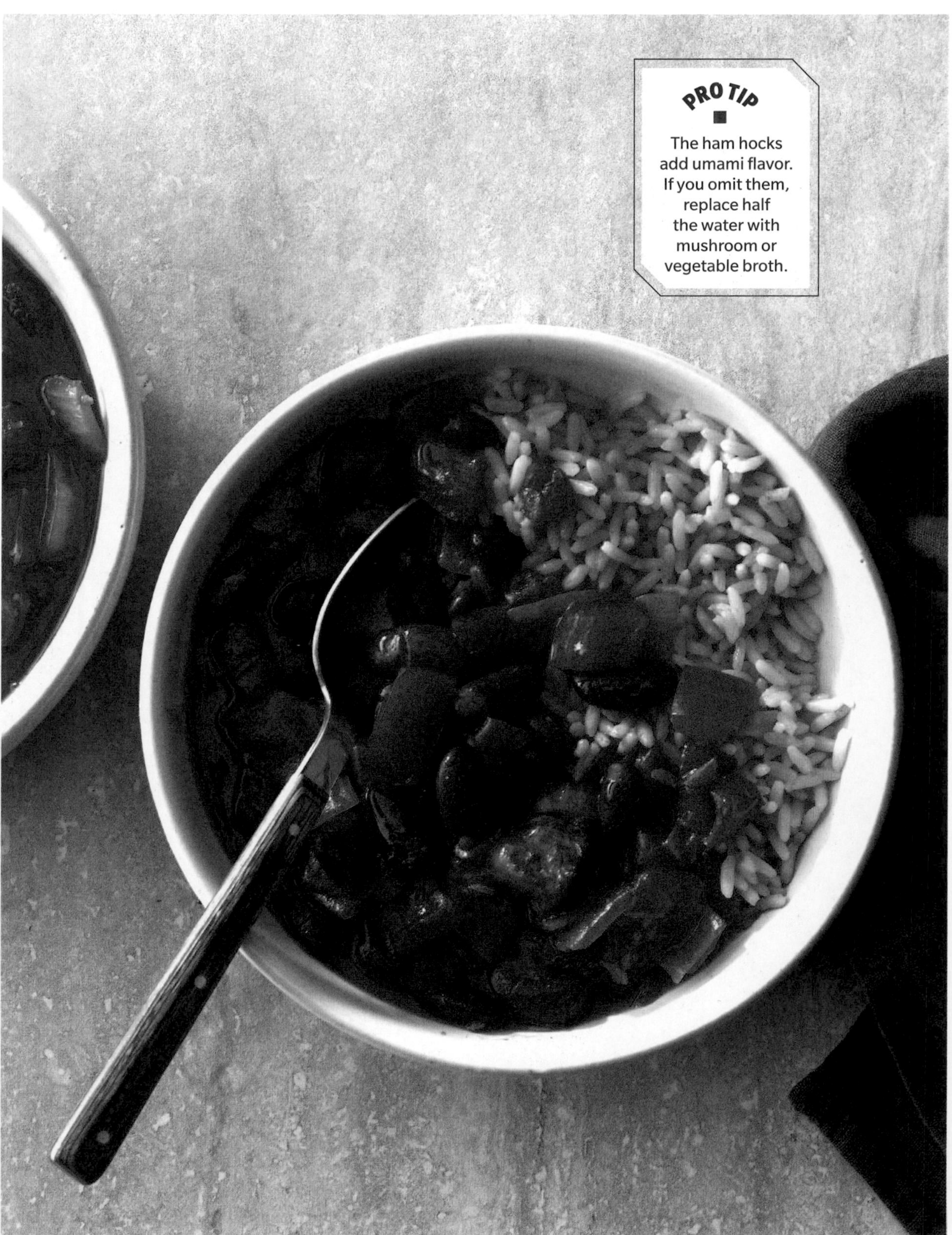
PRO TIP
The ham hocks add umami flavor. If you omit them, replace half the water with mushroom or vegetable broth.

PRESSURE-COOKER RED BEANS & RICE

PREP: 20 min. **COOK:** 45 min. + releasing **MAKES:** 6 servings

- 3 cups water
- 2 smoked ham hocks (about 1 lb.)
- 1 cup dried red beans
- 1 medium onion, chopped
- 1½ tsp. minced garlic
- 1 tsp. ground cumin
- 1 medium tomato, chopped
- 1 medium green pepper, chopped
- 1 tsp. salt
- 4 cups hot cooked rice

1 Place the first 6 ingredients in a 6-qt. electric pressure cooker. Lock lid; close pressure-release valve. Adjust to pressure-cook on high for 35 minutes. Let pressure release naturally.

2 Remove ham hocks; cool slightly. Remove meat from bones. Finely chop meat and return to pressure cooker; discard bones. Stir in tomato, green pepper and salt. Select saute setting and adjust for low heat. Simmer, stirring constantly, 8-10 minutes or until pepper is tender. Serve with rice.

TO FREEZE Freeze the cooled bean mixture in freezer containers. To use, partially thaw in refrigerator overnight. Microwave, covered, on high in a microwave-safe dish until heated through, gently stirring; add water if necessary.

⅓ CUP BEAN MIXTURE WITH ⅔ CUP RICE *216 cal., 2g fat (0 sat. fat), 9mg chol., 671mg sod., 49g carb. (3g sugars, 12g fiber), 12g pro.*

PRESSURE-COOKER CHICKPEA & POTATO CURRY

PREP: 25 min. **COOK:** 5 min. + releasing **MAKES:** 6 servings

- 1 Tbsp. canola oil
- 1 medium onion, chopped
- 2 garlic cloves, minced
- 2 tsp. minced fresh gingerroot
- 2 tsp. ground coriander
- 1 tsp. garam masala
- 1 tsp. chili powder
- ½ tsp. salt
- ½ tsp. ground cumin
- ¼ tsp. ground turmeric
- 2½ cups vegetable stock
- 2 cans (15 oz. each) chickpeas or garbanzo beans, rinsed and drained
- 1 can (15 oz.) crushed tomatoes
- 1 large baking potato, peeled and cut into ¾-in. cubes
- 1 Tbsp. lime juice
- Chopped fresh cilantro
- Hot cooked rice
- Optional: Sliced red onion and lime wedges

1 Select saute setting on a 6-qt. electric pressure cooker. Adjust for medium heat; add oil. When oil is hot, cook and stir onion until crisp-tender, 2-4 minutes. Add garlic, ginger and dry seasonings; cook and stir 1 minute. Add the stock to pressure cooker. Cook for 30 seconds, stirring to loosen browned bits from pan. Press cancel. Stir in the chickpeas, tomatoes and potato.

2 Lock lid; close pressure-release valve. Adjust to pressure-cook on high for 3 minutes. Let pressure release naturally for 10 minutes; quick-release any remaining pressure.

3 Stir in lime juice; sprinkle with cilantro. Serve with rice and, if desired, sliced red onion and lime wedges.

1¼ CUPS *240 cal., 6g fat (0 sat. fat), 0 chol., 767mg sod., 42g carb. (8g sugars, 9g fiber), 8g pro.*

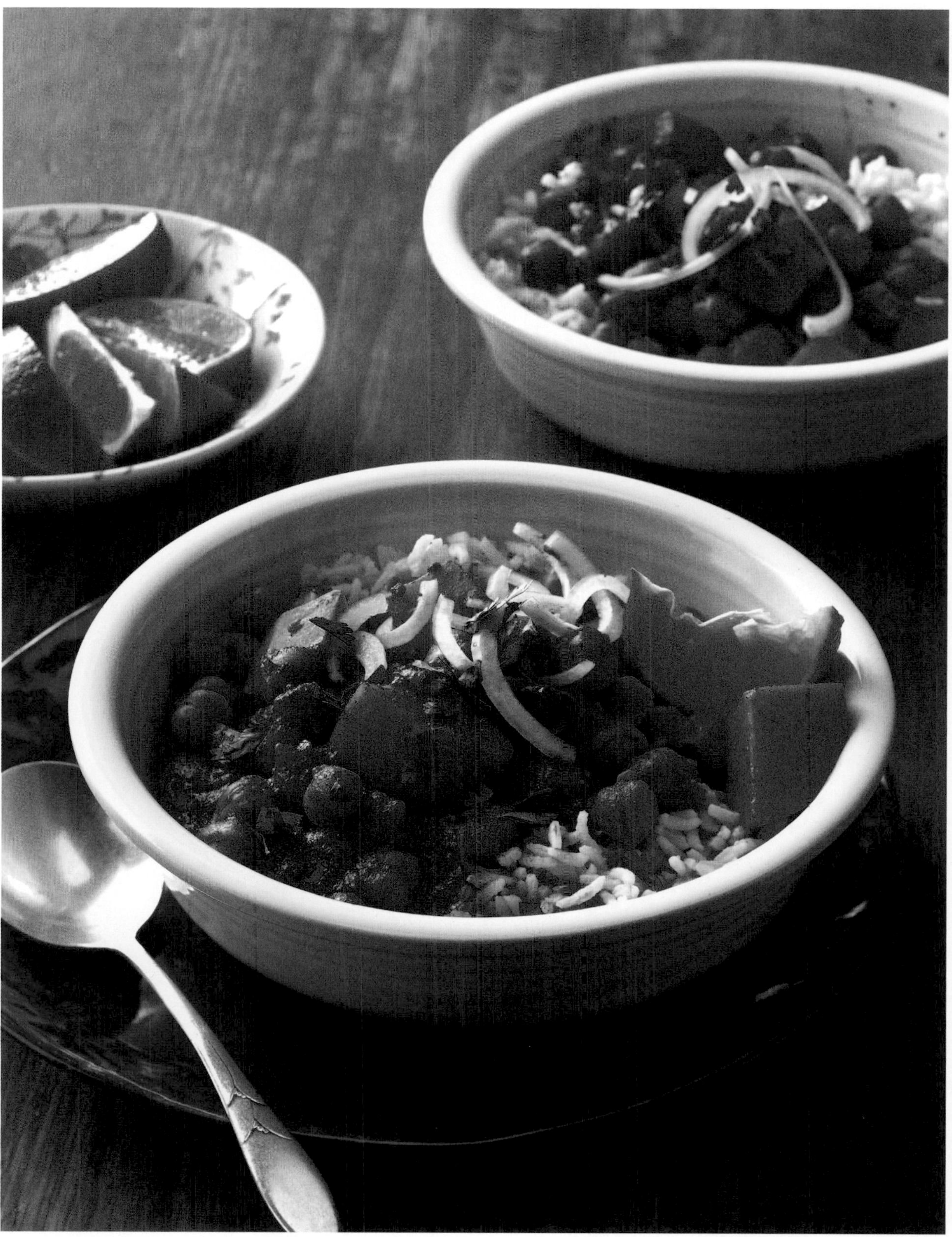

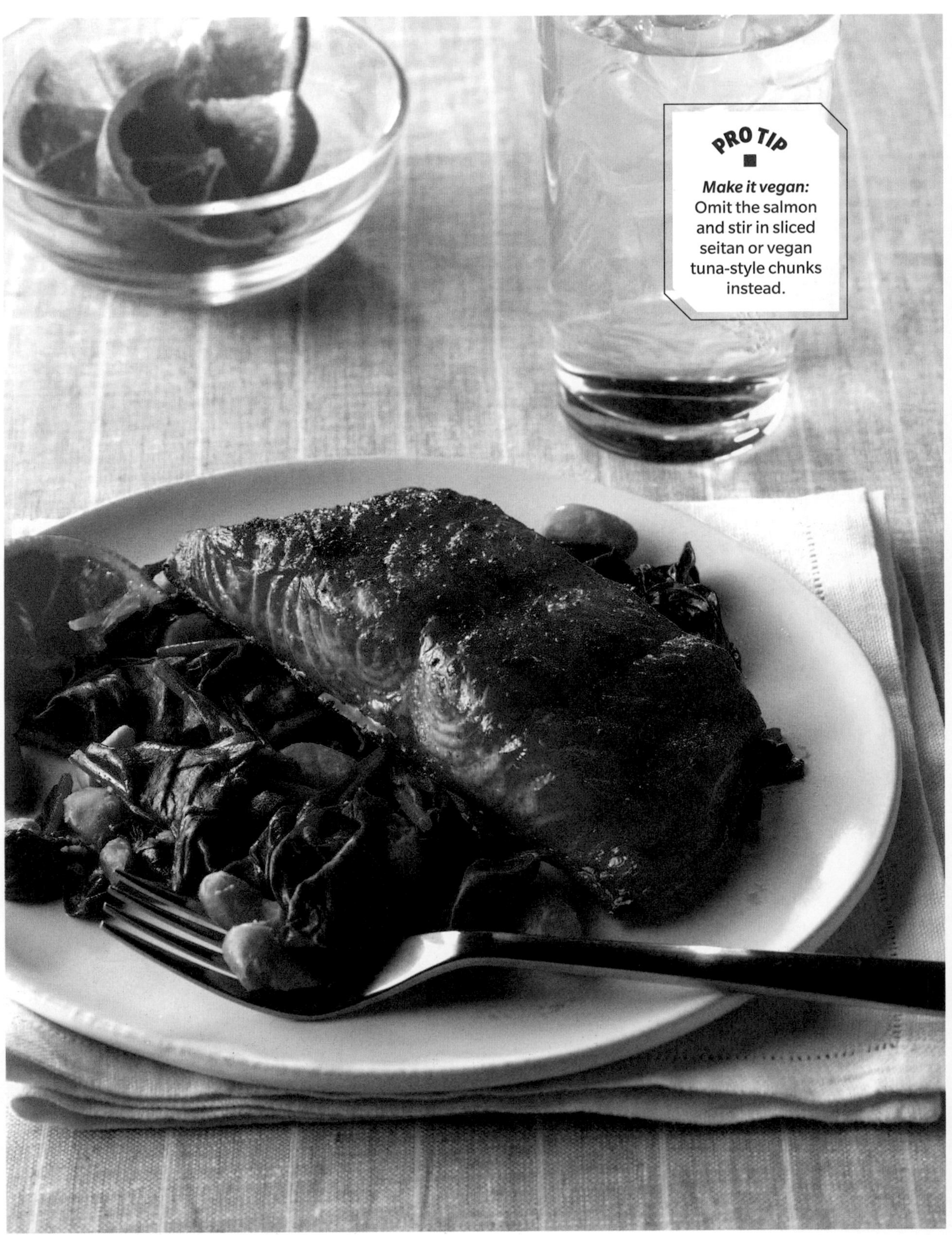

PRO TIP

Make it vegan: Omit the salmon and stir in sliced seitan or vegan tuna-style chunks instead.

SALMON WITH SPINACH & WHITE BEANS

TAKES: 15 min. **MAKES:** 4 servings

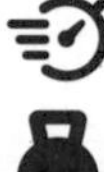

- 4 salmon fillets (4 oz. each)
- 2 tsp. plus 1 Tbsp. olive oil, divided
- 1 tsp. seafood seasoning
- 1 garlic clove, minced
- 1 can (15 oz.) cannellini beans, rinsed and drained
- ¼ tsp. salt
- ¼ tsp. pepper
- 1 pkg. (8 oz.) fresh spinach
- Lemon wedges

1 Preheat broiler. Rub fillets with 2 tsp. oil; sprinkle with seafood seasoning. Place on a greased rack of a broiler pan. Broil 5-6 in. from heat 6-8 minutes or until fish just begins to flake easily with a fork.

2 Meanwhile, in a large skillet, heat remaining oil over medium heat. Add the garlic; cook until fragrant, 15-30 seconds. Add beans, salt and pepper, stirring to coat beans with garlic oil. Stir in spinach until wilted. Serve salmon with spinach mixture and lemon wedges.

1 FILLET WITH ½ CUP SPINACH MIXTURE *317 cal., 17g fat (3g sat. fat), 57mg chol., 577mg sod., 16g carb. (0 sugars, 5g fiber), 24g pro.* ***Diabetic exchanges:*** *3 lean meat, 2 vegetable, 1 fat, ½ starch*

SLOW-COOKER PUMPKIN CHICKEN TAGINE

PREP: 35 min. **COOK:** 5 hours **MAKES:** 4 servings

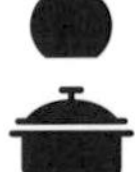

- 1 lb. boneless skinless chicken thighs, cut into ½-in. pieces
- 1 can (15 oz.) garbanzo beans or chickpeas, rinsed and drained
- 1 can (14½ oz.) diced tomatoes, undrained
- 1 medium green pepper, chopped
- 1 cup canned pumpkin
- ¼ cup golden raisins
- 1 Tbsp. maple syrup
- 2 tsp. ground cumin
- 1 tsp. ground cinnamon
- ½ tsp. salt
- ½ tsp. ground coriander
- ¼ tsp. cayenne pepper
- ¼ tsp. ground cloves
- ¼ tsp. ground allspice
- 1 Tbsp. olive oil
- 1 medium onion, chopped
- 2 garlic cloves, minced
- 1 tsp. minced fresh gingerroot
- Hot cooked couscous and chopped fresh cilantro

1 In a 3- or 4-qt. slow cooker, combine the first 14 ingredients. In a small skillet, heat oil over medium heat. Add onion; cook and stir until tender, 5-7 minutes. Add the garlic and ginger; cook 1 minute longer. Stir into slow cooker.

2 Cook, covered, on low until chicken is cooked through and vegetables are tender, 5-6 hours. Serve with couscous; sprinkle with cilantro.

1 SERVING *400 cal., 14g fat (3g sat. fat), 76mg chol., 668mg sod., 42g carb. (18g sugars, 10g fiber), 28g pro.*

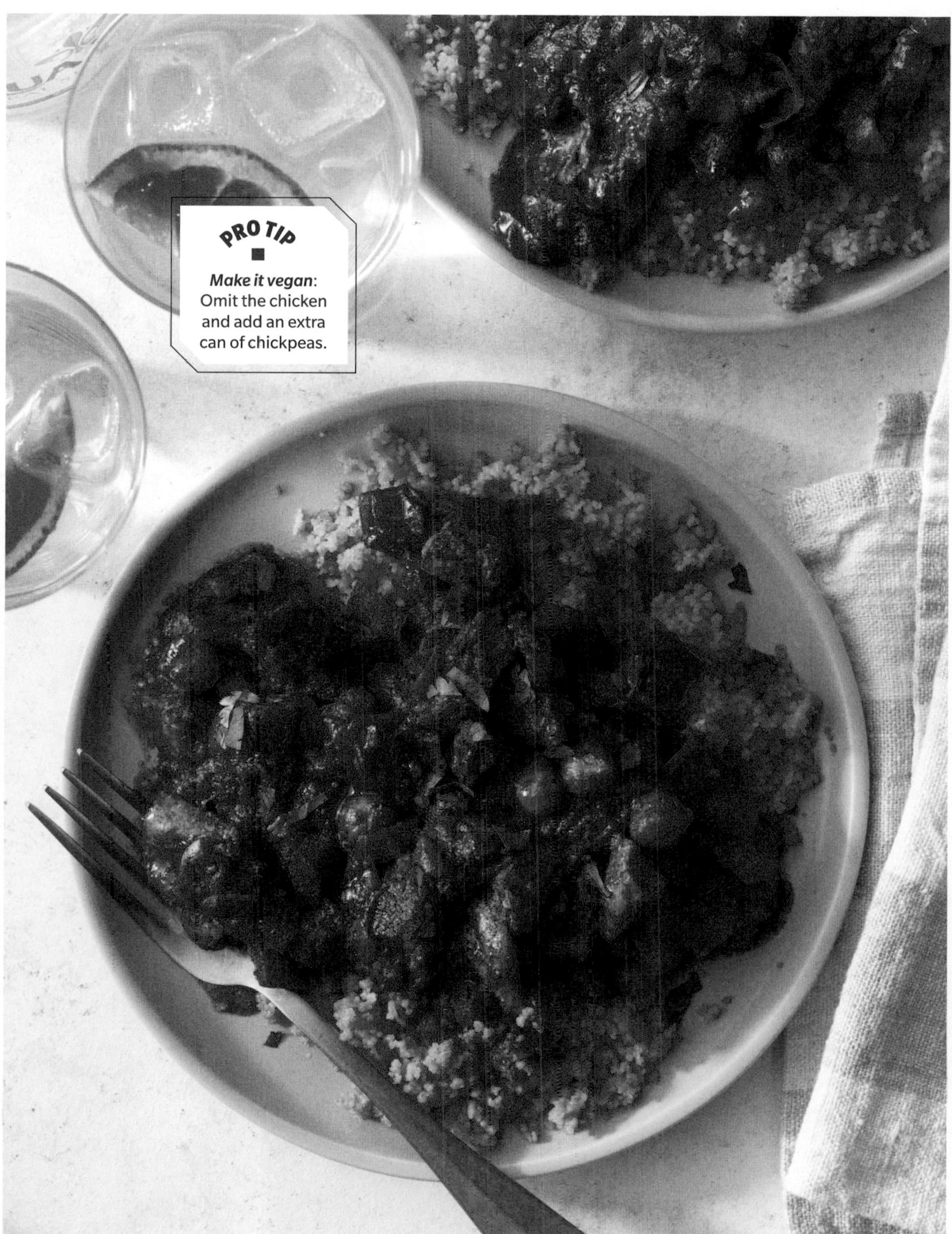
PRO TIP
Make it vegan: Omit the chicken and add an extra can of chickpeas.

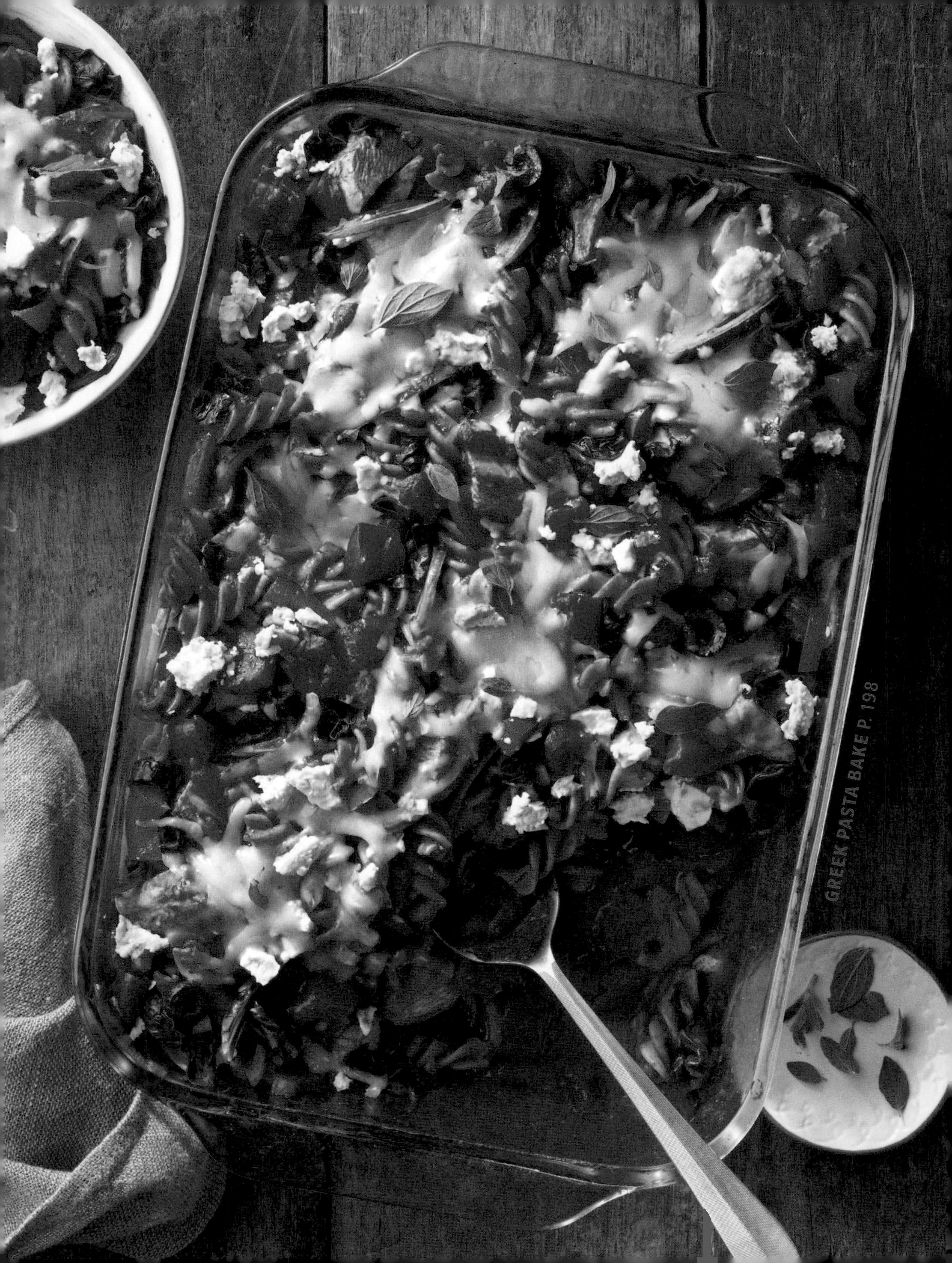

GREEK PASTA BAKE P. 198

CHAPTER 10

PASTA & NOODLES

BUTTERNUT & PORTOBELLO LASAGNA

PREP: 1 hour **BAKE:** 45 min. + standing **MAKES:** 12 servings

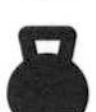

- 1 pkg. (10 oz.) frozen cubed butternut squash, thawed
- 2 tsp. olive oil
- 1 tsp. brown sugar
- ¼ tsp. salt
- ⅛ tsp. pepper

MUSHROOMS

- 4 large portobello mushrooms, coarsely chopped
- 2 tsp. balsamic vinegar
- 2 tsp. olive oil
- ¼ tsp. salt
- ⅛ tsp. pepper

SAUCE

- 2 cans (28 oz. each) whole tomatoes, undrained
- 2 tsp. olive oil
- 2 garlic cloves, minced
- 1 tsp. crushed red pepper flakes
- ½ cup fresh basil leaves, thinly sliced
- ¼ tsp. salt
- ⅛ tsp. pepper

LASAGNA

- 9 no-cook lasagna noodles
- 4 oz. fresh baby spinach (about 5 cups)
- 3 cups part-skim ricotta or vegan ricotta-style cheese
- 1½ cups shredded part-skim mozzarella or vegan mozzarella-style cheese

1 Preheat oven to 350°. In a bowl, combine the first 5 ingredients. In another bowl, combine the ingredients for mushrooms. Transfer to 2 separate foil-lined 15x10x1-in. baking pans. Roast 14-16 minutes or until tender.

2 Drain tomatoes, reserving juices; chop coarsely. In a large saucepan, heat oil over medium heat. Add the garlic and pepper flakes; cook 1 minute. Stir in the chopped tomatoes, reserved tomato juices, basil, salt and pepper. Simmer, uncovered, 35-45 minutes or until thickened.

3 Spread 1 cup sauce into a greased 13x9-in. baking dish. Layer with 3 noodles, 1 cup sauce, spinach and mushrooms. Top with 3 noodles, 1 cup sauce, the ricotta and the roasted squash. Add the remaining noodles and sauce. Sprinkle with mozzarella.

4 Cover; bake 30 minutes. Bake, uncovered, 15-20 minutes, until bubbly. Let stand 15 minutes.

1 PIECE *252 cal., 10g fat (5g sat. fat), 27mg chol., 508mg sod., 25g carb. (5g sugars, 4g fiber), 15g pro.* ***Diabetic exchanges:*** *2 starch, 1 medium-fat meat, ½ fat*

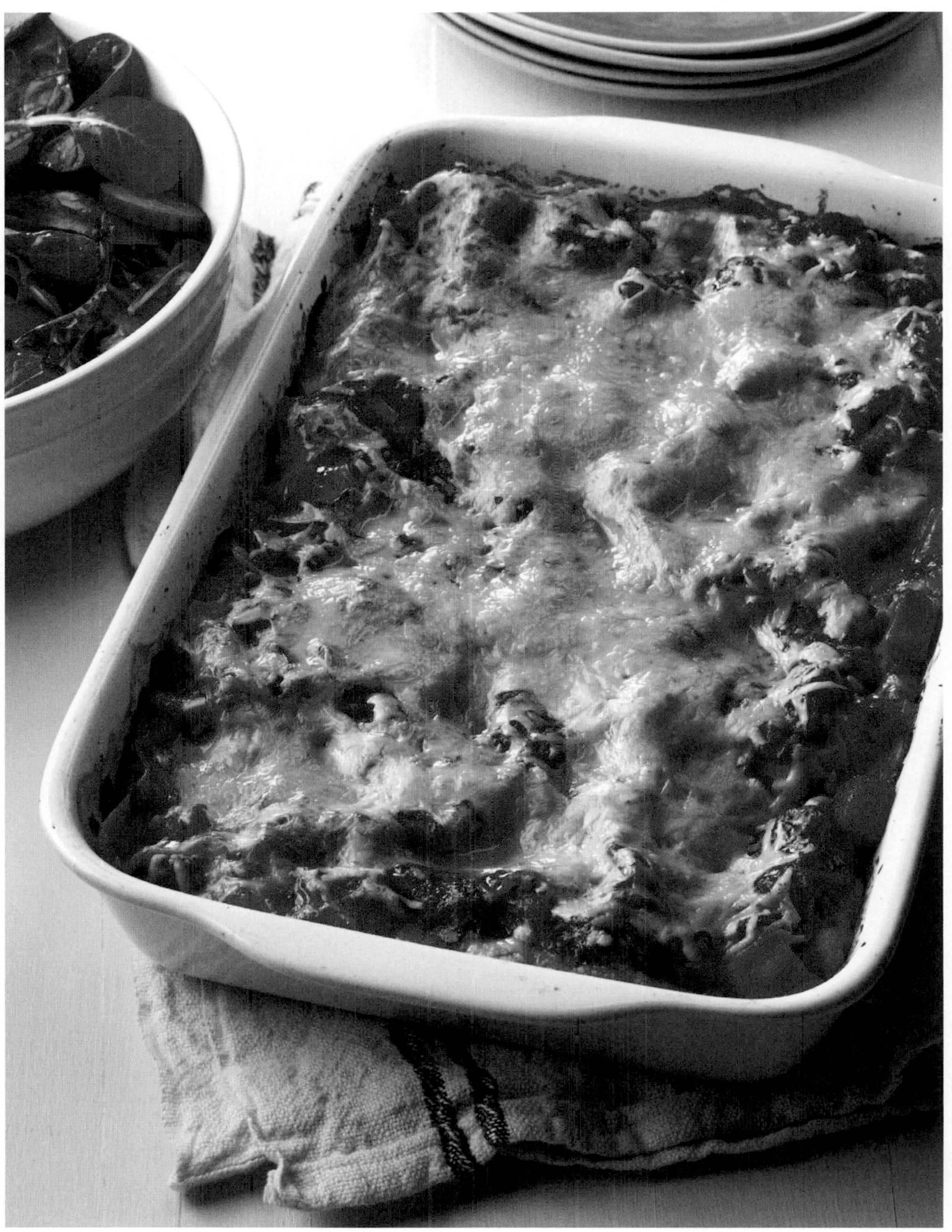

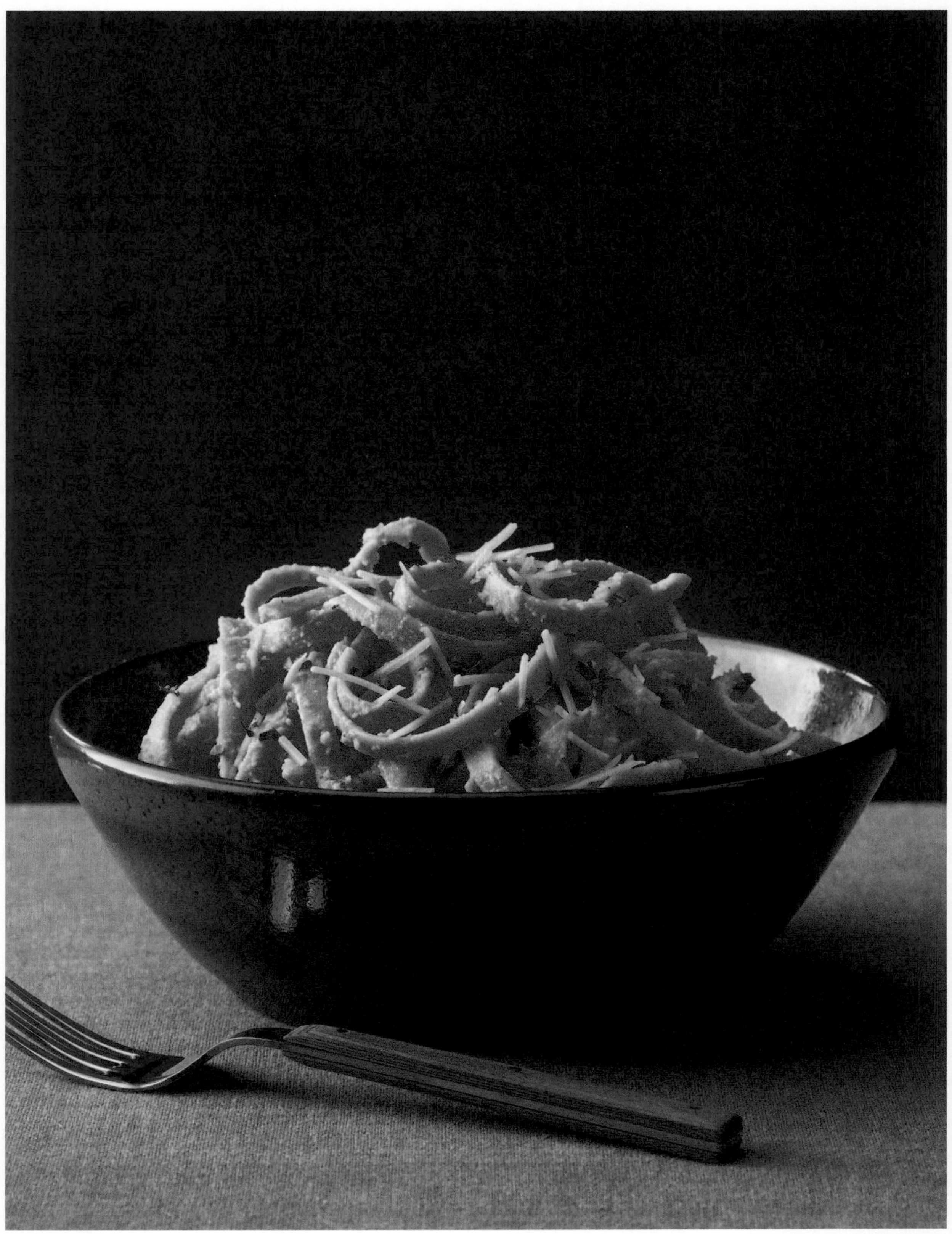

CAULIFLOWER ALFREDO

PREP: 20 min. **COOK:** 20 min. **MAKES:** 6 servings

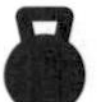

- 2 Tbsp. extra virgin olive oil
- 3 garlic cloves, minced
- 1 shallot, minced
- 1 medium head cauliflower, chopped
- 2 vegetable bouillon cubes
- ⅔ cup shredded vegan Parmesan-style cheese, plus additional for garnish
- ¼ tsp. crushed red pepper flakes
- 1 pkg. (16 oz.) fettuccine
- Chopped fresh parsley

1 In a Dutch oven, heat oil over medium-high heat. Add garlic and shallot; cook and stir until fragrant, 1-2 minutes. Add cauliflower, 4 cups water and bouillon; bring to a boil. Cook, covered, until tender, 5-6 minutes. Drain; cool slightly. Transfer to a food processor; add ⅔ cup Parmesan and the pepper flakes. Process until pureed smooth.

2 Meanwhile, cook fettuccine according to package directions for al dente. Drain fettuccine; place in a large bowl. Add cauliflower mixture; toss to coat. Sprinkle with parsley and additional Parmesan.

1⅓ CUPS *440 cal., 15g fat (1g sat. fat), 0 chol., 1100mg sod., 65g carb. (5g sugars, 5g fiber), 18g pro.*

GREEK PASTA BAKE

PREP: 20 min. **BAKE:** 25 min. **MAKES:** 8 servings

- 3⅓ cups uncooked whole grain spiral or penne pasta

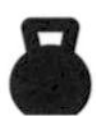
- 4 cups cubed cooked chicken breast
- 1 can (29 oz.) tomato sauce
- 1 can (14½ oz.) no-salt-added diced tomatoes, drained
- 1 pkg. (10 oz.) frozen chopped spinach, thawed and squeezed dry
- 2 cans (2¼ oz. each) sliced ripe olives, drained
- ¼ cup thinly sliced red onion
- ¼ cup chopped green pepper
- 1 tsp. dried basil
- 1 tsp. dried oregano
- 1 cup shredded mozzarella or vegan mozzarella-style cheese
- ½ cup crumbled feta or vegan feta-style cheese
- Optional toppings: Chopped fresh oregano or fresh basil

1 Preheat oven to 400°. Cook pasta according to the package directions; drain. In a large bowl, combine pasta, chicken, tomato sauce, tomatoes, spinach, ripe olives, onion, green pepper, basil and oregano.

2 Transfer to a 13x9-in. baking dish coated with cooking spray. Sprinkle with cheeses. Bake, uncovered, until heated through and the cheese is melted, about 25 minutes. If desired, sprinkle with oregano or basil.

TO FREEZE Cool unbaked casserole; cover and freeze. To use, partially thaw in refrigerator overnight. Remove from the refrigerator 30 minutes before baking. Preheat oven to 400°. Bake the casserole as directed, increasing time as necessary to heat through and for a thermometer inserted in center to read 165°.

1½ CUPS *398 cal., 10g fat (3g sat. fat), 67mg chol., 832mg sod., 47g carb. (5g sugars, 9g fiber), 34g pro.* ***Diabetic exchanges:*** *3 very lean meat, 3 lean meat, 2½ starch, 1 vegetable, ½ fat*

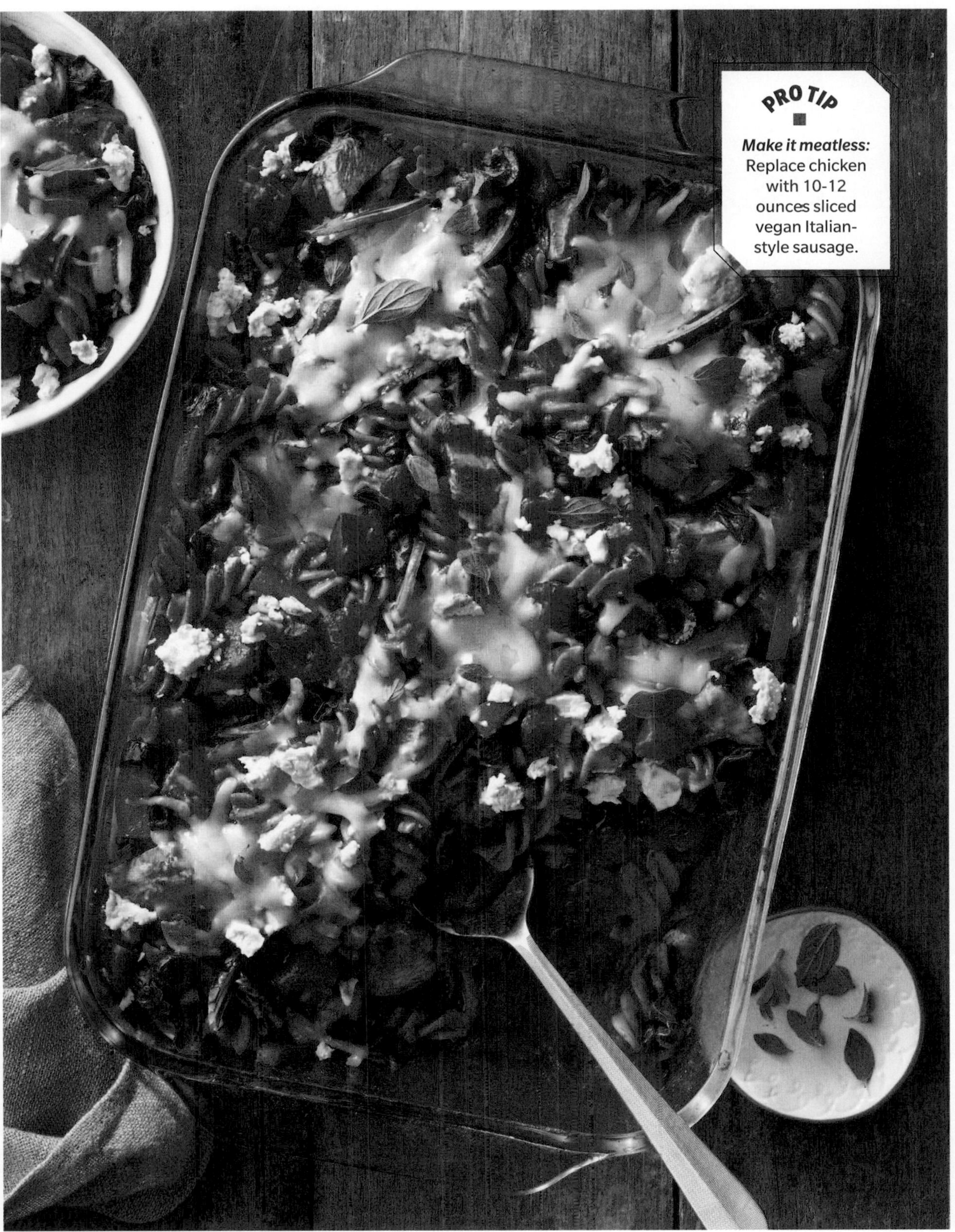

PRO TIP

Make it meatless: Replace chicken with 10-12 ounces sliced vegan Italian-style sausage.

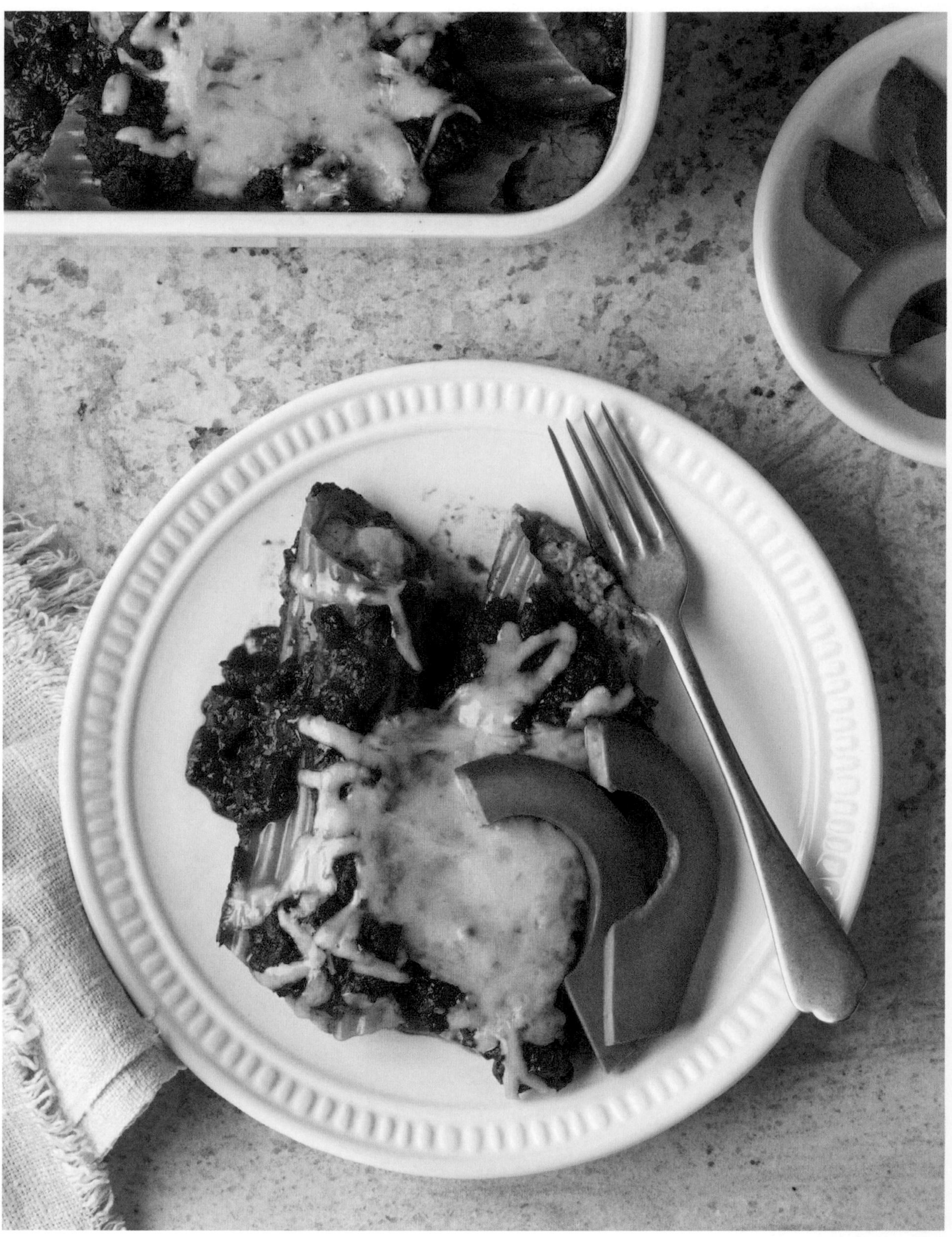

CREAMY AVOCADO MANICOTTI

PREP: 25 min. **BAKE:** 45 min. **MAKES:** 7 servings

- 1 pkg. (8 oz.) manicotti shells
- 1 small onion, finely chopped
- 1 Tbsp. olive oil
- 2 garlic cloves, minced
- 1 can (28 oz.) crushed tomatoes
- ½ cup minced fresh basil or 3 Tbsp. dried basil
- ⅓ cup dry red wine or vegetable broth
- 1 Tbsp. brown sugar
- ½ tsp. salt
- ½ tsp. pepper

FILLING

- 1 container (15 oz.) reduced-fat ricotta or vegan ricotta-style cheese
- 1 medium ripe avocado, peeled and mashed
- ½ cup grated Parmesan or vegan Parmesan-style cheese
- ¼ tsp. salt
- ¼ tsp. pepper
- 1 cup shredded part-skim mozzarella or vegan mozzarella-style cheese
- 1 medium ripe avocado, sliced, optional

1 Cook manicotti according to package directions. Meanwhile, in a large skillet, saute onion in oil until tender. Add garlic; cook 1 minute longer. Stir in tomatoes, basil, wine, brown sugar, salt and pepper. Bring to a boil. Reduce heat; simmer, uncovered, for 10-15 minutes, stirring occasionally.

2 Drain manicotti. In a small bowl, combine ricotta cheese, avocado, Parmesan cheese, salt and pepper. Stuff the cheese mixture into manicotti shells. Spread 1 cup sauce into a greased 13x9-in. baking dish. Arrange manicotti over sauce. Pour remaining sauce over top.

3 Cover; bake at 350° until bubbly, 35 minutes. Uncover; sprinkle with mozzarella cheese. Bake 10-15 minutes longer or until cheese is melted. If desired, garnish with avocado slices.

2 PIECES *359 cal., 13g fat (5g sat. fat), 29mg chol., 625mg sod., 41g carb. (7g sugars, 5g fiber), 18g pro.* ***Diabetic exchanges:*** *2 starch, 2 vegetable, 2 medium-fat meat, 1 fat*

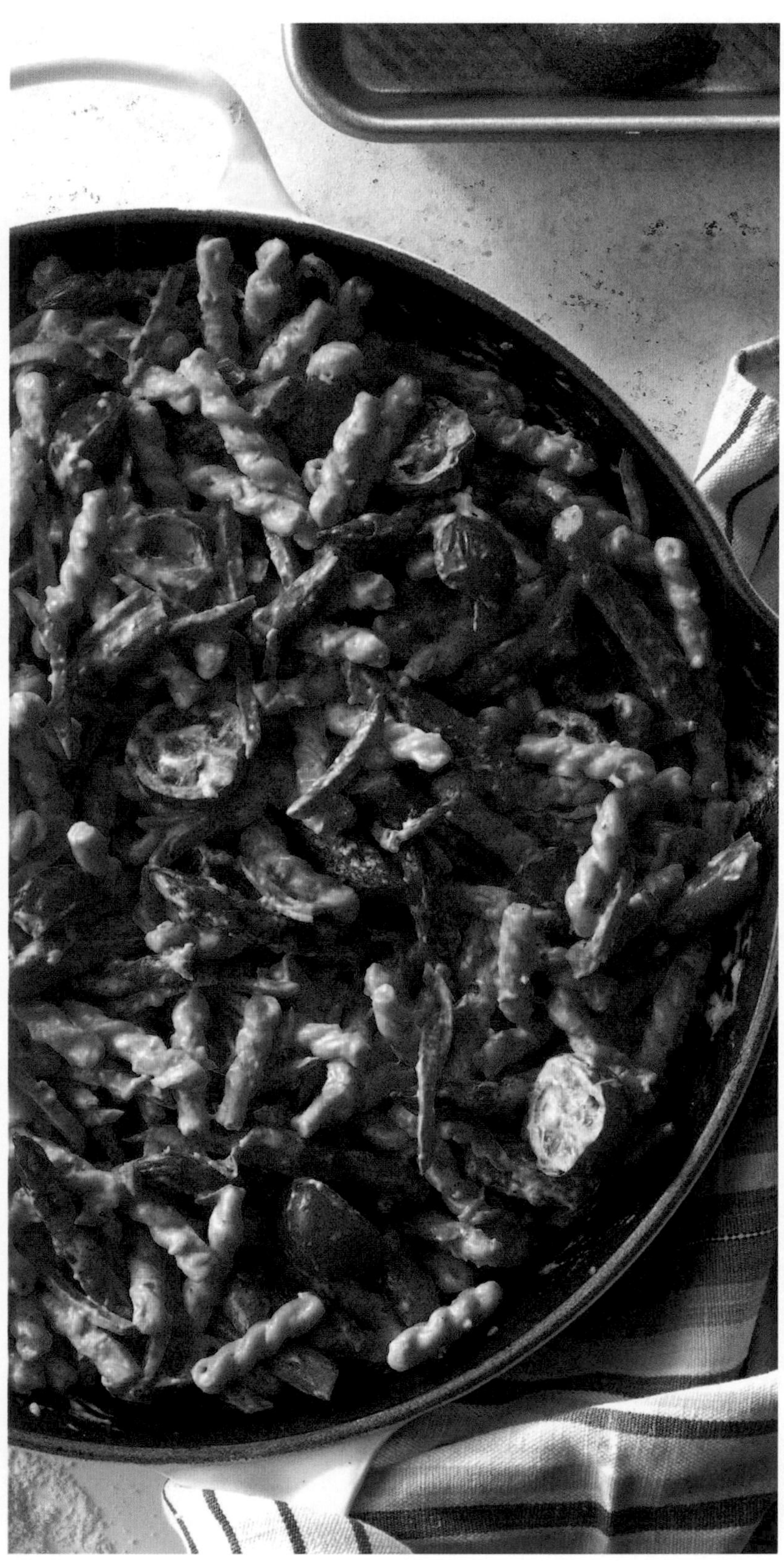

CREAMY PASTA PRIMAVERA

TAKES: 30 min.
MAKES: 6 servings

- 2 cups uncooked gemelli or spiral pasta
- 1 lb. fresh asparagus, trimmed and cut into 2-in. pieces
- 3 medium carrots, shredded
- 2 tsp. canola oil
- 2 cups cherry tomatoes, halved
- 1 garlic clove, minced
- ½ cup grated Parmesan or vegan Parmesan-style cheese
- ½ cup dairy or vegan heavy whipping cream
- ¼ tsp. pepper

1 Cook pasta according to package directions. In a large skillet over medium-high heat, saute asparagus and carrots in oil until crisp-tender. Add tomatoes and garlic; cook 1 minute longer.

2 Stir in the cheese, cream and pepper. Drain pasta; toss with asparagus mixture.

1⅓ CUPS *275 cal., 12g fat (6g sat. fat), 33mg chol., 141mg sod., 35g carb. (5g sugars, 3g fiber), 10g pro.* ***Diabetic exchanges:*** *2 starch, 2 fat, 1 vegetable.*

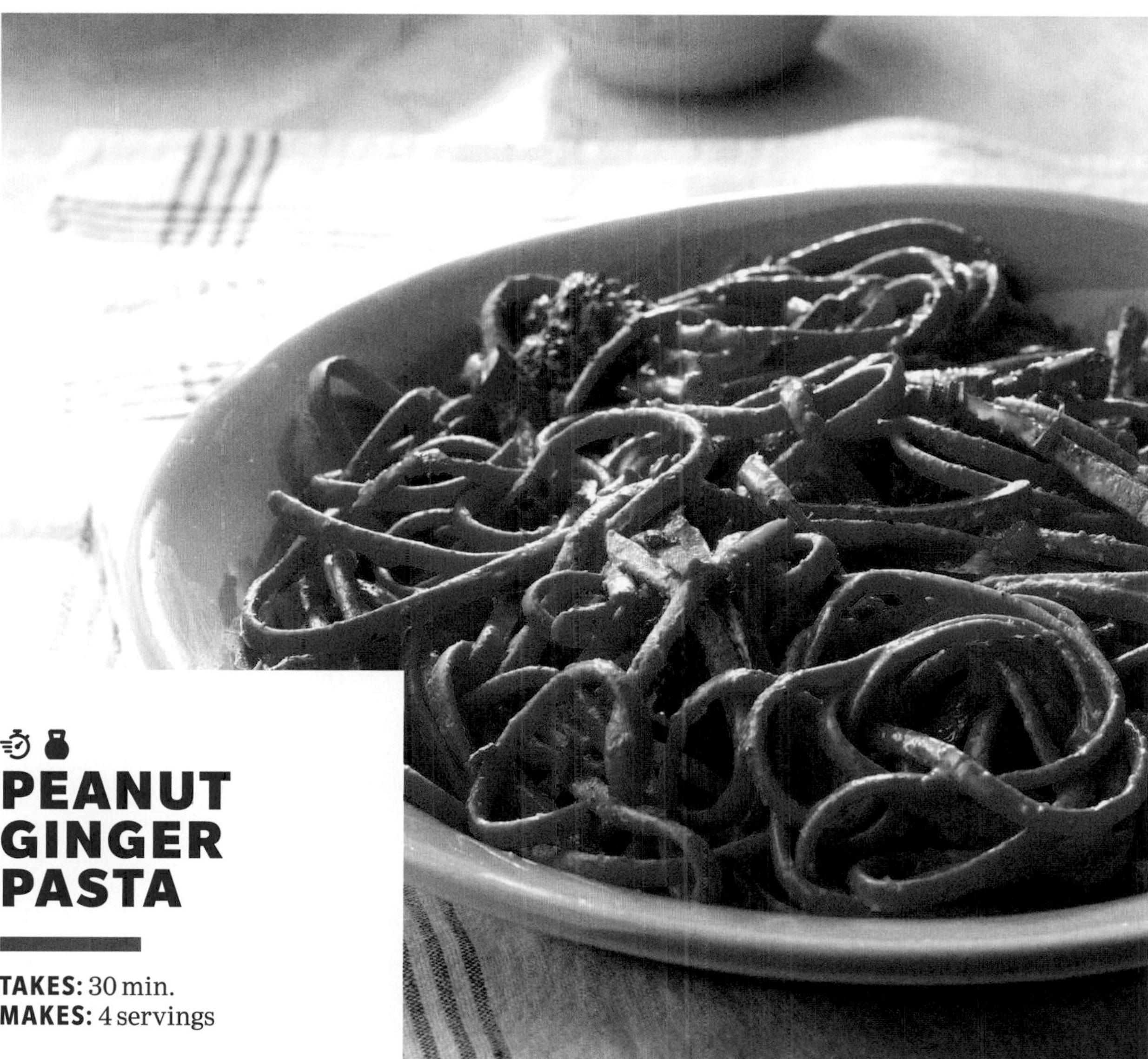

PEANUT GINGER PASTA

TAKES: 30 min.
MAKES: 4 servings

2½ tsp. grated lime zest
¼ cup lime juice
2 Tbsp. reduced-sodium soy sauce
2 tsp. water
1 tsp. sesame oil
⅓ cup creamy peanut butter
2½ tsp. minced fresh gingerroot
2 garlic cloves, minced
¼ tsp. salt
¼ tsp. pepper
8 oz. uncooked whole wheat linguine
2 cups small fresh broccoli florets
2 medium carrots, grated
1 medium sweet red pepper, julienned
2 green onions, chopped
2 Tbsp. minced fresh basil

1 Place the first 10 ingredients in a blender; cover and process until blended. Cook linguine according to the package directions, adding broccoli during the last 5 minutes of cooking; drain.

2 Transfer linguine and broccoli to a large bowl. Add remaining ingredients. Add peanut butter mixture and toss to combine.

2 CUPS *365 cal., 13g fat (2g sat. fat), 0 chol., 567mg sod., 57g carb. (6g sugars, 10g fiber), 14g pro.*

CURRIED SQUASH & SAUSAGE

PREP: 15 min. **COOK:** 20 min. **MAKES:** 8 servings

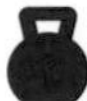

- 1 lb. mild bulk Italian sausage or frozen vegan Italian sausage-style crumbles
- 1 Tbsp. olive oil
- 1 medium onion, chopped
- 1 medium green pepper, chopped
- 1 large acorn squash or 6 cups butternut squash, seeded, peeled and cubed (½ in.)
- 1 large unpeeled apple, cubed (½ in.)
- 2 to 3 tsp. curry powder
- 1 tsp. salt
- 3 cups cooked small pasta shells
- ¼ cup water

1 In a stockpot, cook and crumble sausage over medium heat until no longer pink, 5-6 minutes; remove from pan.

2 In same pan, heat oil; cook and stir onion and pepper 3 minutes. Add squash; cook 5 minutes. Stir in apple, curry powder and salt until vegetables are crisp-tender, 3-4 minutes.

3 Return sausage to pan; add pasta and water. Heat through.

1⅓ CUPS *385 cal., 18g fat (5g sat. fat), 38mg chol., 735mg sod., 44g carb. (7g sugars, 4g fiber), 14g pro.*

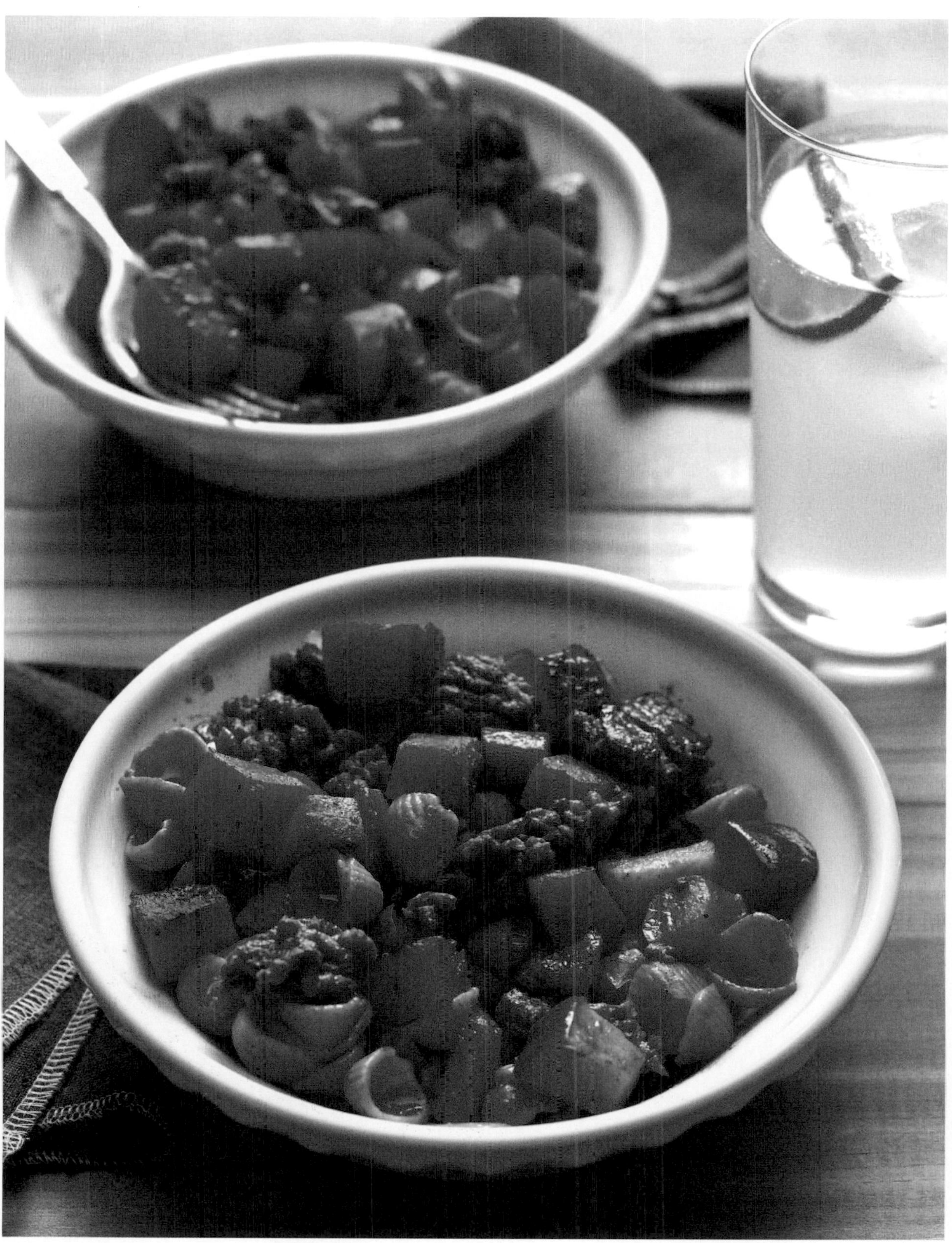

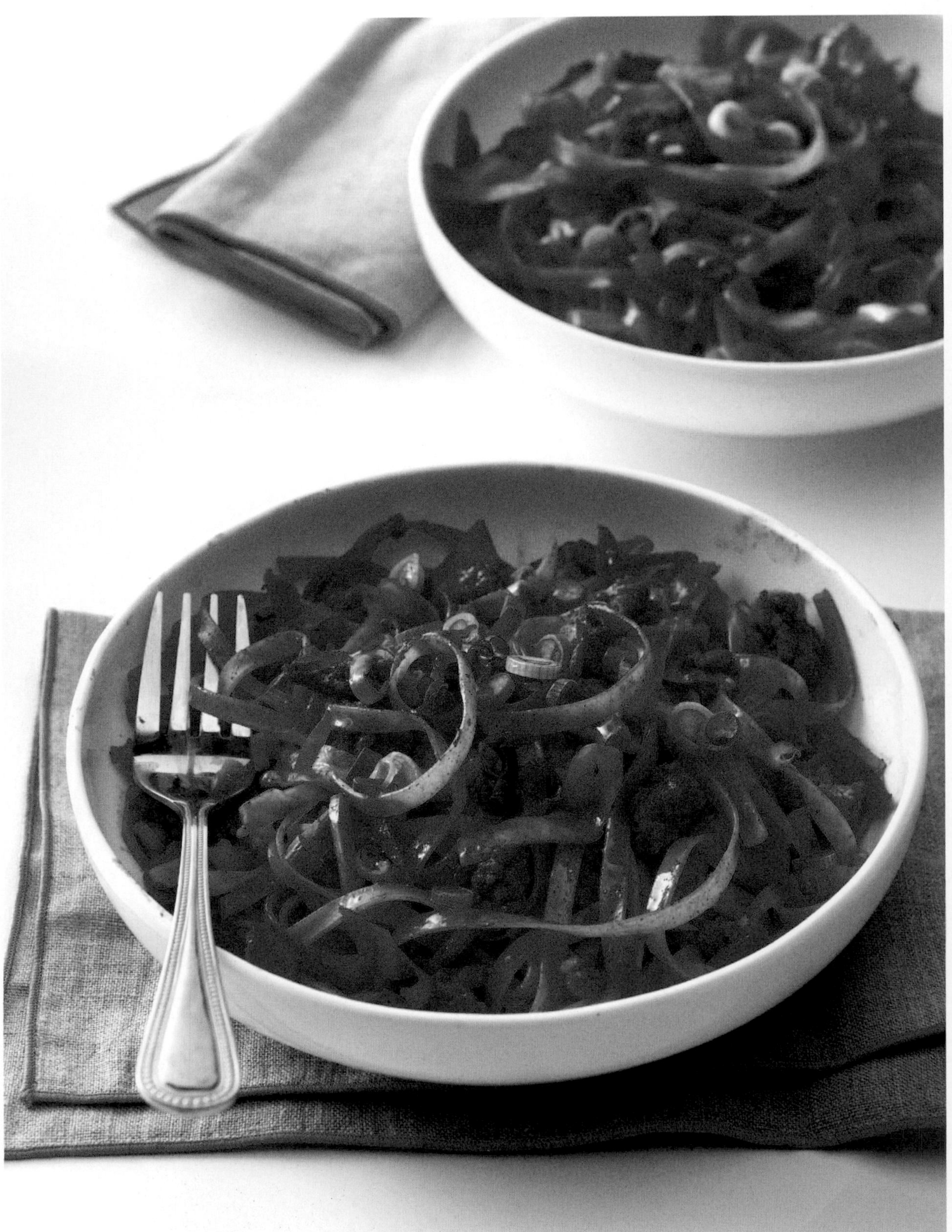

EGG ROLL NOODLES

TAKES: 30 min. **MAKES:** 4 servings

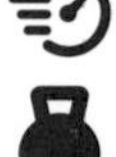

- 1 Tbsp. sesame oil
- ½ lb. ground pork or frozen vegetarian meat crumbles
- 1 Tbsp. soy sauce
- 1 garlic clove, minced
- 1 tsp. ground ginger
- ½ tsp. salt
- ¼ tsp. ground turmeric
- ¼ tsp. pepper
- 6 cups shredded cabbage (about 1 small head)
- 2 large carrots, shredded (about 2 cups)
- 4 oz. rice noodles
- 3 green onions, thinly sliced

1 In a large cast-iron or other heavy skillet, heat oil over medium-high heat; cook and crumble pork until browned, 4-6 minutes. Stir in soy sauce, garlic and seasonings. Add cabbage and carrots; cook until vegetables are tender, stirring occasionally, 4-6 minutes longer.

2 Cook rice noodles according to package directions; drain and immediately add to pork mixture, tossing to combine. Sprinkle with green onions.

1½ CUPS: *302 cal., 12g fat (4g sat. fat), 38mg chol., 652mg sod., 33g carb. (2g sugars, 4g fiber), 14g pro.* ***Diabetic exchanges:*** *2 vegetable, 2 medium-fat meat, 1½ starch, ½ fat*

HARVEST BOW TIES

PREP: 25 min. **COOK:** 15 min. **MAKES:** 8 servings

- 1 small spaghetti squash (about 1½ lbs.)
- 12 oz. uncooked bow tie pasta (about 4½ cups)
- 2 Tbsp. olive oil
- 1 lb. sliced fresh mushrooms
- 1 cup chopped sweet onion
- 2 garlic cloves, minced
- 1 can (14½ oz.) diced tomatoes, undrained
- 6 oz. fresh baby spinach (about 8 cups)
- ¾ tsp. salt
- ½ tsp. pepper
- 2 Tbsp. vegan butter
- 2 Tbsp. vegan sour cream

1 Halve squash lengthwise; discard seeds. Place squash on a microwave-safe plate, cut side down. Microwave, uncovered, on high until tender, 9-11 minutes. Cool slightly. Meanwhile, in a 6-qt. Dutch oven or stockpot, cook pasta according to package directions. Drain; return to pot.

2 In a large skillet, heat oil over medium-high heat; saute mushrooms and onion until tender. Add garlic; cook and stir 1 minute. Separate strands of squash with a fork; add to skillet. Stir in tomatoes, spinach, salt and pepper; cook until spinach is wilted, stirring occasionally. Stir in butter and sour cream until blended.

3 Add to pasta. Heat through, tossing to coat.

1½ CUPS *279 cal., 9g fat (2g sat. fat), 0 chol., 364mg sod., 44g carb. (5g sugars, 5g fiber), 9g pro.*

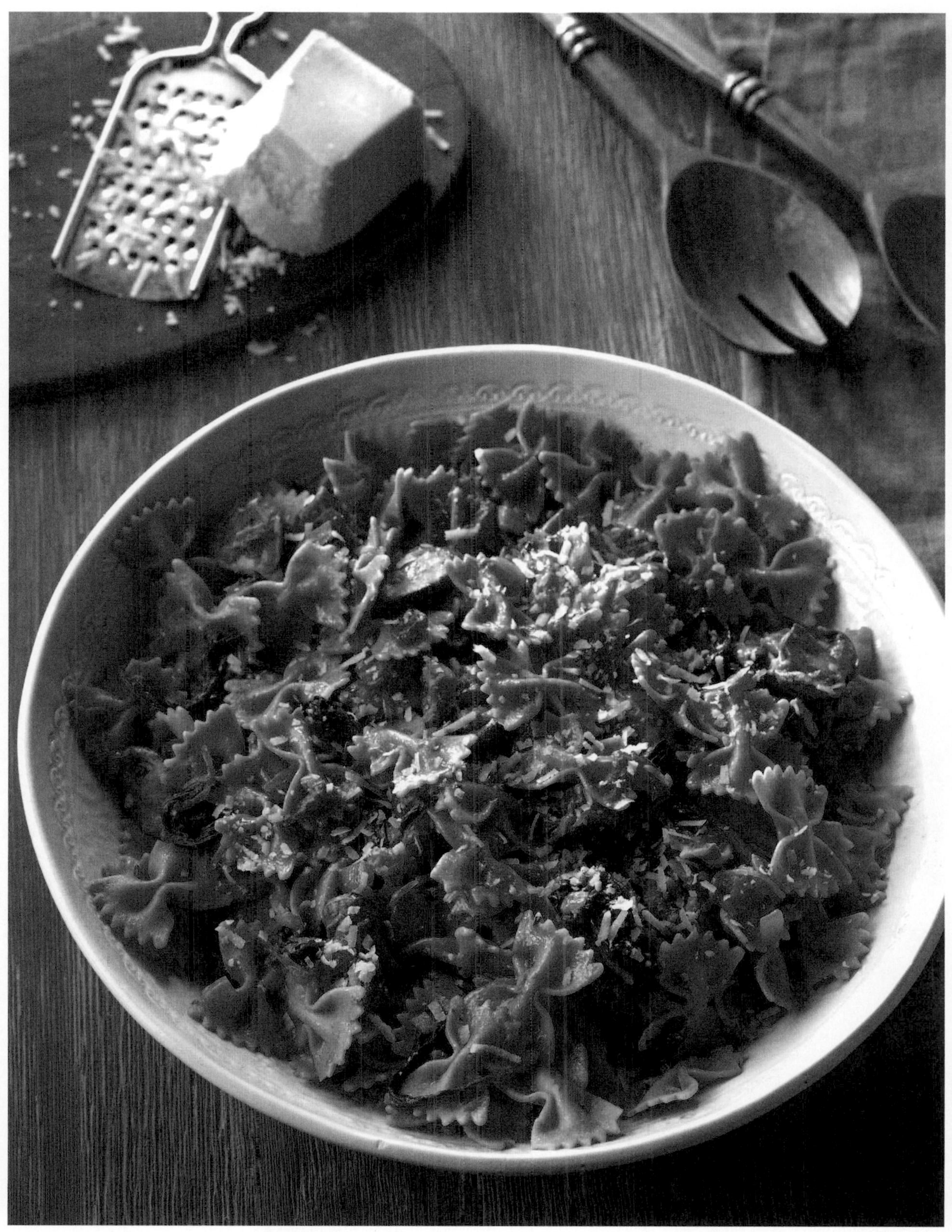

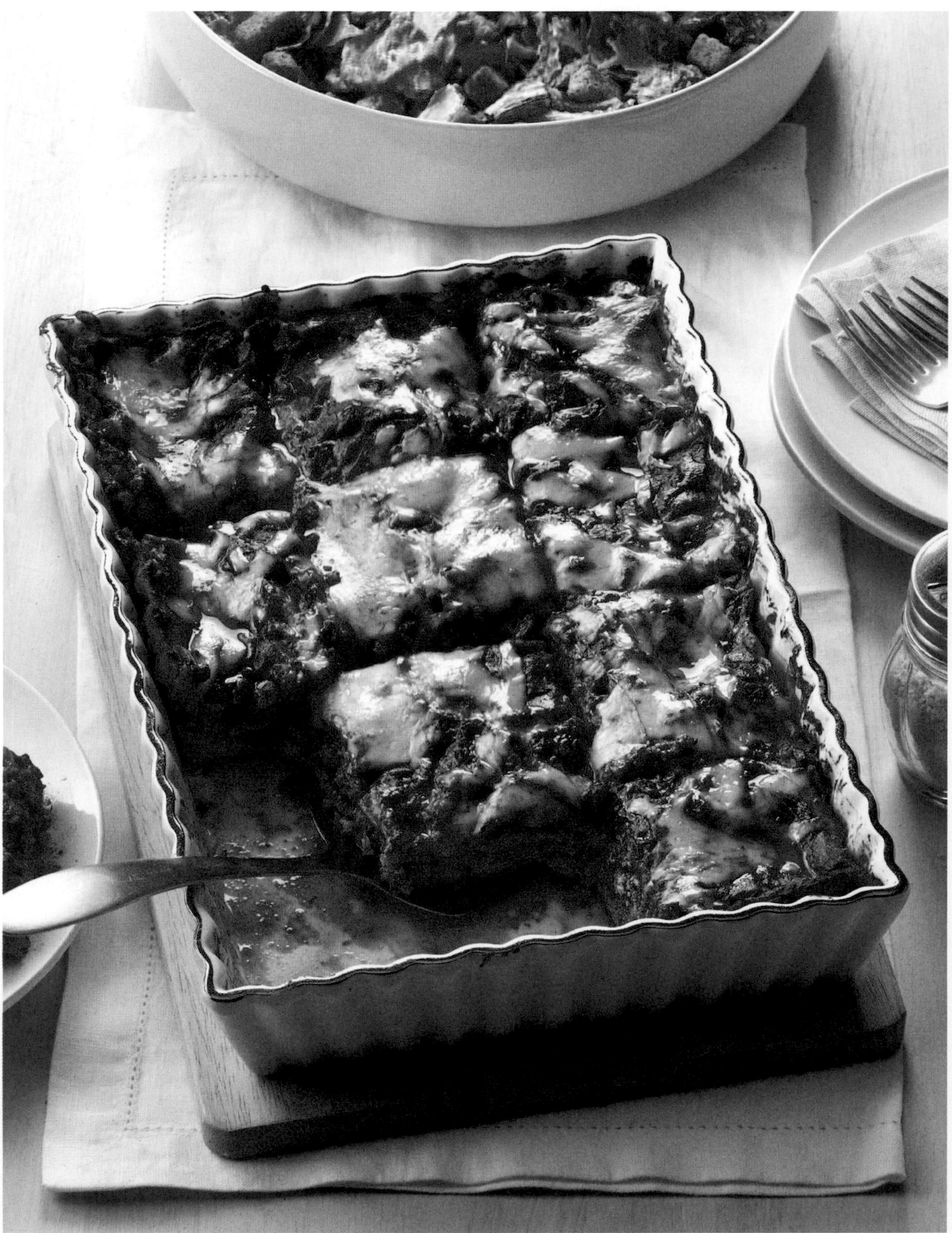

MUSHROOM LASAGNA

PREP: 30 min. **BAKE:** 45 min. + standing **MAKES:** 12 servings

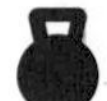

- 10 uncooked whole wheat lasagna noodles
- 1½ cups sliced fresh mushrooms
- ¼ cup chopped onion
- 2 garlic cloves, minced
- 1 can (14½ oz.) Italian diced tomatoes, undrained
- 1 can (12 oz.) tomato paste
- 1 pkg. (14 oz.) firm tofu, drained and cubed
- 2 large eggs, lightly beaten, or vegan liquid egg substitute
- 3 cups 2% cottage or vegan cottage-style cheese
- ½ cup grated Parmesan or vegan Parmesan-style cheese
- ½ cup packed fresh parsley leaves
- ½ tsp. pepper
- 2 cups shredded part-skim mozzarella or vegan mozzarella-style cheese, divided

1 Preheat oven to 375°. Cook the noodles according to the package directions for al dente. Meanwhile, in a large saucepan, cook mushrooms and onion over medium heat until tender. Add garlic; cook 1 minute. Add tomatoes and tomato paste; cook and stir until heated through.

2 Pulse tofu in a food processor until smooth. Add the next 5 ingredients; pulse until combined. Drain noodles.

3 Place 5 noodles into a 13x9-in. baking dish coated with cooking spray, overlapping as needed. Layer with half the tofu mixture, half the sauce and half the mozzarella. Top with remaining noodles, tofu mixture and sauce.

4 Bake, covered, 35 minutes. Sprinkle with the remaining mozzarella. Bake, uncovered, until the cheese is melted, 10-15 minutes. Let stand 10 minutes before serving.

1 PIECE *258 cal., 9g fat (4g sat. fat), 48mg chol., 498mg sod., 26g carb. (9g sugars, 3g fiber), 19g pro.* ***Diabetic exchanges:*** *2 medium-fat meat, 1½ starch*

STUFFED SHELLS WITH BROCCOLI

PREP: 20 min. **BAKE:** 30 min. **MAKES:** 8 servings

- 24 uncooked jumbo pasta shells
- 1 carton (15 oz.) part-skim ricotta or vegan ricotta-style cheese
- 3 cups frozen chopped broccoli, thawed and drained
- 1 cup shredded part-skim mozzarella or vegan mozzarella-style cheese
- 2 large egg whites or vegan liquid egg substitute
- 1 Tbsp. minced fresh basil or 1 tsp. dried basil
- ½ tsp. garlic salt
- ¼ tsp. pepper
- 1 jar (26 oz.) meatless spaghetti sauce
- 2 Tbsp. shredded Parmesan or vegan Parmesan-style cheese

1 Cook pasta according to package directions. In a large bowl, combine ricotta, broccoli, mozzarella, egg whites and seasonings. Drain pasta and rinse in cold water.

2 Spread half the spaghetti sauce into a 13x9-in. baking dish coated with cooking spray. Stuff pasta shells with ricotta mixture; arrange over spaghetti sauce. Pour remaining sauce over pasta shells.

3 Cover and bake at 375° for 25 minutes. Uncover; sprinkle with Parmesan cheese. Bake until heated through, about 5 minutes longer.

3 STUFFED SHELLS *279 cal., 8g fat (5g sat. fat), 26mg chol., 725mg sod., 36g carb. (8g sugars, 4g fiber), 18g pro.* ***Diabetic exchanges:*** *2½ starch, 2 lean meat*

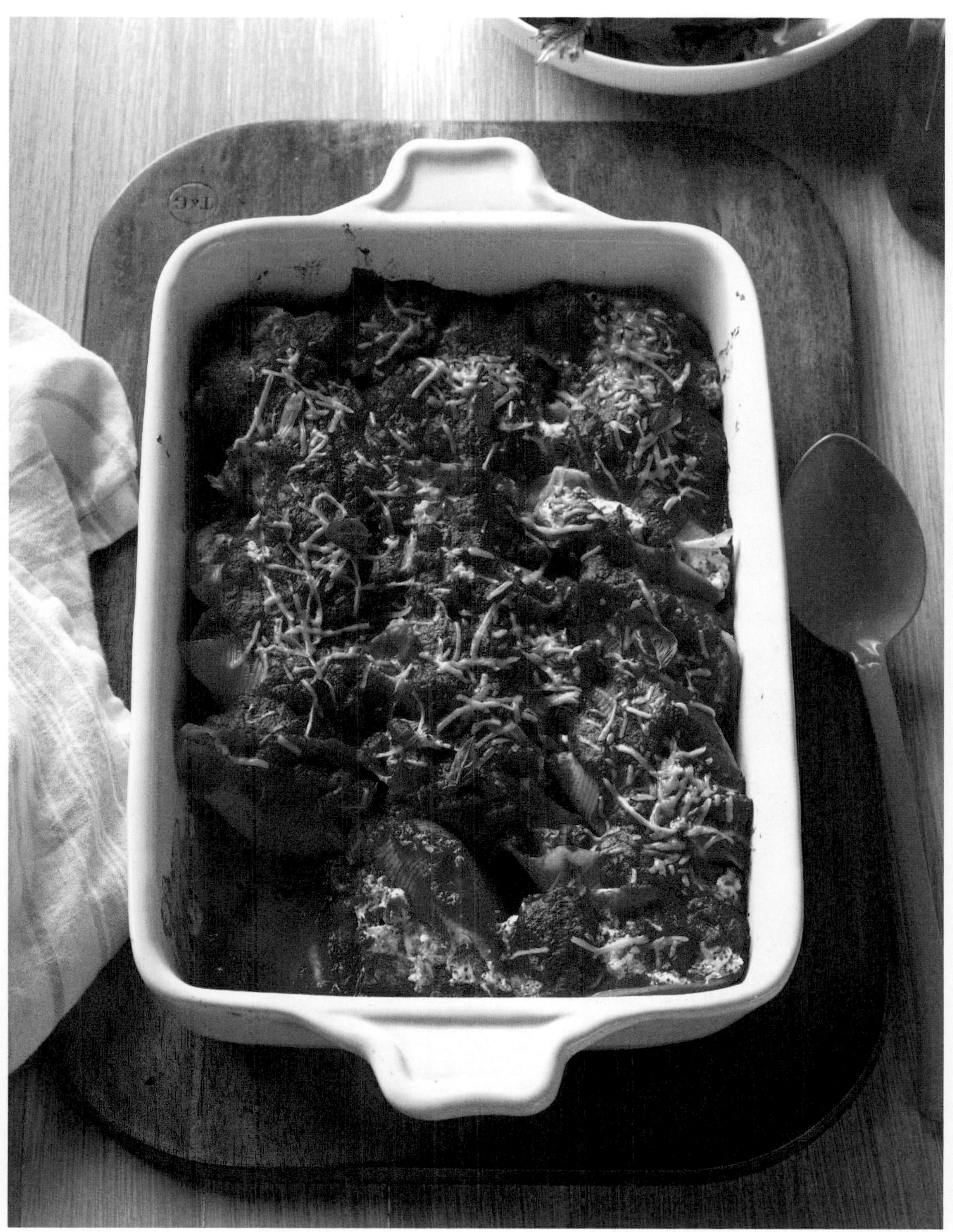

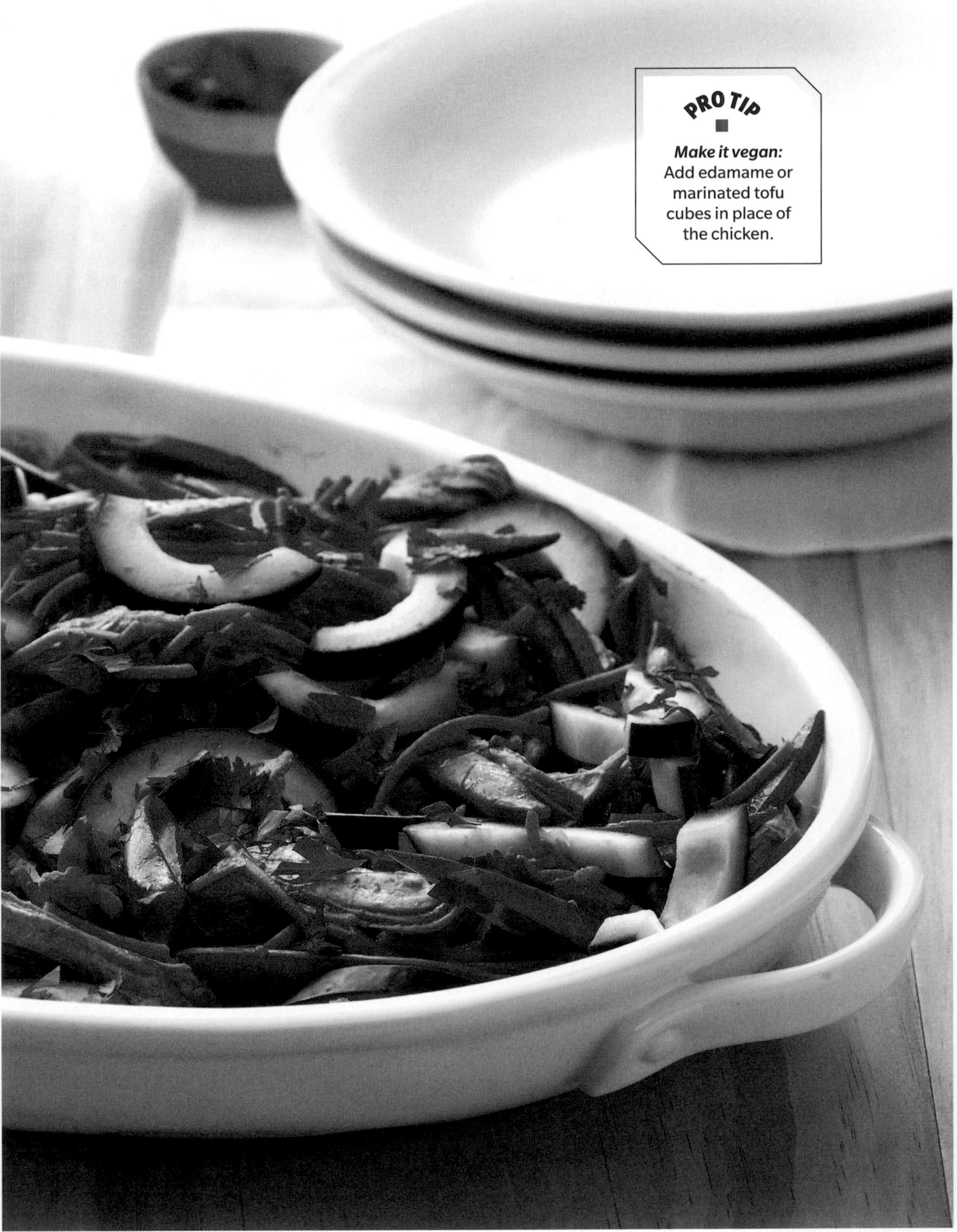

PRO TIP

Make it vegan: Add edamame or marinated tofu cubes in place of the chicken.

THAI CHICKEN PASTA SKILLET

TAKES: 30 min. **MAKES:** 6 servings

- 6 oz. uncooked whole wheat spaghetti
- 2 tsp. canola oil
- 1 pkg. (10 oz.) fresh sugar snap peas, trimmed and cut diagonally into thin strips
- 2 cups julienned carrots (about 8 oz.)
- 2 cups shredded cooked chicken
- 1 cup Thai peanut sauce
- 1 medium cucumber, halved lengthwise, seeded and sliced diagonally
- Chopped fresh cilantro, optional

1 Cook spaghetti according to package directions; drain.

2 Meanwhile, in a large skillet, heat the oil over medium-high heat. Add snap peas and carrots; stir-fry 6-8 minutes or until crisp-tender. Add the chicken, peanut sauce and spaghetti; heat through, tossing to combine.

3 Transfer to a serving plate. Top with the cucumber and, if desired, cilantro.

1⅓ CUPS *403 cal., 15g fat (3g sat. fat), 42mg chol., 432mg sod., 43g carb. (15g sugars, 6g fiber), 25g pro.* ***Diabetic exchanges:*** *3 lean meat, 2½ starch, 2 fat, 1 vegetable*

TOFU CHOW MEIN

PREP: 15 min. + standing **COOK:** 15 min. **MAKES:** 4 servings

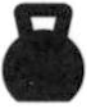

- 8 oz. uncooked whole wheat angel hair pasta
- 3 Tbsp. sesame oil, divided
- 1 pkg. (16 oz.) extra-firm tofu
- 2 cups sliced fresh mushrooms
- 1 medium sweet red pepper, julienned
- ¼ cup reduced-sodium soy sauce
- 3 green onions, thinly sliced

1 Cook pasta according to the package directions. Drain; rinse with cold water and drain again. Toss with 1 Tbsp. oil; spread onto a baking sheet and let stand about 1 hour.

2 Meanwhile, cut tofu into ½-in. cubes and blot dry. Wrap in a clean kitchen towel; place on a plate and refrigerate until ready to cook.

3 In a large skillet, heat 1 Tbsp. oil over medium heat. Add pasta, spreading evenly; cook until bottom is lightly browned, about 5 minutes. Remove from pan.

4 In same skillet, heat remaining oil over medium-high heat; stir-fry mushrooms, pepper and tofu until mushrooms are tender, 3-4 minutes. Add pasta and soy sauce; toss and heat through. Sprinkle with green onions.

1½ CUPS *417 cal., 17g fat (2g sat. fat), 0 chol., 588mg sod., 48g carb. (3g sugars, 8g fiber), 21g pro.* ***Diabetic exchanges:*** *3 fat, 2½ starch, 2 lean meat, 1 vegetable*

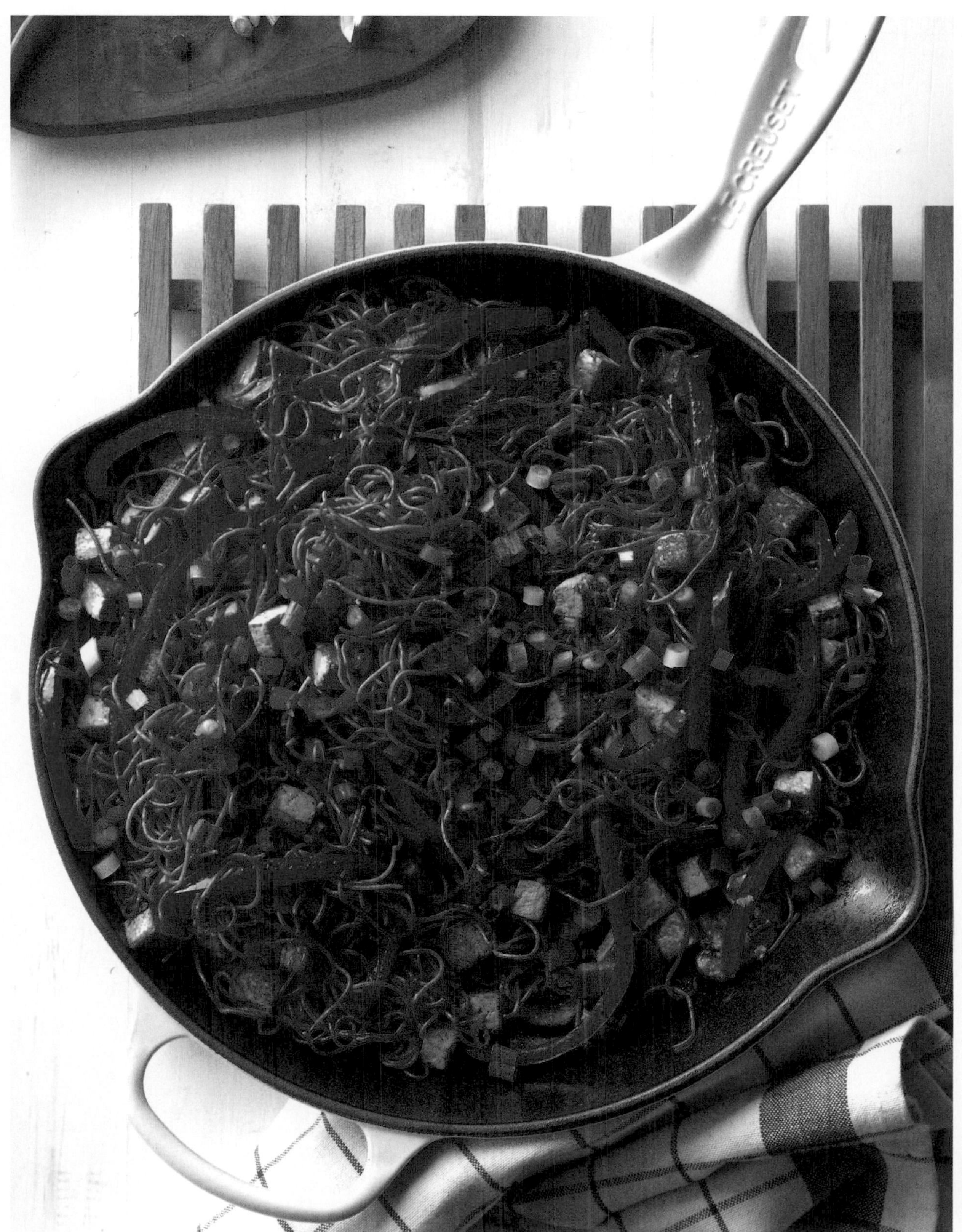
LE CREUSET

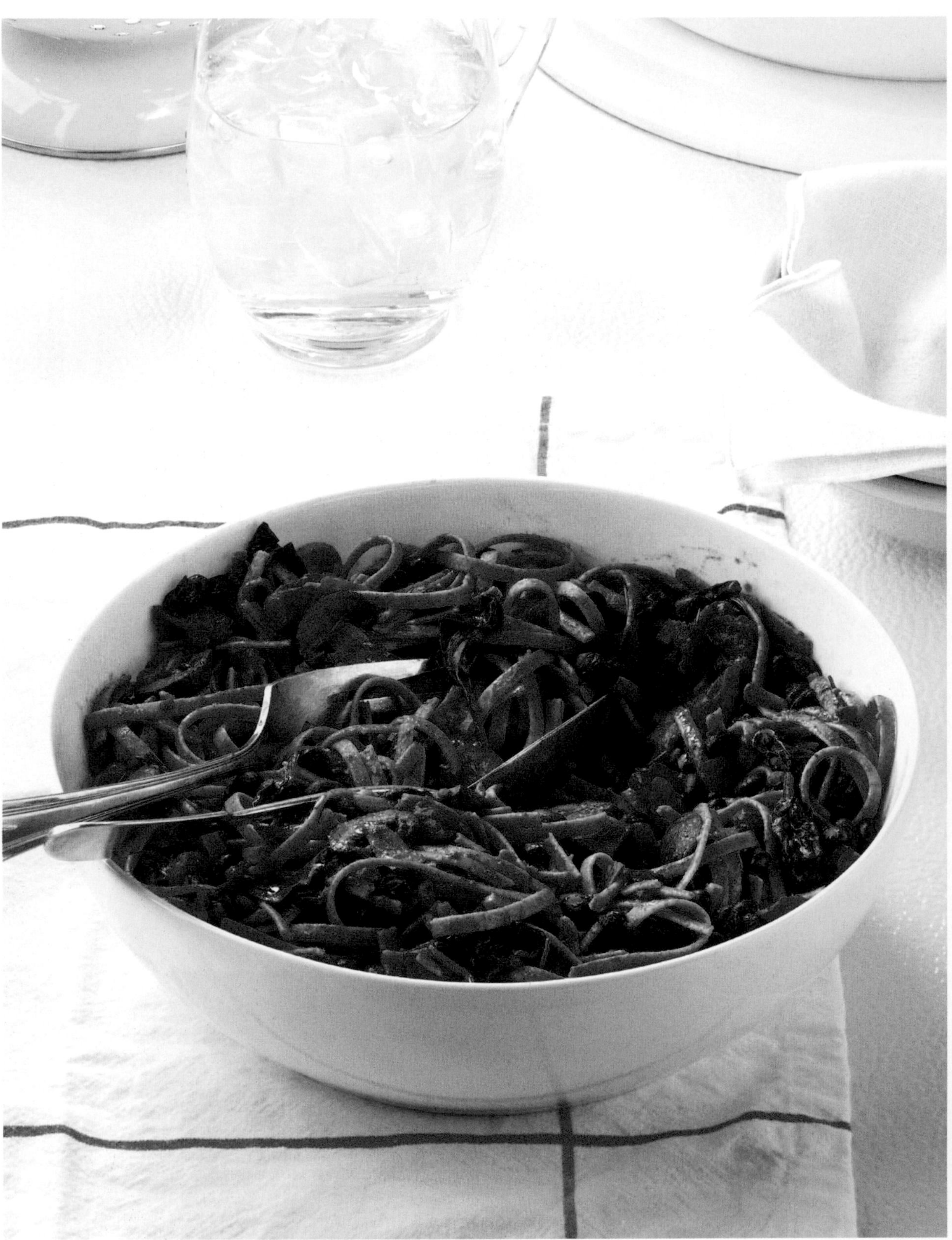

BLACK BEAN PASTA

TAKES: 25 min. **MAKES:** 6 servings

- 9 oz. uncooked whole wheat fettuccine
- 1 Tbsp. olive oil
- 1¾ cups sliced baby portobello mushrooms
- 1 garlic clove, minced
- 1 can (15 oz.) black beans, rinsed and drained
- 1 can (14½ oz.) diced tomatoes, undrained
- 1 tsp. dried rosemary, crushed
- ½ tsp. dried oregano
- 2 cups fresh baby spinach

1 Cook fettuccine according to package directions. Meanwhile, in a large skillet, heat oil over medium-high heat. Add the mushrooms; cook and stir 4-6 minutes or until tender. Add garlic; cook 1 minute longer.

2 Stir in black beans, tomatoes, rosemary and oregano; heat through. Stir in spinach until wilted. Drain fettuccine; add to the bean mixture and toss to combine.

1¼ CUPS *255 cal., 3g fat (0 sat. fat), 0 chol., 230mg sod., 45g carb. (4g sugars, 9g fiber), 12g pro.* ***Diabetic exchanges:*** *3 starch, 1 lean meat, ½ fat*

UDON NOODLES WITH PINEAPPLE VINAIGRETTE

TAKES: 30 min. **MAKES:** 8 servings

- 1 pkg. (12.8 oz.) dried Japanese udon noodles
- ½ cup unsweetened pineapple juice
- ¼ cup sesame oil
- 2 Tbsp. white wine vinegar
- 2 tsp. grated fresh gingerroot
- 2 tsp. minced seeded jalapeno pepper
- 3 cups fresh arugula or baby spinach
- 2 cups chopped peeled mango
- 1 cup salted peanuts
- ½ cup coarsely chopped fresh cilantro leaves
- ¼ cup coarsely chopped fresh mint leaves
- 2 Tbsp. black sesame seeds

1 Cook noodles according to package directions. Rinse with cold water; drain well. Whisk together the next 5 ingredients. Pour over noodles; toss to coat. Refrigerate until serving.

2 To serve, top the noodles with the arugula, mango, peanuts, cilantro and mint; toss to combine. Sprinkle with sesame seeds.

1⅓ CUPS *370 cal., 19g fat (3g sat. fat), 0 chol., 590mg sod., 42g carb. (12g sugars, 5g fiber), 13g pro.*

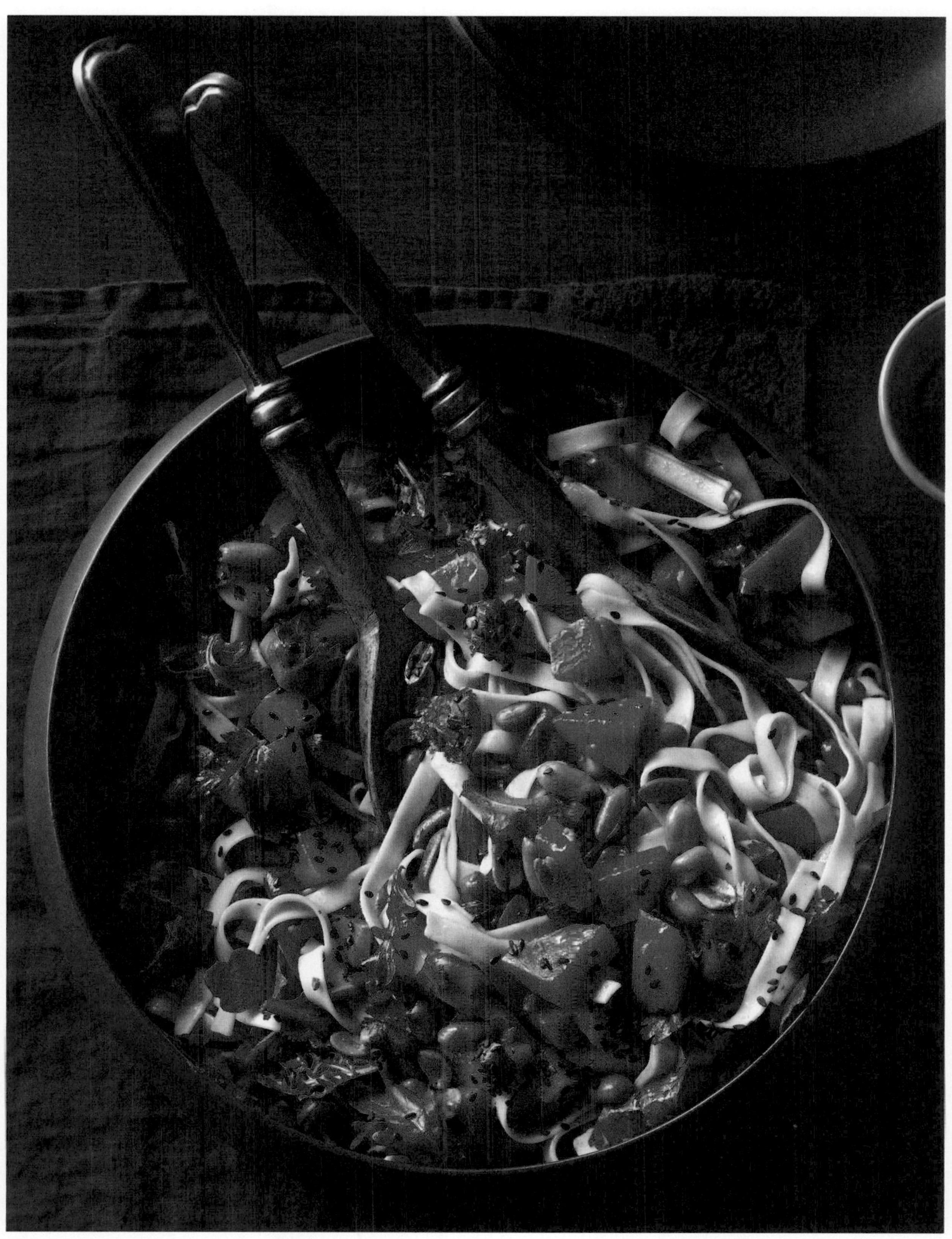

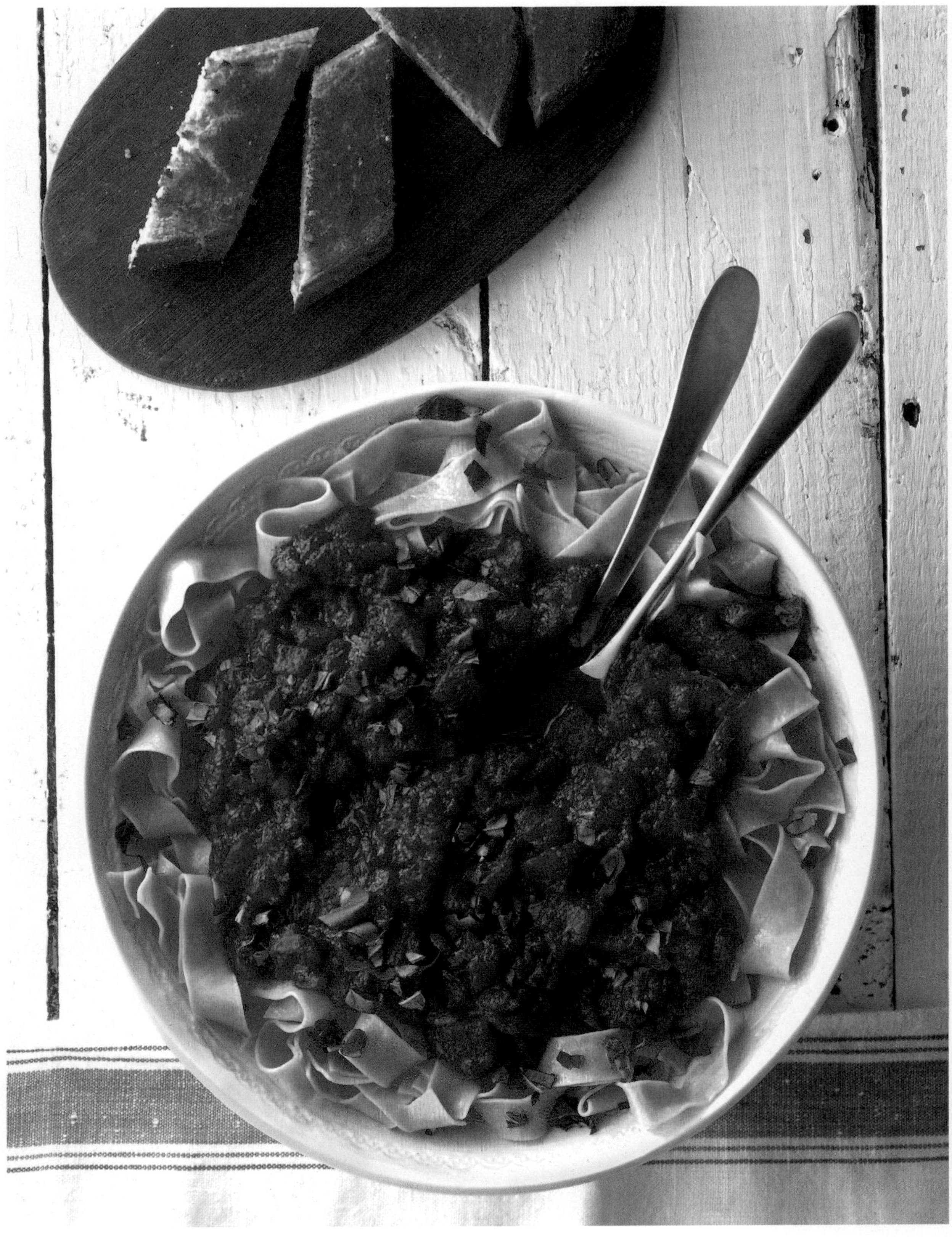

HOMEMADE SPAGHETTI SAUCE

PREP: 20 min. **COOK:** 3¼ hours **MAKES:** 2 qt.

- 4 medium onions, chopped
- ½ cup canola oil
- 12 cups chopped peeled fresh tomatoes
- 4 garlic cloves, minced
- 3 bay leaves
- 4 tsp. salt
- 2 tsp. dried oregano
- 1¼ tsp. pepper
- ½ tsp. dried basil
- 2 cans (6 oz. each) tomato paste
- ⅓ cup packed brown sugar
- Hot cooked pasta
- Minced fresh basil, optional

1 In a Dutch oven, saute onions in oil until tender. Add tomatoes, garlic, bay leaves, salt, oregano, pepper and basil. Bring to a boil. Reduce heat; cover and simmer for 2 hours, stirring occasionally.

2 Add tomato paste and brown sugar; simmer, uncovered, for 1 hour. Discard bay leaves. Serve with pasta and, if desired, basil.

½ CUP *133 cal., 7g fat (1g sat. fat), 0 chol., 614mg sod., 17g carb. (12g sugars, 3g fiber), 2g pro.*

VEGAN MAC & CHEESE

PREP: 20 min. + standing **COOK:** 10 min. **MAKES:** 6 servings

- 2 cups raw cashews
- 16 oz. uncooked elbow macaroni
- 1½ cups water
- ⅓ cup nutritional yeast
- 2 tsp. lemon juice
- 2 tsp. salt
- 2 tsp. onion powder
- 1½ tsp. paprika
- 1 tsp. pepper
- ⅛ tsp. cayenne pepper

1 Rinse cashews in cold water. Place in a large bowl; add water to cover by 3 in. Cover and let stand overnight.

2 Cook macaroni according to package directions. Drain and rinse cashews, discarding liquid. Transfer to a food processor. Add 1½ cups water, nutritional yeast, lemon juice and seasonings; cover and process until pureed, 3-4 minutes, scraping down sides as needed.

3 Drain macaroni; return to pan. Stir in cashew mixture. Cook and stir over medium-low heat until heated through. Sprinkle with additional paprika if desired.

1⅔ CUPS *497 cal., 18g fat (3g sat. fat), 0 chol., 803mg sod., 67g carb. (5g sugars, 5g fiber), 18g pro.*

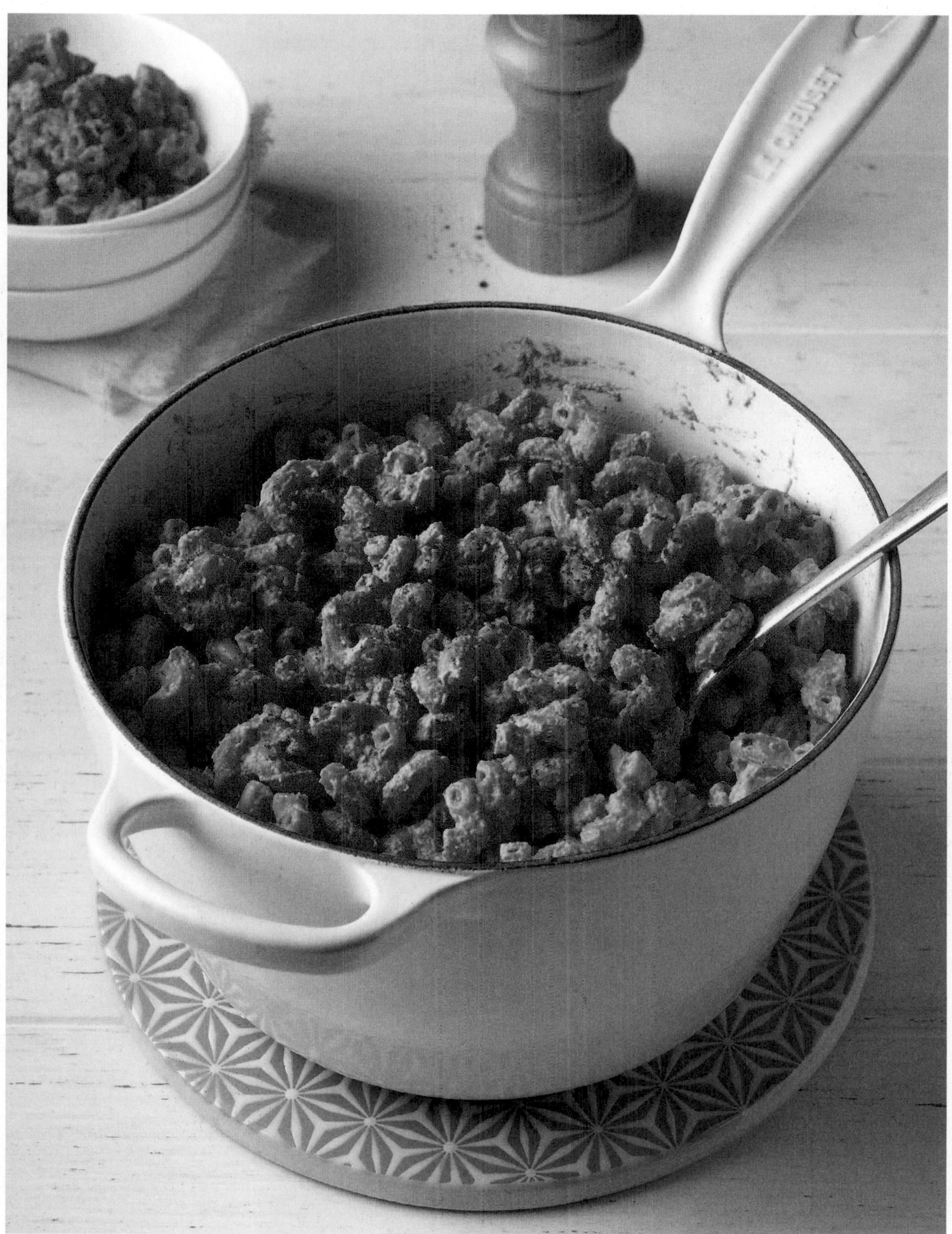
LE CREUSET

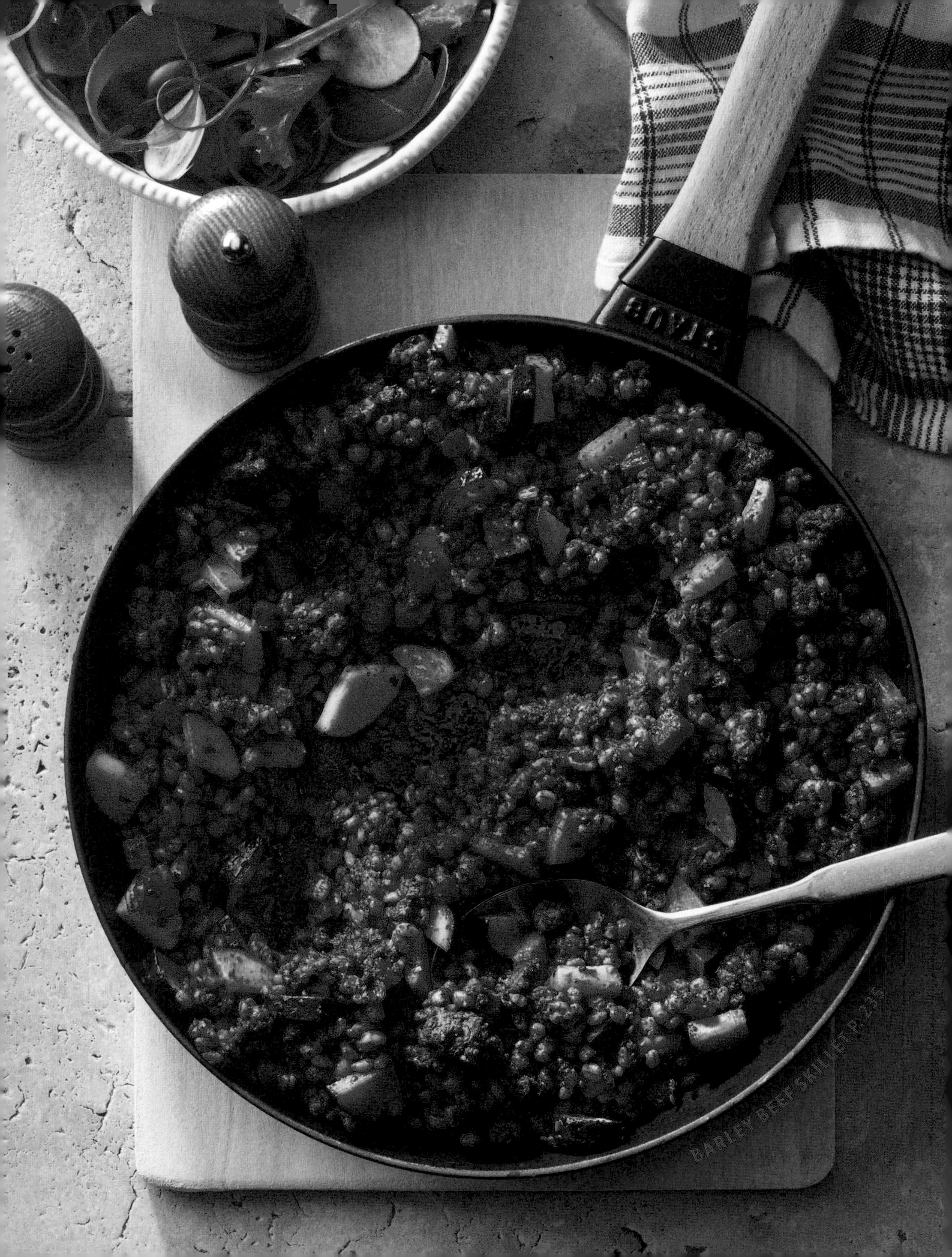

BARLEY BEEF SKILLET P. 235

CHAPTER 11

RICE & GRAINS

QUINOA PEPPER SAUTE

TAKES: 30 min. **MAKES:** 4 servings

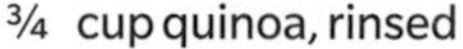

- 1½ cups vegetable stock
- ¾ cup quinoa, rinsed
- 1 lb. Italian turkey sausage links, casings removed or frozen vegan Italian sausage-style crumbles
- 1 medium sweet red pepper, chopped
- 1 medium green pepper, chopped
- ¾ cup chopped sweet onion
- 1 garlic clove, minced
- ¼ tsp. garam masala
- ¼ tsp. pepper
- ⅛ tsp. salt

1 In a small saucepan, bring stock to a boil. Add quinoa. Reduce heat; simmer, covered, 12-15 minutes or until liquid is absorbed. Remove from heat.

2 In a large skillet, cook and crumble sausage with peppers and onion over medium-high heat 8-10 minutes or until no longer pink. Add garlic and seasonings; cook and stir 1 minute. Stir in the quinoa.

TO FREEZE Place cooled quinoa mixture in freezer containers. To use, partially thaw in refrigerator overnight. Microwave, covered, on high in a microwave-safe dish until heated through, stirring occasionally.

1 CUP *261 cal., 9g fat (2g sat. fat), 42mg chol., 760mg sod., 28g carb. (3g sugars, 4g fiber), 17g pro.* ***Diabetic exchanges****: 2 starch, 2 medium-fat meat*

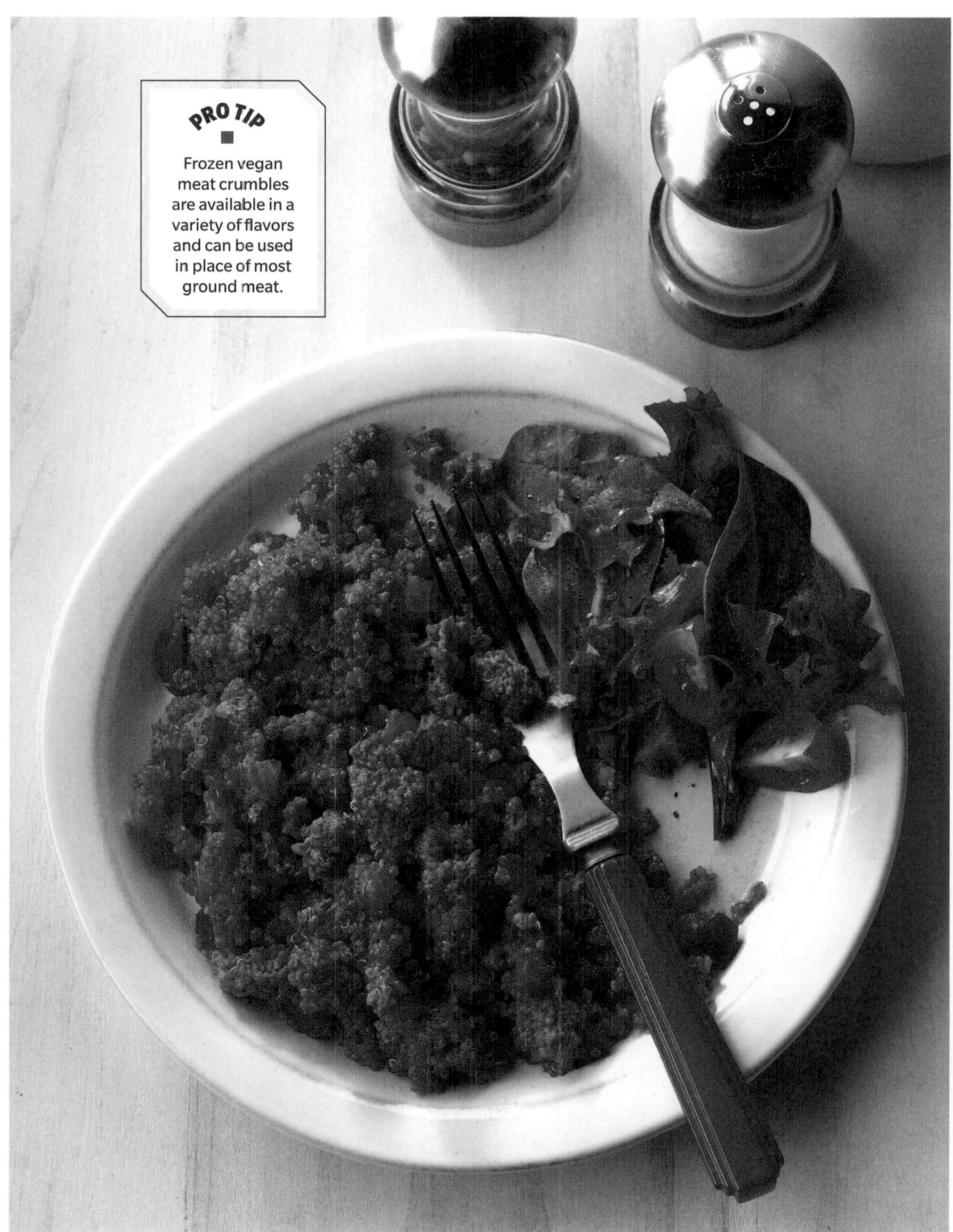
PRO TIP
Frozen vegan meat crumbles are available in a variety of flavors and can be used in place of most ground meat.

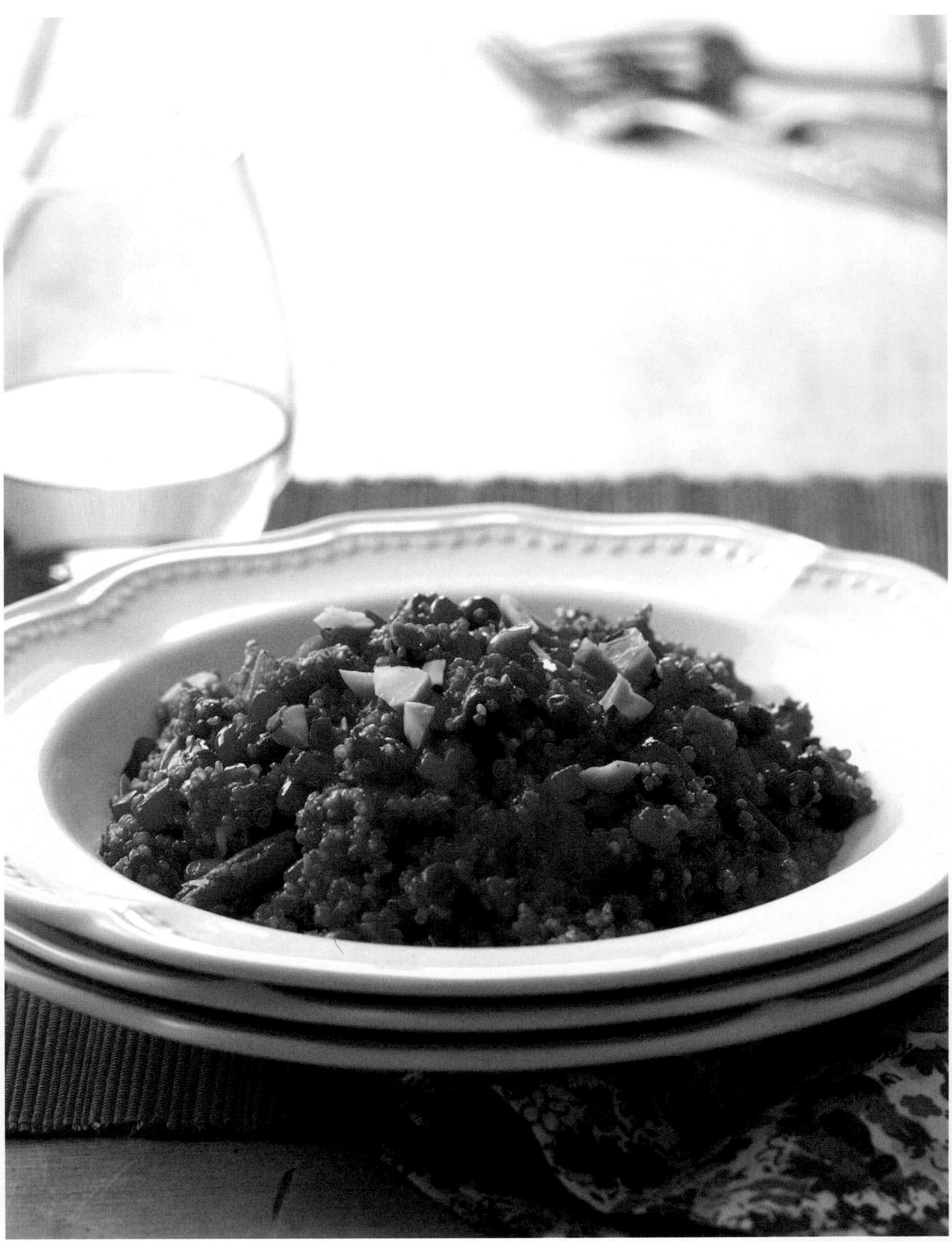

SPICY ORANGE QUINOA

PREP: 30 min. **COOK:** 25 min. **MAKES:** 4 servings

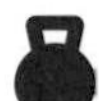

- 1 serrano pepper, halved and seeded
- 1½ cups vegetable broth
- ¼ cup orange juice
- ¼ tsp. cayenne pepper
- ¼ tsp. saffron threads or 1 tsp. ground turmeric
- 1 cup quinoa, rinsed
- 1 Tbsp. olive oil
- 1 Tbsp. vegan spreadable margarine
- 1 large onion, chopped
- 1 cup chopped fresh mushrooms
- ½ cup plus 2 Tbsp. chopped Brazil nuts, divided
- 2 bay leaves
- 1 pkg. (16 oz.) frozen mixed vegetables, thawed
- 7 garlic cloves, minced
- 1 medium orange, sectioned and chopped
- 3 Tbsp. lemon juice
- 2 tsp. grated lemon zest
- 2 tsp. grated orange zest
- ½ tsp. pepper
- ¼ tsp. salt

1 Broil pepper halves 4 in. from the heat until skin blisters. Cool slightly; finely chop pepper; set aside.

2 In a large saucepan, bring the broth, orange juice, cayenne and saffron to a boil. Add quinoa. Reduce heat; simmer, covered, 12-15 minutes or until liquid is absorbed. Remove from heat; fluff with a fork.

3 Meanwhile, in a Dutch oven, heat oil and buttery spread over medium-high heat. Add onion, mushrooms, ½ cup nuts and bay leaves; cook and stir until onion is tender. Add mixed vegetables, garlic and reserved serrano pepper; cook 4-5 minutes longer. Stir in orange, lemon juice, zests, pepper and salt.

4 Gently stir quinoa into the vegetable mixture; discard bay leaves. Sprinkle with remaining Brazil nuts.

1¾ CUPS *480 cal., 23g fat (5g sat. fat), 0 chol., 583mg sod., 60g carb. (10g sugars, 11g fiber), 14g pro.*

CUMIN QUINOA PATTIES

TAKES: 30 min. **MAKES:** 4 servings

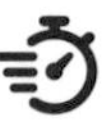

- 1 cup water
- ½ cup quinoa, rinsed
- 1 medium carrot, cut into 1-in. pieces
- 1 cup canned cannellini beans, rinsed and drained
- ¼ cup panko bread crumbs
- 3 green onions, chopped
- 1 large egg, lightly beaten or vegan egg substitute
- 3 tsp. ground cumin
- ¼ tsp. salt
- ⅛ tsp. pepper
- 2 Tbsp. olive oil
- Optional toppings: Vegan sour cream, salsa and minced fresh cilantro

1 In a small saucepan, bring water to a boil. Add quinoa. Reduce heat; simmer, covered, 12-15 minutes or until liquid is absorbed. Remove from heat; fluff with a fork.

2 Meanwhile, place carrot in a food processor; pulse until coarsely chopped. Add beans; process until chopped. Transfer mixture to a large bowl. Mix in cooked quinoa, bread crumbs, green onions, egg and seasonings. Shape mixture into 8 patties.

3 In a large skillet, heat oil over medium heat. Add patties; cook until a thermometer reads 160°, 3-4 minutes on each side, turning carefully. If desired, serve with optional toppings.

2 PATTIES *235 cal., 10g fat (1g sat. fat), 47mg chol., 273mg sod., 28g carb. (2g sugars, 5g fiber), 8g pro.* ***Diabetic exchanges:*** *2 starch, 1½ fat, 1 lean meat*

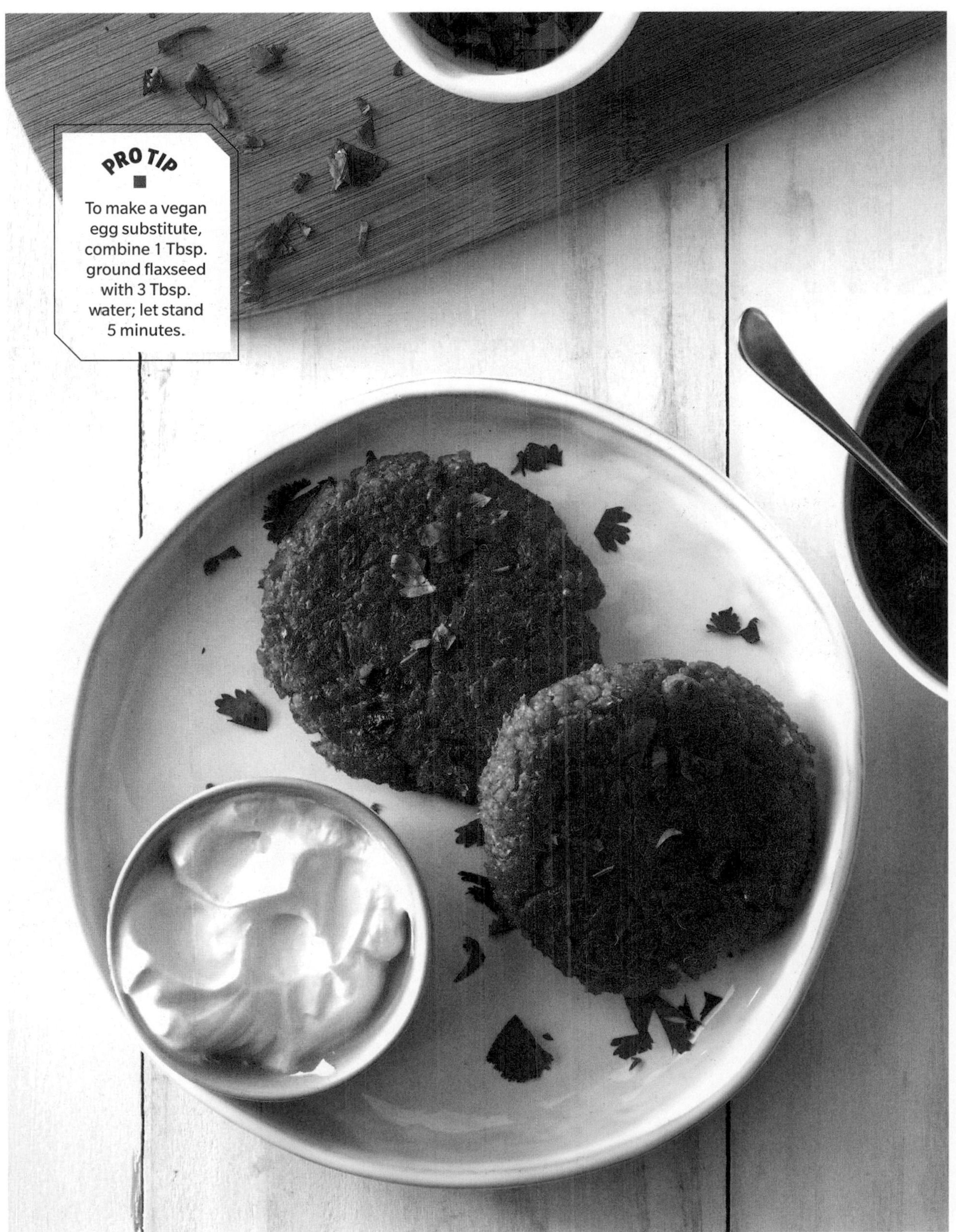

PRO TIP

To make a vegan egg substitute, combine 1 Tbsp. ground flaxseed with 3 Tbsp. water; let stand 5 minutes.

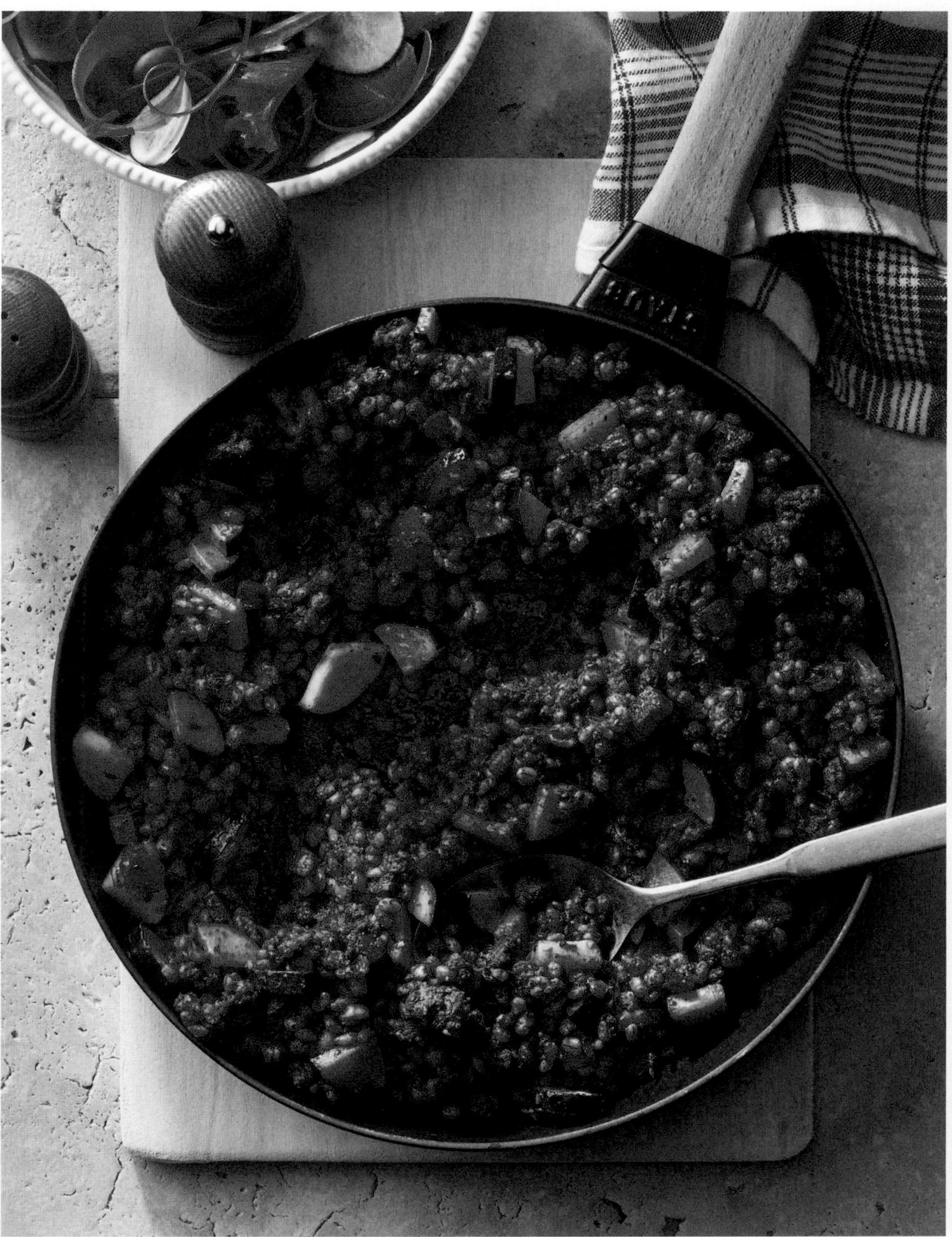

BARLEY BEEF SKILLET

PREP: 20 min. **COOK:** 20 min. **MAKES:** 4 servings

- 1 lb. lean ground beef (90% lean) or frozen vegetarian meat crumbles
- ¼ cup chopped onion
- 1 garlic clove, minced
- 1 can (14½ oz.) reduced-sodium beef or vegetable broth
- 1 can (8 oz.) tomato sauce
- 1 cup water
- 2 small carrots, chopped
- 1 small tomato, seeded and chopped
- 1 small zucchini, chopped
- 1 cup medium pearl barley
- 2 tsp. Italian seasoning
- ¼ tsp. salt
- ⅛ tsp. pepper

In a large skillet, cook beef and onion over medium heat until meat is no longer pink. Add garlic; cook 1 minute longer. Drain. Add the broth, tomato sauce and water; bring to a boil. Stir in the remaining ingredients. Reduce heat; cover and simmer until barley is tender, 20-25 minutes.

1½ CUPS *400 cal., 10g fat (4g sat. fat), 73mg chol., 682mg sod., 48g carb. (4g sugars, 10g fiber), 30g pro.*

CHICKEN BULGUR SKILLET

PREP: 15 min. **COOK:** 30 min. **MAKES:** 4 servings

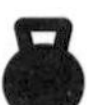

- 1 lb. boneless skinless chicken breasts, cut into 1-in. cubes
- 2 tsp. olive oil
- 2 medium carrots, chopped
- ⅔ cup chopped onion
- 3 Tbsp. chopped walnuts
- ½ tsp. caraway seeds
- ¼ tsp. ground cumin
- 1½ cups bulgur
- 2 cups reduced-sodium chicken or vegetable broth
- 2 Tbsp. raisins
- ¼ tsp. salt
- ⅛ tsp. ground cinnamon

1 In a large cast-iron or other heavy skillet, cook chicken in oil over medium-high heat until meat is no longer pink. Remove and keep warm. In the same skillet, cook and stir the carrots, onion, nuts, caraway seeds and cumin until the onion starts to brown, 3-4 minutes.

2 Stir in bulgur. Gradually add the broth; bring to a boil over medium heat. Reduce heat; add the raisins, salt, cinnamon and chicken. Cover and simmer until bulgur is tender, 12-15 minutes.

1½ CUPS *412 cal., 8g fat (1g sat. fat), 66mg chol., 561mg sod., 51g carb. (8g sugars, 12g fiber), 36g pro.*

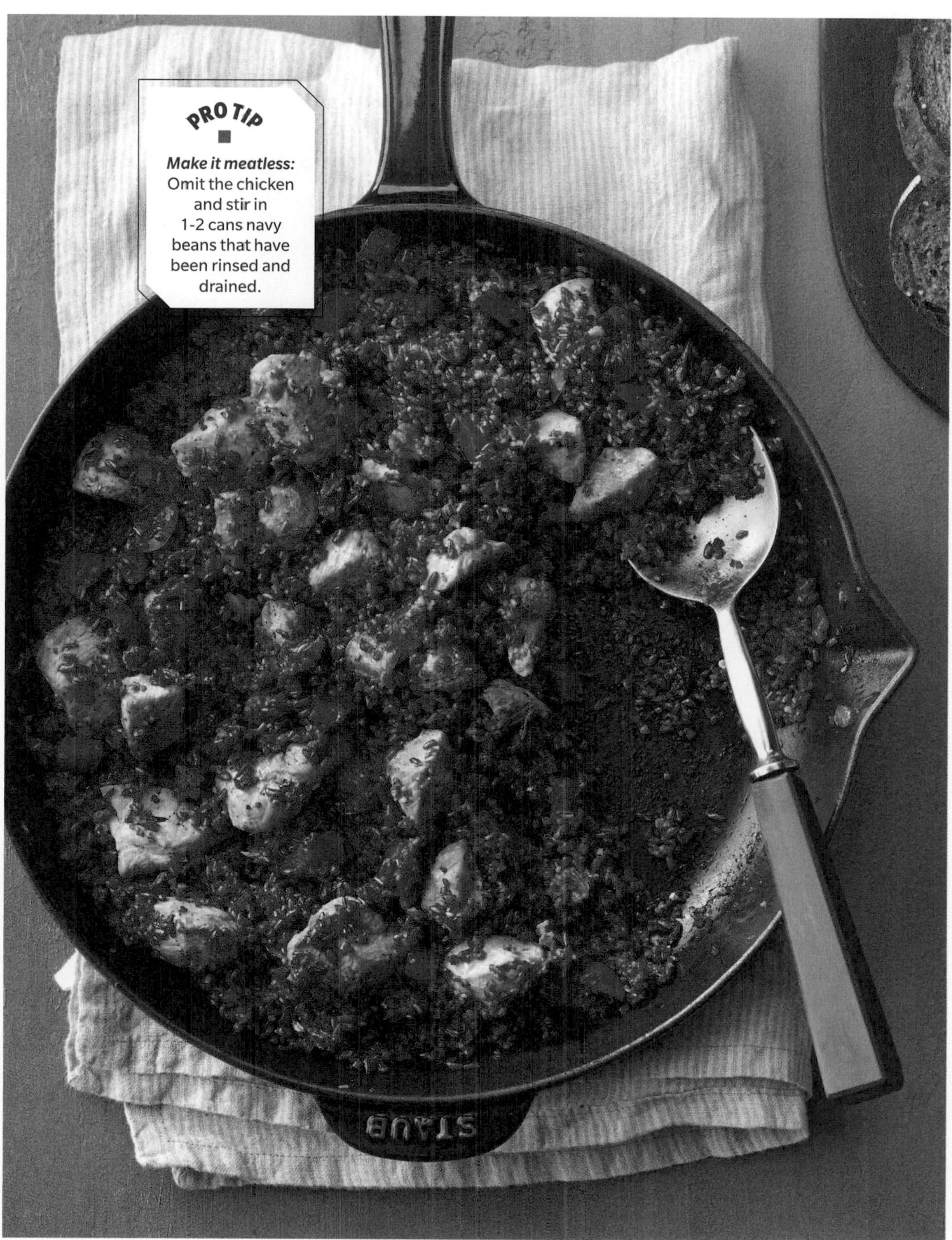
PRO TIP
Make it meatless: Omit the chicken and stir in 1-2 cans navy beans that have been rinsed and drained.
STAUB

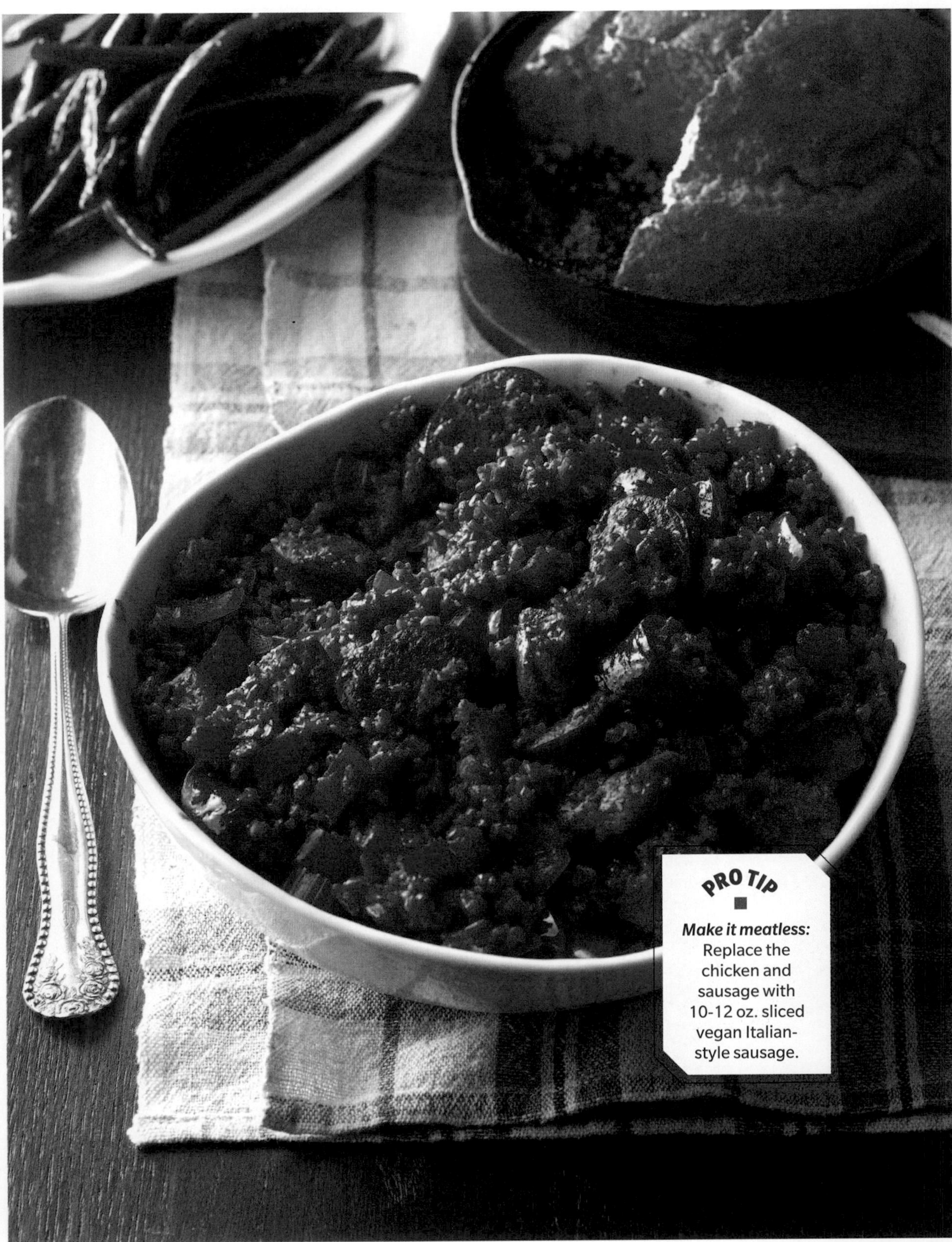

PRO TIP

Make it meatless: Replace the chicken and sausage with 10-12 oz. sliced vegan Italian-style sausage.

BULGUR JAMBALAYA

TAKES: 30 min. **MAKES:** 4 servings

- 8 oz. boneless skinless chicken breasts, cut into ¾-in. pieces
- 1 tsp. Cajun seasoning
- 2 tsp. olive oil
- 6 oz. smoked turkey sausage, sliced
- 1 medium sweet red pepper, diced
- 2 celery ribs, diced
- 1 small onion, chopped
- ½ cup no-salt-added tomato sauce
- 1 cup bulgur
- 1 cup reduced-sodium chicken or vegetable broth
- ¾ cup water
- ¼ tsp. cayenne pepper, optional

1 Toss chicken with Cajun seasoning. In a large saucepan, heat oil over medium heat; saute chicken 2-3 minutes or until browned. Remove from pan.

2 In same pan, saute sausage until browned, 1-2 minutes. Add red pepper, celery and onion; cook and stir 2 minutes. Stir in tomato sauce; cook 30 seconds. Stir in the bulgur, broth, water, chicken and, if desired, cayenne; bring to a boil. Reduce heat; simmer, covered, until bulgur is tender and liquid is almost absorbed, about 10 minutes, stirring occasionally.

1 CUP *287 cal., 6g fat (2g sat. fat), 58mg chol., 751mg sod., 34g carb. (5g sugars, 6g fiber), 24g pro.* ***Diabetic exchanges:*** *3 lean meat, 2 starch, ½ fat*

PORTOBELLO POLENTA STACKS

TAKES: 30 min. **MAKES:** 4 servings

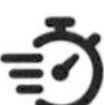

- 1 Tbsp. olive oil
- 3 garlic cloves, minced
- 2 Tbsp. balsamic vinegar
- 4 large portobello mushrooms (about 5 in.), stems removed
- ¼ tsp. salt
- ¼ tsp. pepper
- 1 tube (18 oz.) polenta, cut into 12 slices
- 4 slices tomato
- ½ cup grated Parmesan or vegan Parmesan-style cheese
- 2 Tbsp. minced fresh basil

1 Preheat oven to 400°. In a small saucepan, heat oil over medium heat. Add garlic; cook and stir until tender, 1-2 minutes (do not allow to brown). Stir in vinegar; remove from heat.

2 Place mushrooms in a 13x9-in. baking dish, gill side up. Brush with vinegar mixture; sprinkle with salt and pepper. Top with polenta and tomato slices; sprinkle with cheese.

3 Bake, uncovered, until the mushrooms are tender, 20-25 minutes. Sprinkle with fresh basil.

1 SERVING *219 cal., 6g fat (2g sat. fat), 9mg chol., 764mg sod., 32g carb. (7g sugars, 3g fiber), 7g pro.* ***Diabetic exchanges:*** *1½ starch, 1 vegetable, 1 lean meat, 1 fat*

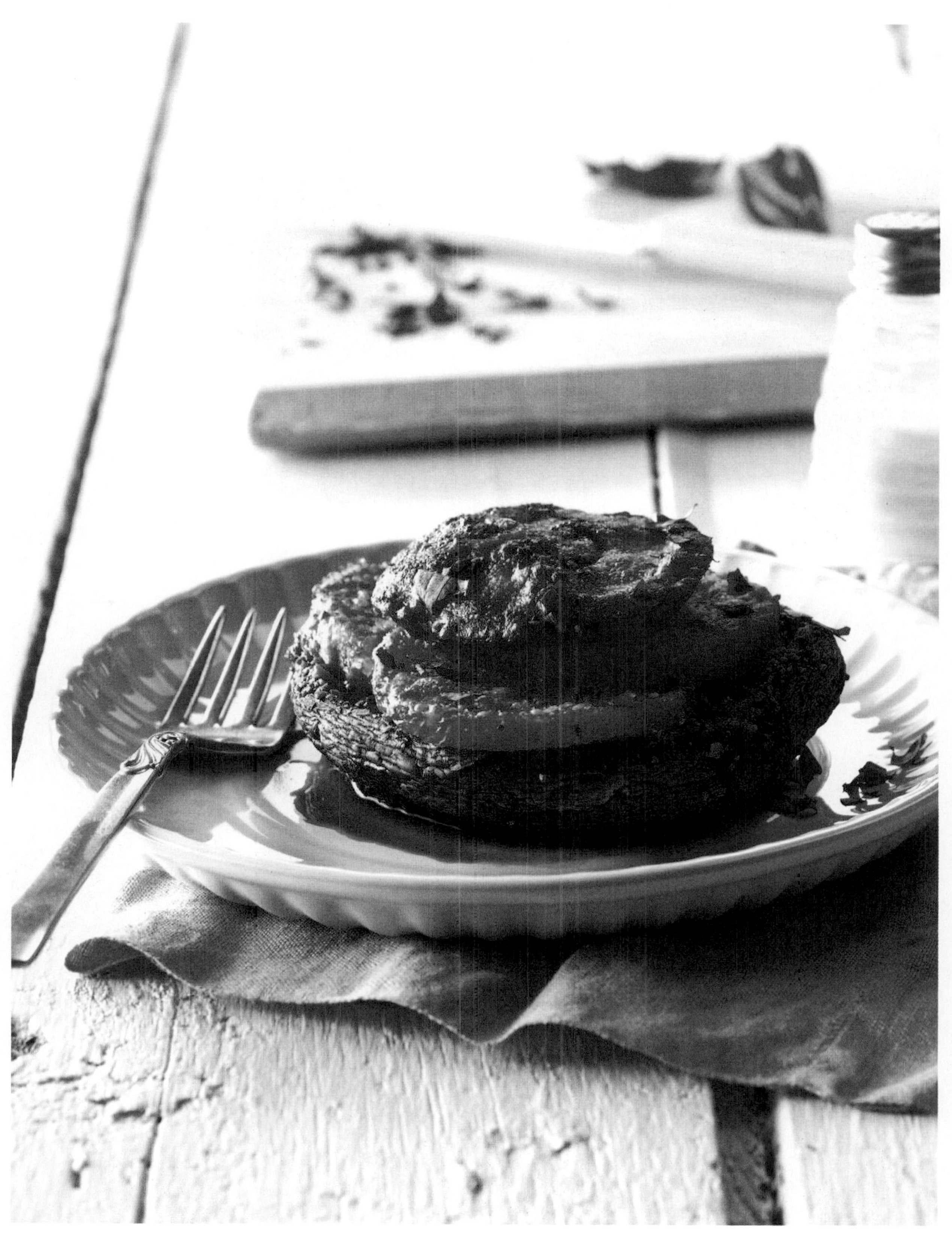

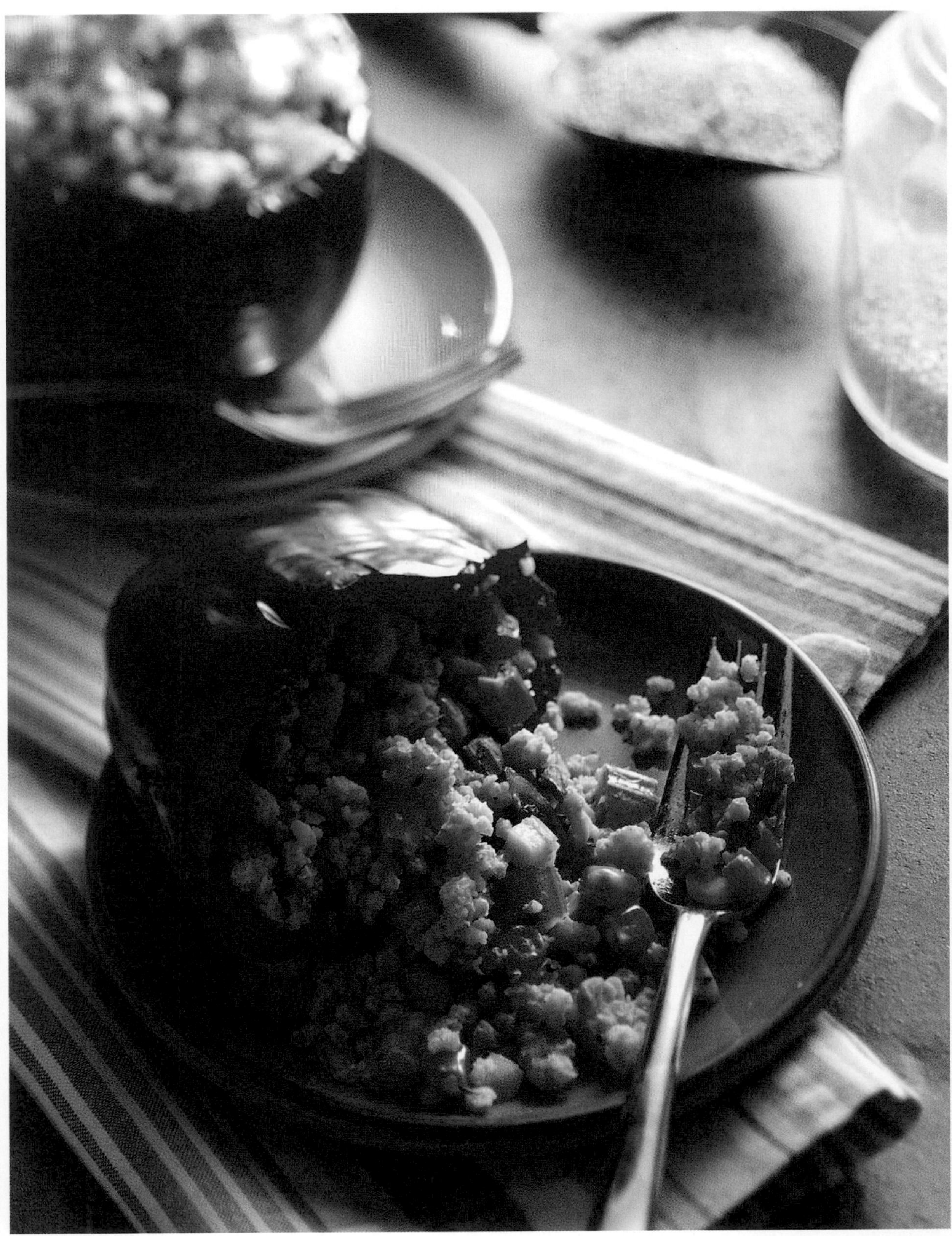

STUFFED RED PEPPERS

PREP: 40 min. **BAKE:** 55 min. **MAKES:** 2 servings

- ¼ cup uncooked millet, rinsed and drained
- ¾ cup vegetable broth
- 2 medium sweet red peppers
- ⅓ cup frozen corn, thawed
- ¼ cup finely chopped onion
- 3 Tbsp. finely chopped celery
- 2 Tbsp. chopped walnuts
- 1 green onion, finely chopped
- 1½ tsp. chopped fresh mint or ½ tsp. dried mint flakes
- 1 tsp. shredded lemon peel
- ¾ tsp. fresh chopped oregano or ¼ tsp. dried oregano
- 1 small garlic clove, minced
- ¼ tsp. salt
- ⅛ tsp. pepper
- 1 Tbsp. olive oil

1 In a saucepan, bring millet and broth to a boil. Reduce heat; simmer, covered, until millet is tender and broth is absorbed, 30-35 minutes. Transfer to a large bowl and cool.

2 Meanwhile, cut the tops off peppers and remove seeds. In a large saucepan, cook peppers in boiling water for 3-5 minutes. Drain and rinse in cold water; set aside.

3 With a fork, fluff cooled millet. Add the corn, onion, celery, nuts, green onion and seasonings; blend well. Spoon into the sweet peppers. Drizzle with oil. Place in a baking dish coated with cooking spray. Cover and bake at 350° for 55-60 minutes or until tender.

1 SERVING *278 cal., 13g fat (2g sat. fat), 0 chol., 666mg sod., 37g carb. (8g sugars, 7g fiber), 7g pro.*

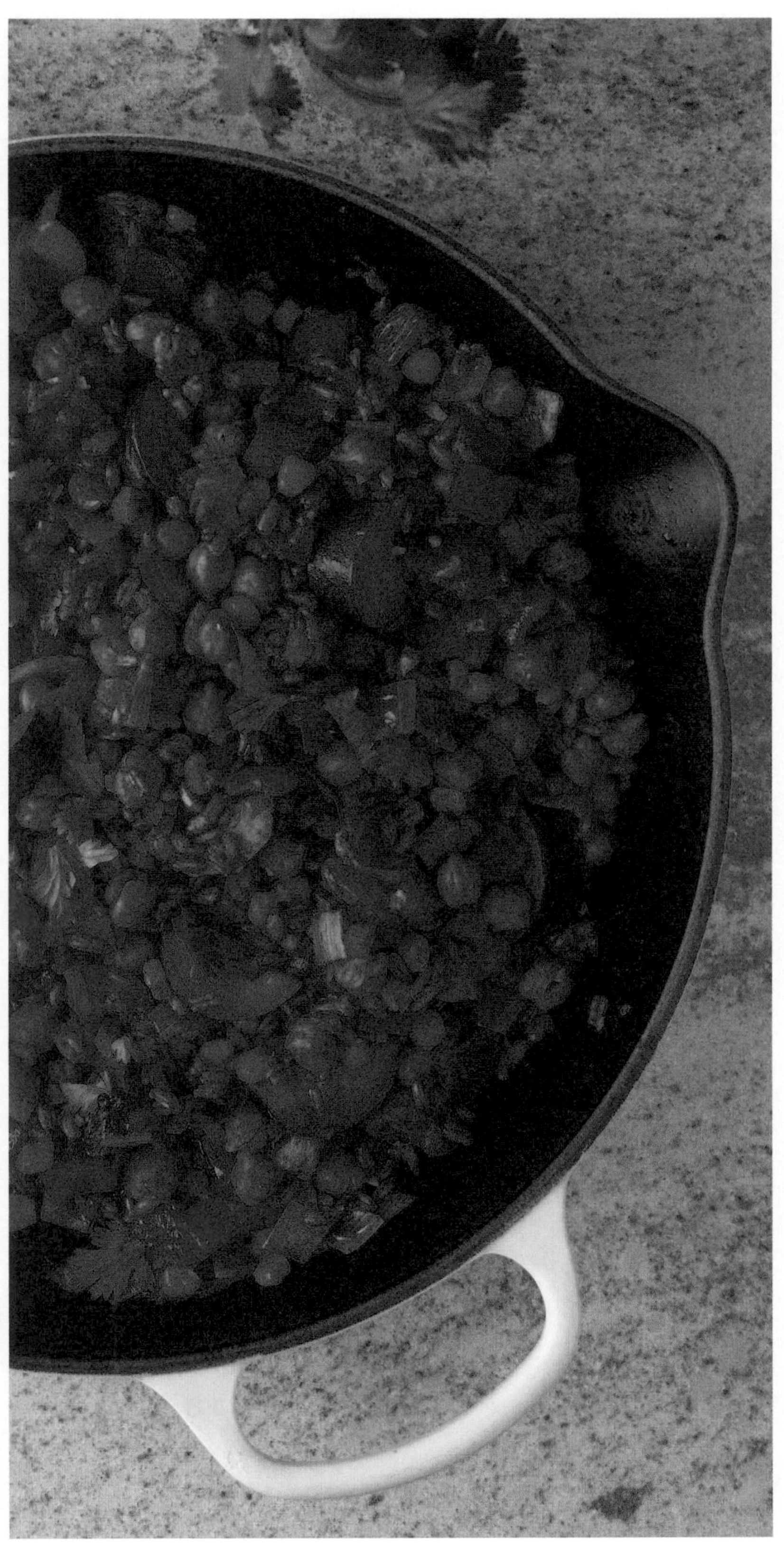

FARRO SKILLET

PREP: 20 min.
COOK: 30 min.
MAKES: 4 servings

- 1 Tbsp. canola oil
- 1 medium onion, chopped
- 1 medium sweet red pepper, chopped
- 3 garlic cloves, minced
- 1 can (14½ oz.) vegetable broth
- 1 can (14½ oz.) diced tomatoes
- 1 can (15 oz.) garbanzo beans or chickpeas, rinsed and drained
- 1 small zucchini, halved and cut into ½-in. slices
- 1 cup farro, rinsed
- 1 cup frozen corn
- ¾ tsp. ground cumin
- ¼ tsp. salt
- ¼ tsp. pepper
- Chopped fresh cilantro

Heat oil in a large skillet over medium-high heat. Add onion and pepper; cook and stir until tender, 2-3 minutes. Add garlic; cook 1 minute longer. Stir in the broth, tomatoes, beans, zucchini, farro, corn, cumin, salt and pepper. Bring to a boil. Reduce heat; cover and simmer until farro is tender, 25-30 minutes. Sprinkle with cilantro.

1½ CUPS *416 cal., 8g fat (0 sat. fat), 0 chol., 757mg sod., 73g carb. (10g sugars, 15g fiber), 14g pro.*

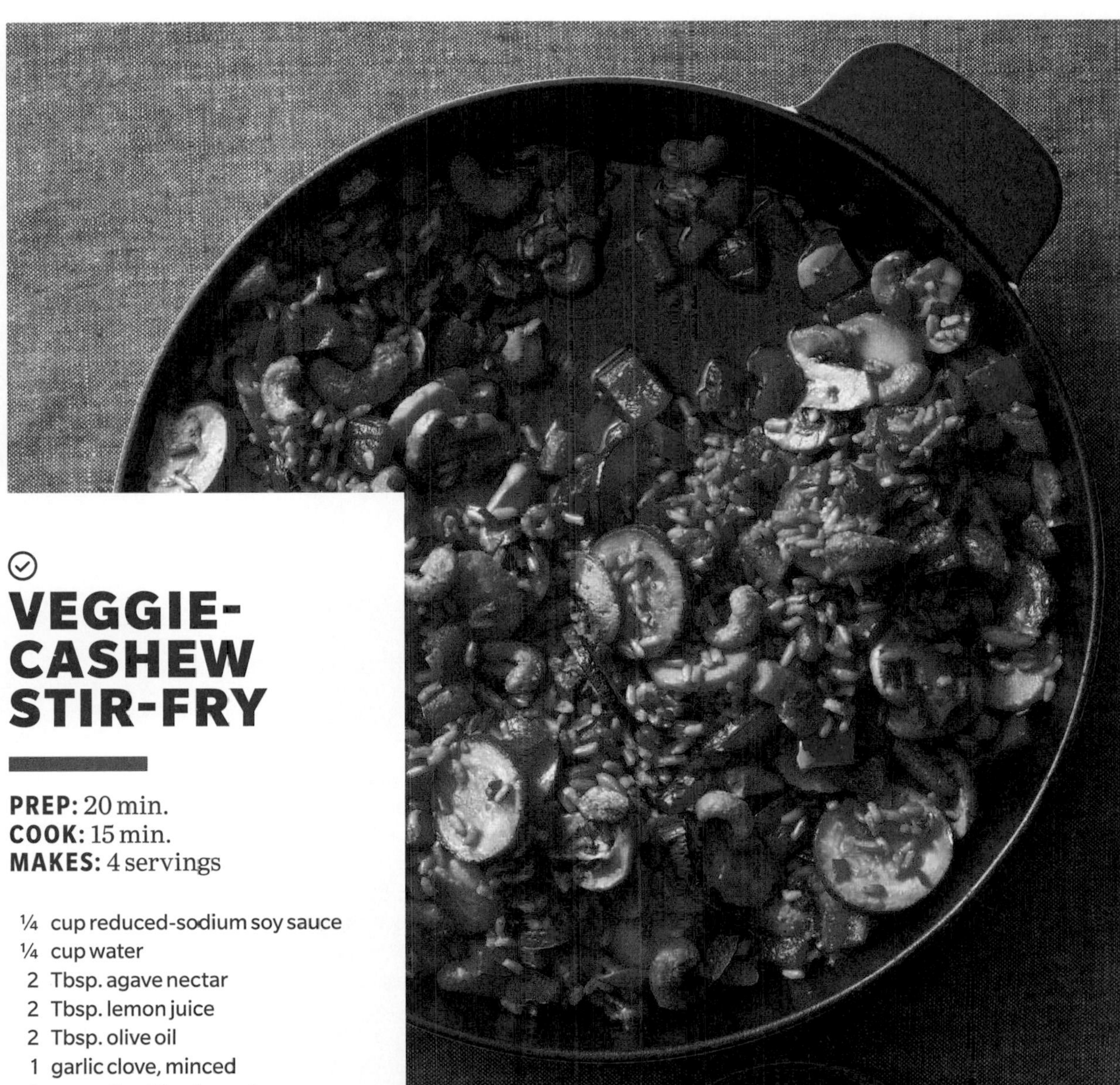

VEGGIE-CASHEW STIR-FRY

PREP: 20 min.
COOK: 15 min.
MAKES: 4 servings

- ¼ cup reduced-sodium soy sauce
- ¼ cup water
- 2 Tbsp. agave nectar
- 2 Tbsp. lemon juice
- 2 Tbsp. olive oil
- 1 garlic clove, minced
- 2 cups sliced fresh mushrooms
- 1 cup coarsely chopped fresh baby carrots
- 1 small zucchini, cut into ¼-in. slices
- 1 small sweet red pepper, coarsely chopped
- 1 small green pepper, coarsely chopped
- 4 green onions, sliced
- 2 cups cooked brown rice
- 1 can (8 oz.) sliced water chestnuts, drained
- ½ cup roasted cashews

1 In a small bowl, mix soy sauce, water, agave and lemon juice until smooth; set aside.

2 In a large skillet, heat oil over medium-high heat. Stir-fry garlic for 1 minute. Add vegetables; cook until vegetables are crisp-tender, 6-8 minutes.

3 Stir soy sauce mixture and add to pan. Bring to a boil. Add the rice and water chestnuts; heat through. Top with cashews.

1½ CUPS *385 cal., 16g fat (3g sat. fat), 0 chol., 671mg sod., 56g carb. (15g sugars, 6g fiber), 9g pro.*

MUSHROOM & BROWN RICE HASH WITH POACHED EGGS

TAKES: 30 min. **MAKES:** 4 servings

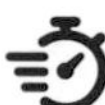

- 2 Tbsp. olive oil
- 1 lb. sliced baby portobello mushrooms
- ½ cup chopped sweet onion
- 1 pkg. (8.8 oz.) ready-to-serve brown rice
- 1 large carrot, grated
- 2 green onions, thinly sliced
- ½ tsp. salt
- ¼ tsp. pepper
- ¼ tsp. caraway seeds
- 4 large eggs, cold

1 In a large skillet, heat olive oil over medium-high heat; saute the mushrooms until lightly browned, 5-7 minutes. Add sweet onion; cook 1 minute. Add rice and carrot; cook and stir for 4-5 minutes or until vegetables are tender. Stir in green onions, salt, pepper and caraway seeds; heat through.

2 Meanwhile, place 2-3 in. of water in a large saucepan or skillet with high sides. Bring to a boil; adjust heat to maintain a gentle simmer. Break cold eggs, 1 at a time, into a small bowl; holding bowl close to surface of water, slip egg into water.

3 Cook, uncovered, until the whites are completely set and yolks begin to thicken but are not hard, 3-5 minutes. Using a slotted spoon, lift eggs out of water. Serve over rice mixture.

1 SERVING *282 cal., 13g fat (3g sat. fat), 186mg chol., 393mg sod., 26g carb. (4g sugars, 3g fiber), 13g pro.* ***Diabetic exchanges:*** *1½ starch, 1½ fat, 1 medium-fat meat*

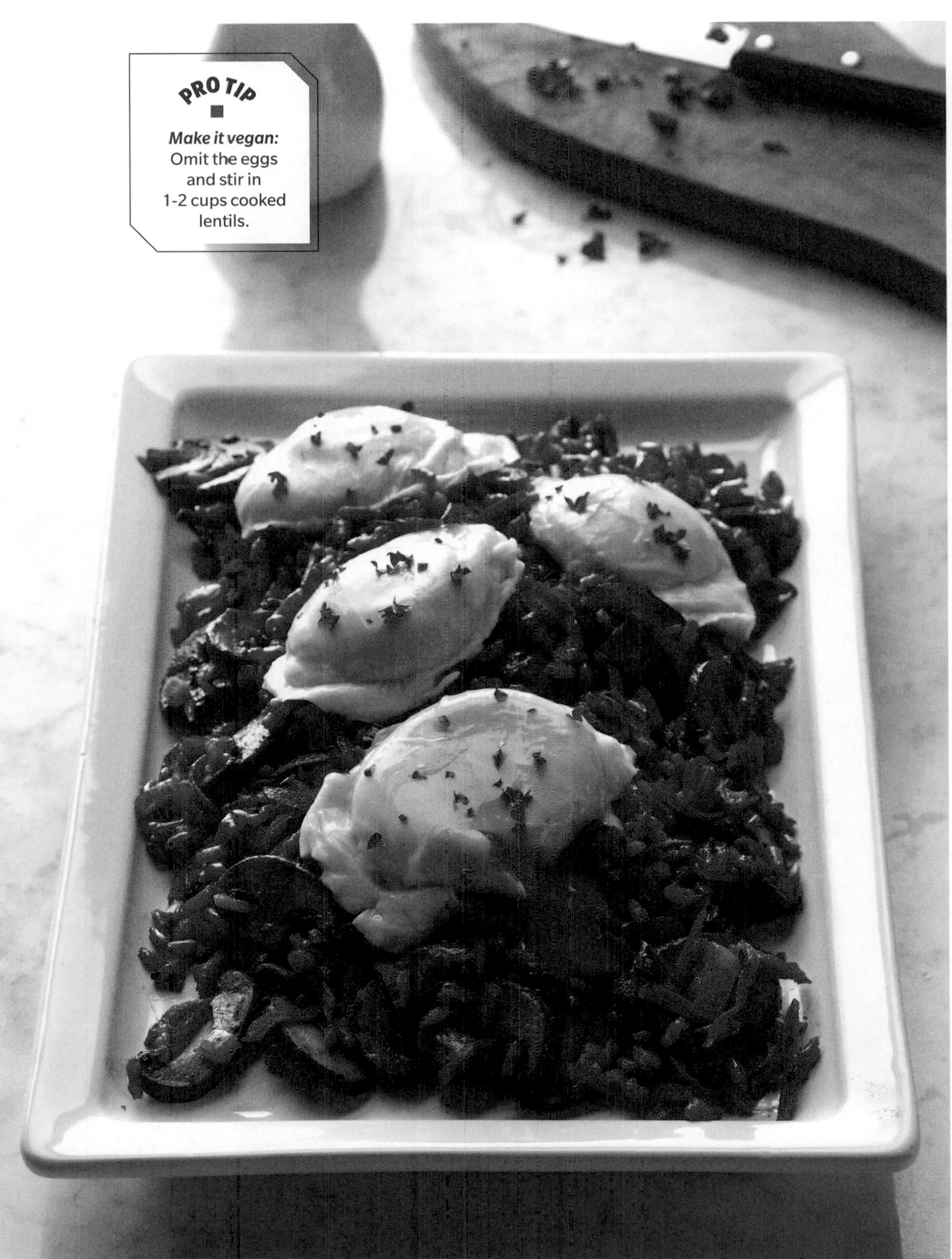

PRO TIP

Make it vegan: Omit the eggs and stir in 1-2 cups cooked lentils.

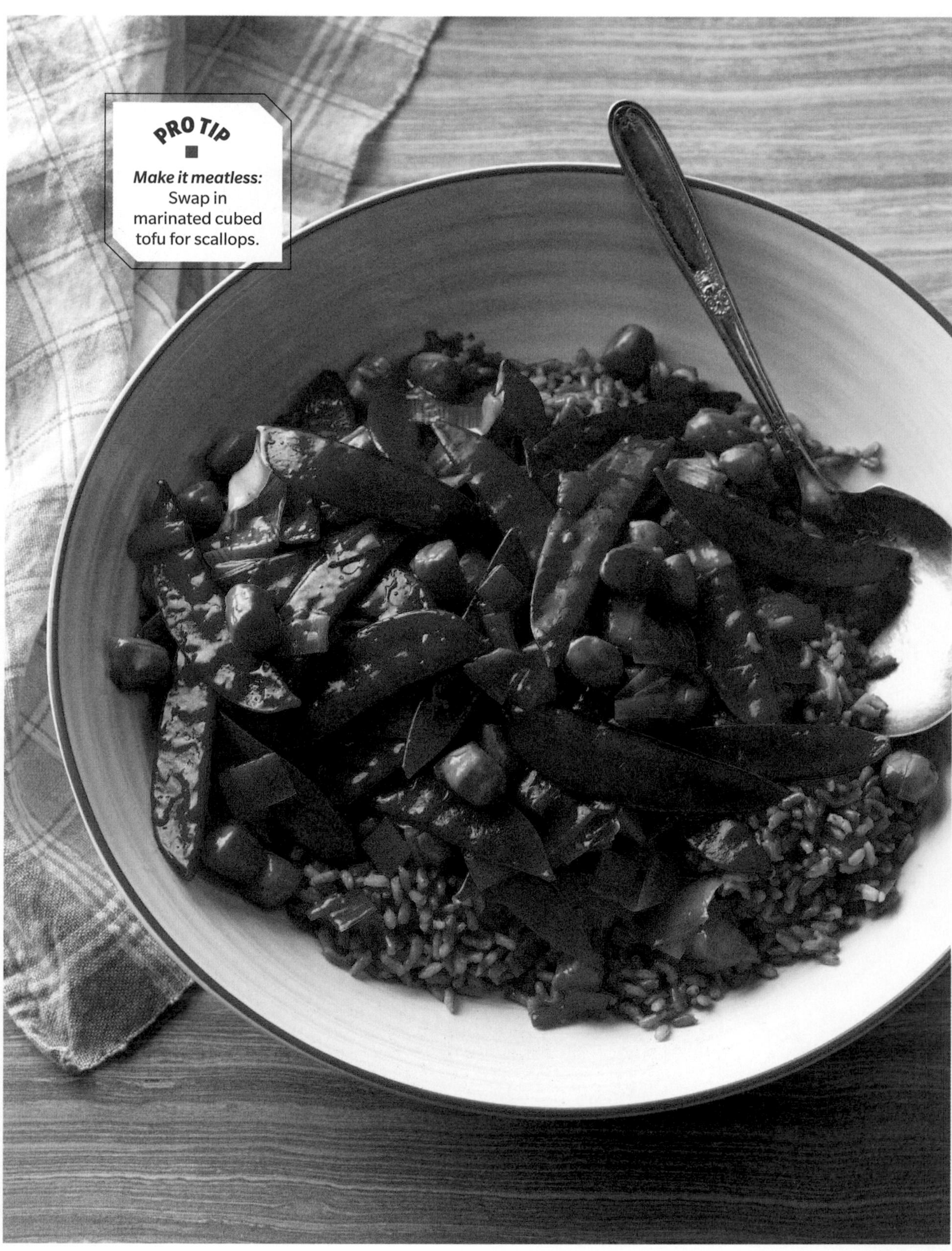
PRO TIP
Make it meatless: Swap in marinated cubed tofu for scallops.

SCALLOPS WITH SNOW PEAS

TAKES: 30 min. **MAKES:** 4 servings

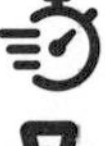

- 2 Tbsp. cornstarch
- 2 Tbsp. reduced-sodium soy sauce
- ⅔ cup water
- 4 tsp. canola oil, divided
- 1 lb. bay scallops
- ½ lb. fresh snow peas, halved diagonally
- 2 medium leeks (white portion only), cut into 3x½-in. strips
- 1½ tsp. minced fresh gingerroot
- 3 cups hot cooked brown rice

1 Mix cornstarch, soy sauce and water. In a large nonstick skillet, heat 2 tsp. oil over medium-high heat; stir-fry scallops until firm and opaque, 1-2 minutes. Remove from pan.

2 In same pan, heat remaining oil over medium-high heat; stir-fry the snow peas, leeks and ginger until peas are just crisp-tender, 4-6 minutes. Stir cornstarch mixture; add to pan. Cook and stir until the sauce is thickened, about 1 minute. Add scallops; heat through. Serve with rice.

1 CUP STIR-FRY WITH ¾ CUP RICE
378 cal., 7g fat (1g sat. fat), 27mg chol., 750mg sod., 57g carb. (4g sugars, 5g fiber), 21g pro.

GENERAL TSO'S CAULIFLOWER

PREP: 25 min. **COOK:** 20 min. **MAKES:** 4 servings

Oil for deep-fat frying
½ cup all-purpose flour
½ cup cornstarch
1 tsp. salt
1 tsp. baking powder
¾ cup club soda
1 medium head cauliflower, cut into 1-in. florets (about 6 cups)

SAUCE
¼ cup orange juice
3 Tbsp. sugar
3 Tbsp. soy sauce
3 Tbsp. vegetable broth
2 Tbsp. rice vinegar
2 tsp. sesame oil
2 tsp. cornstarch
2 Tbsp. canola oil
2 to 6 dried pasilla or other hot chiles, chopped
3 green onions, white part minced, green part thinly sliced
3 garlic cloves, minced
1 tsp. grated fresh gingerroot
½ tsp. grated orange zest
4 cups hot cooked rice

1 In an electric skillet or deep fryer, heat oil to 375°. Combine flour, cornstarch, salt and baking powder. Stir in club soda just until blended (batter will be thin). Dip florets, a few at a time, into batter and fry until the cauliflower is tender and coating is light brown, 8-10 minutes. Drain on paper towels.

2 For sauce, whisk together first 6 ingredients; whisk in cornstarch until smooth.

3 In a large saucepan, heat canola oil over medium-high heat. Add the chiles; cook and stir until fragrant, 1-2 minutes. Add white part of onions, garlic, ginger and orange zest; cook until fragrant, about 1 minute. Stir soy sauce mixture; add to saucepan. Bring to a boil; cook and stir until thickened, 2-4 minutes.

4 Add cauliflower to sauce; toss to coat. Serve with rice; sprinkle with thinly sliced green onions.

1 CUP WITH 1 CUP RICE *584 cal., 17g fat (2g sat. fat), 0 chol., 1628mg sod., 97g carb. (17g sugars, 5g fiber), 11g pro.*

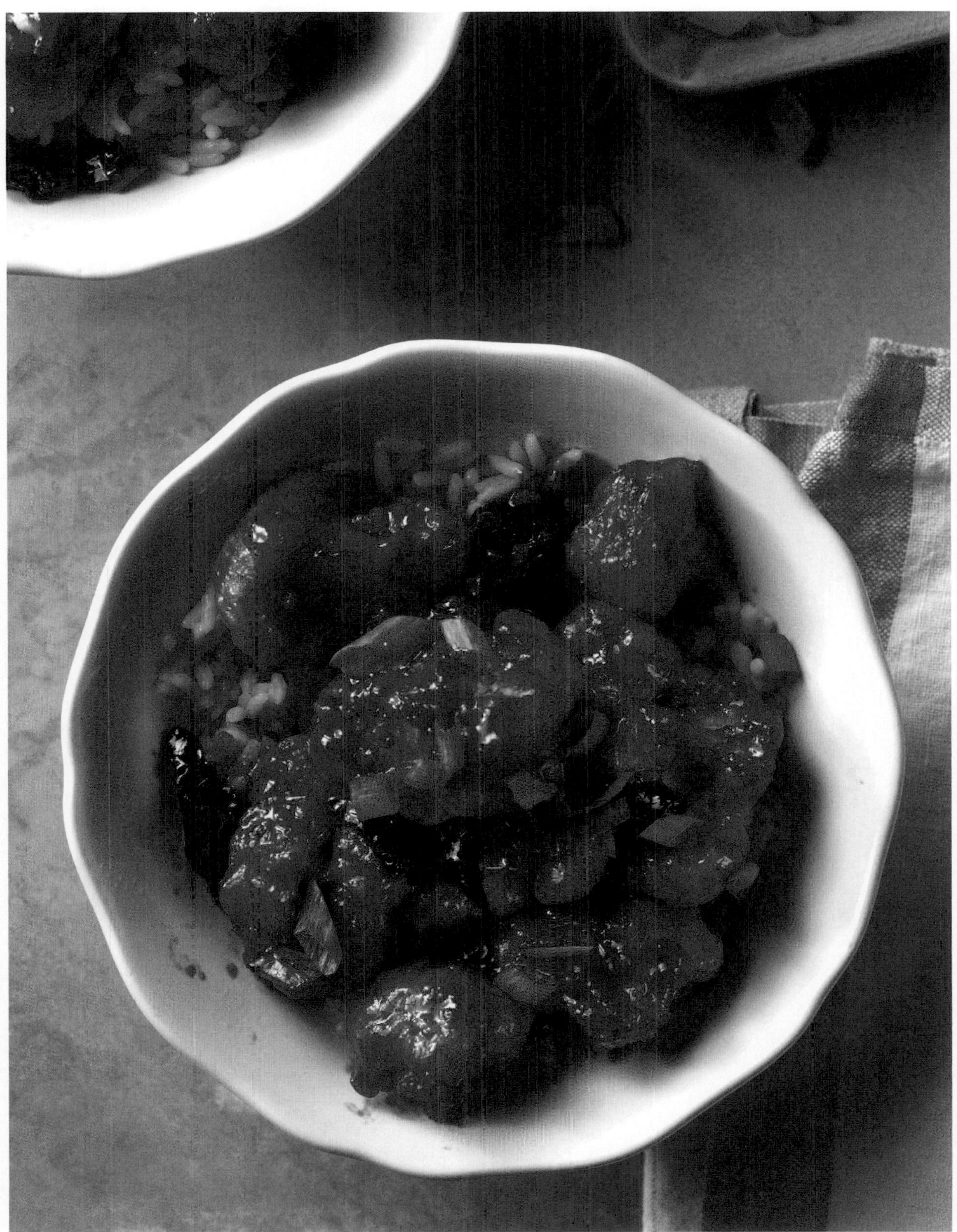

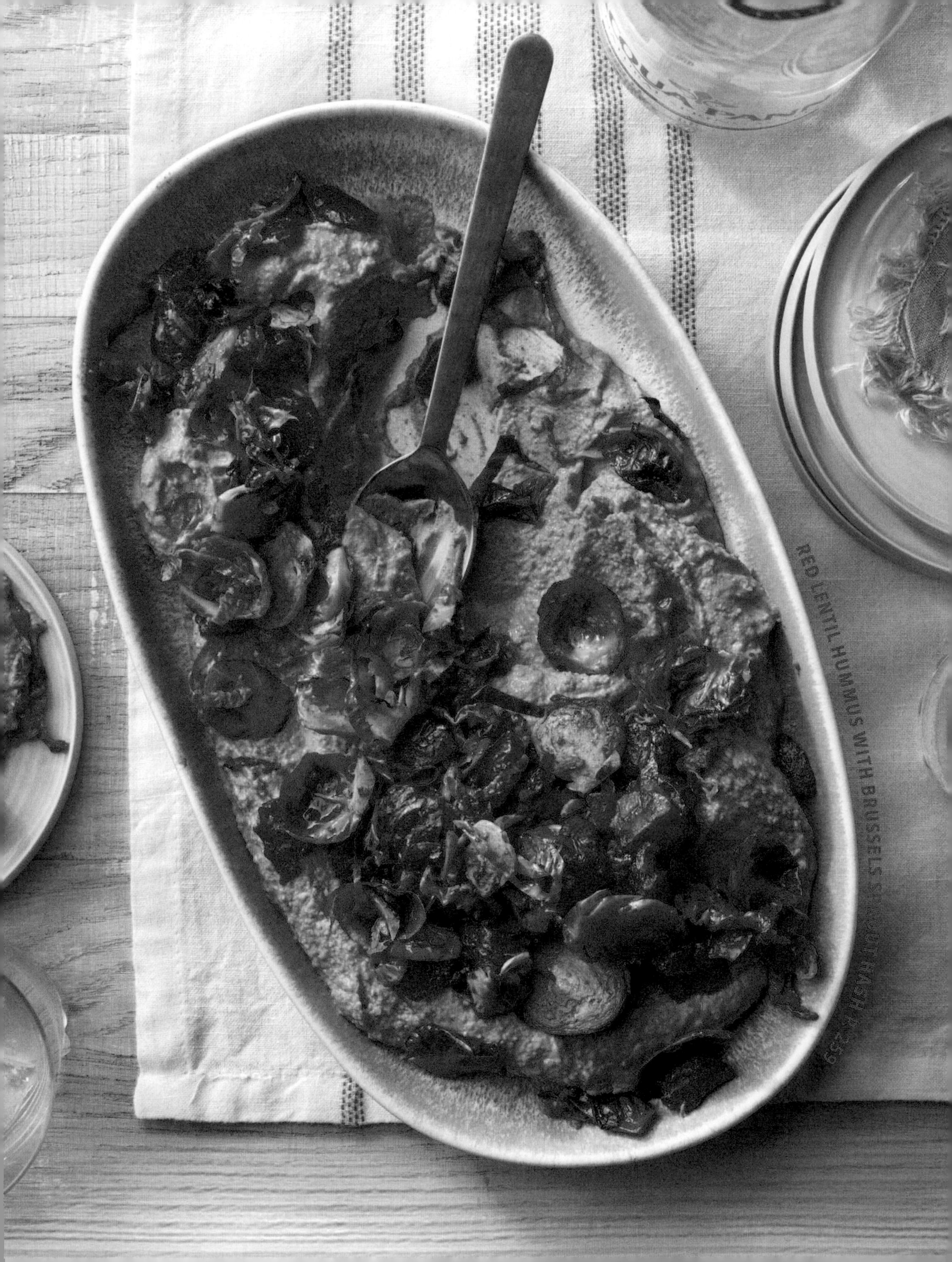

RED LENTIL HUMMUS WITH BRUSSELS SPROUT HASH P. 259

CHAPTER 12

STARTERS, SIDES & SNACKS

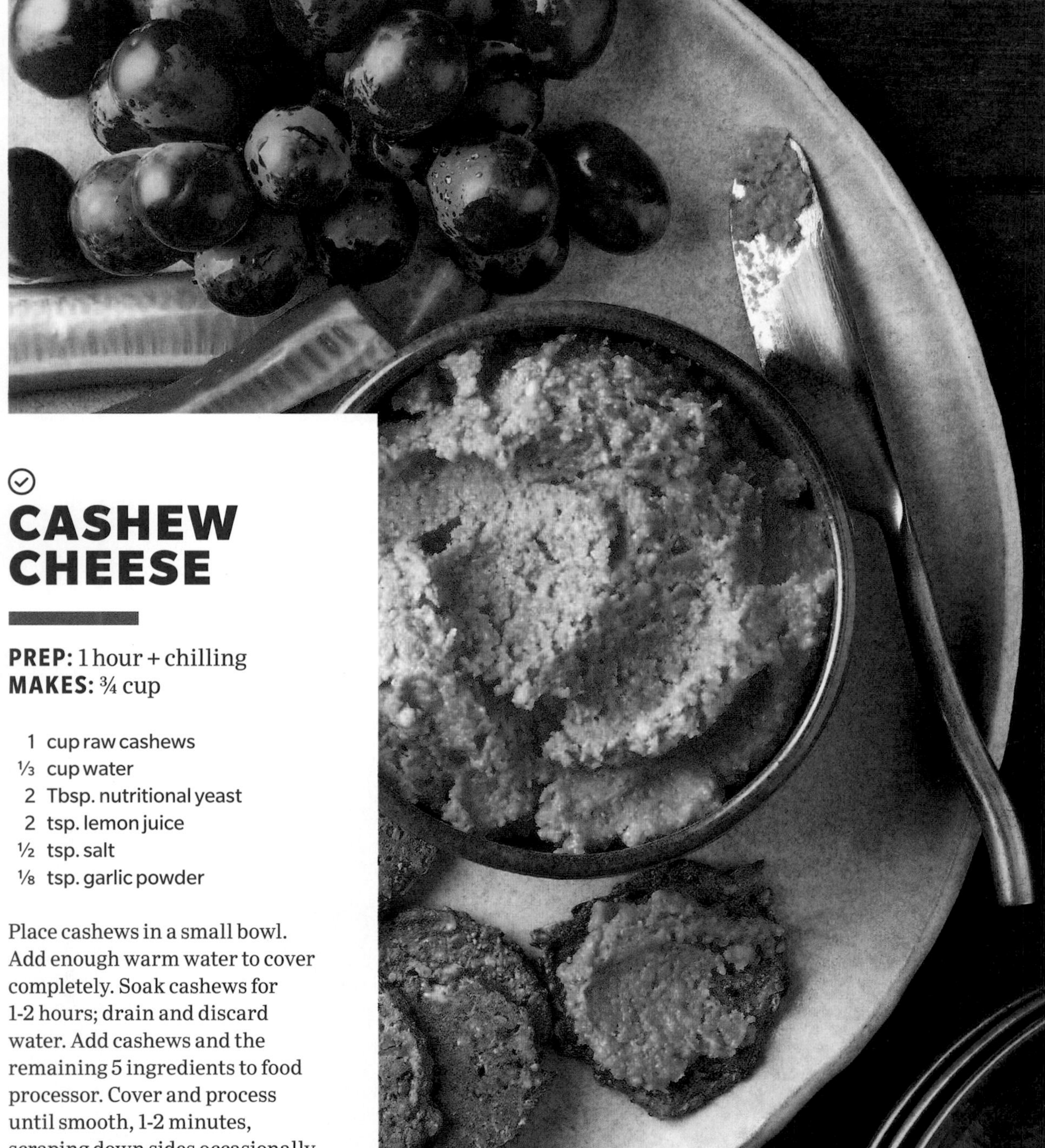

CASHEW CHEESE

PREP: 1 hour + chilling
MAKES: ¾ cup

- 1 cup raw cashews
- ⅓ cup water
- 2 Tbsp. nutritional yeast
- 2 tsp. lemon juice
- ½ tsp. salt
- ⅛ tsp. garlic powder

Place cashews in a small bowl. Add enough warm water to cover completely. Soak cashews for 1-2 hours; drain and discard water. Add cashews and the remaining 5 ingredients to food processor. Cover and process until smooth, 1-2 minutes, scraping down sides occasionally. Transfer to serving dish. Cover and refrigerate for at least 1 hour.

1 TBSP. *56 cal., 4g fat (1g sat. fat), 0 chol., 101mg sod., 3g carb. (1g sugars, 0 fiber), 2g pro.* ***Diabetic exchanges:*** *1 fat*

GARLIC PUMPKIN SEEDS

TAKES: 25 min.
MAKES: 2 cups

- 1 Tbsp. canola oil
- ½ tsp. celery salt
- ½ tsp. garlic powder
- ½ tsp. seasoned salt
- 2 cups fresh pumpkin seeds

1 In a small bowl, combine the oil, celery salt, garlic powder and seasoned salt. Add pumpkin seeds; toss to coat. Spread a quarter of the seeds in a single layer on a microwave-safe plate. Microwave, uncovered, on high for 1 minute; stir.

2 Microwave 2-3 minutes longer or until seeds are crunchy and lightly browned, stirring after each minute. Repeat with the remaining pumpkin seeds. Serve warm, or cool before storing in an airtight container.

¼ CUP *87 cal., 5g fat (1g sat. fat), 0 chol., 191mg sod., 9g carb. (0 sugars, 1g fiber), 3g pro.*
Diabetic exchanges: *1 fat, ½ starch*

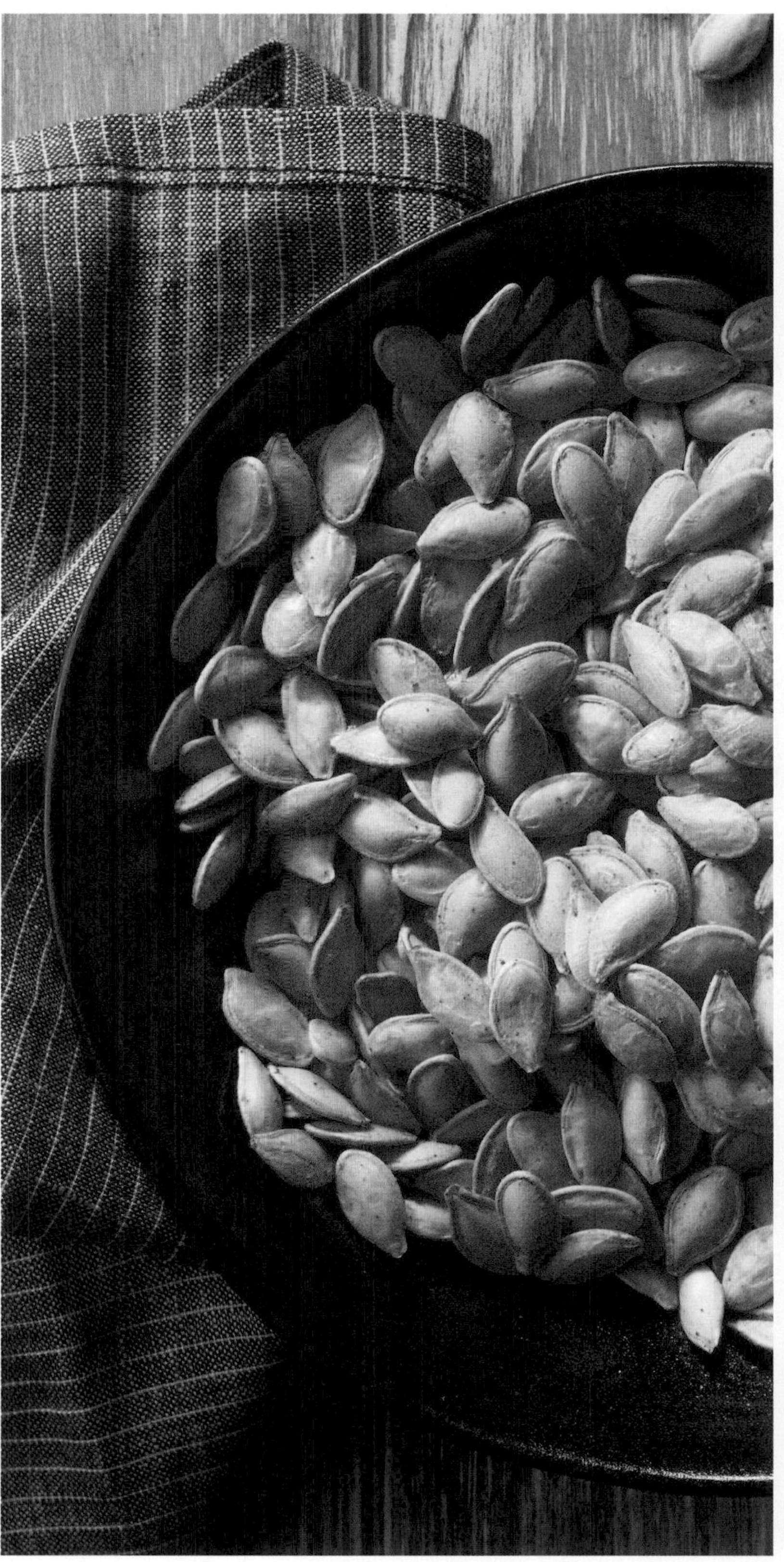

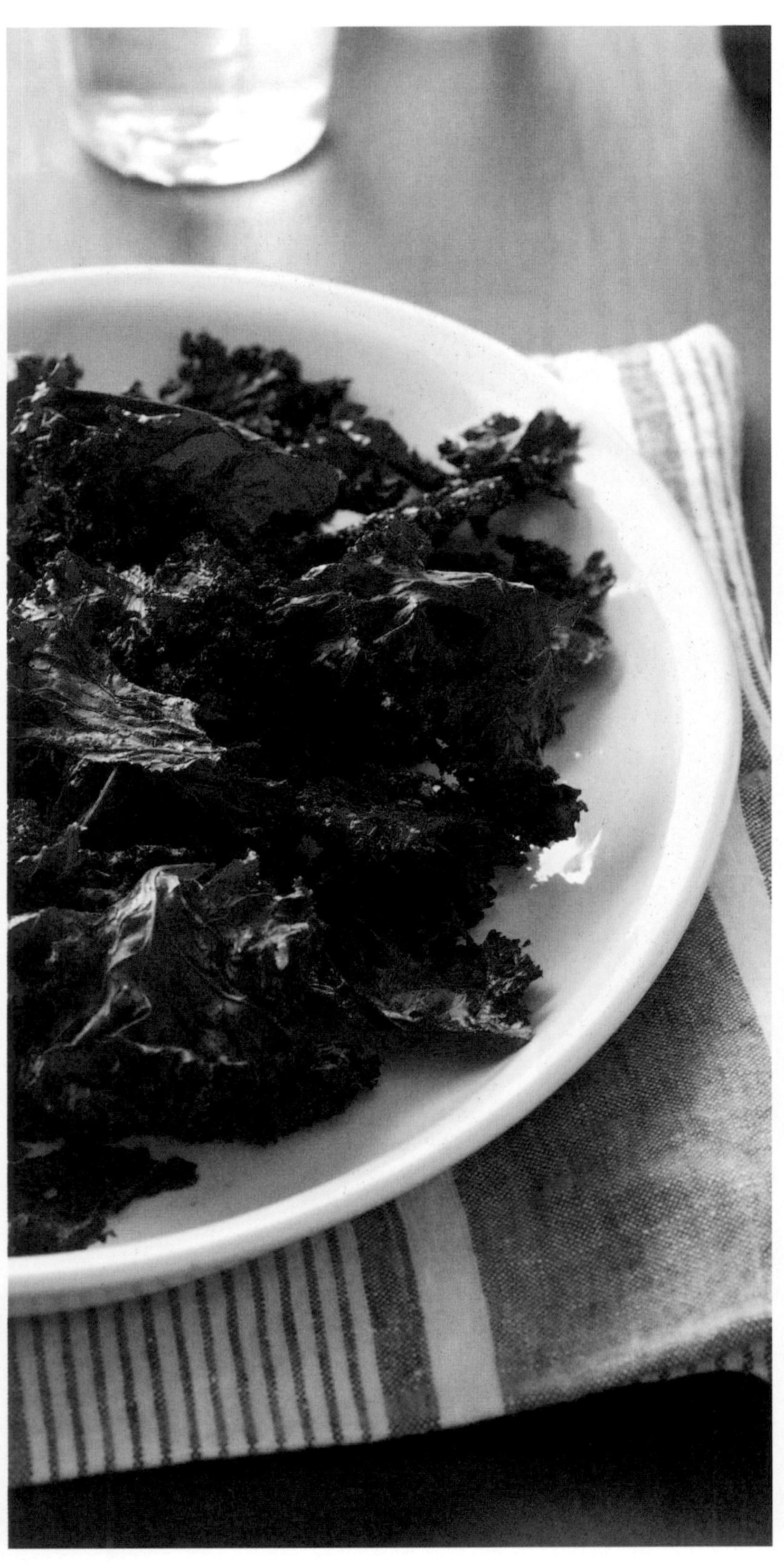

OLD BAY CRISPY KALE CHIPS

PREP: 10 min. **COOK:** 30 min.
MAKES: 4 servings

- 1 bunch kale, washed
- 2 Tbsp. olive oil
- 1 to 3 tsp. Old Bay Seasoning
- Sea salt, to taste

1 Preheat oven to 300°. Remove tough stems from kale and tear leaves into large pieces. Place in a large bowl. Toss with olive oil and seasonings. Arrange leaves in a single layer on greased baking sheets.

2 Bake, uncovered, 10 minutes, and then rotate pans. Continue baking until crisp and just starting to brown, about 15 minutes longer. Let stand at least 5 minutes before serving.

1 SERVING *101 cal., 7g fat (1g sat. fat), 0 chol., 202mg sod., 8g carb. (0 sugars, 2g fiber), 3g pro.* ***Diabetic exchanges:*** *1½ fat, 1 vegetable*

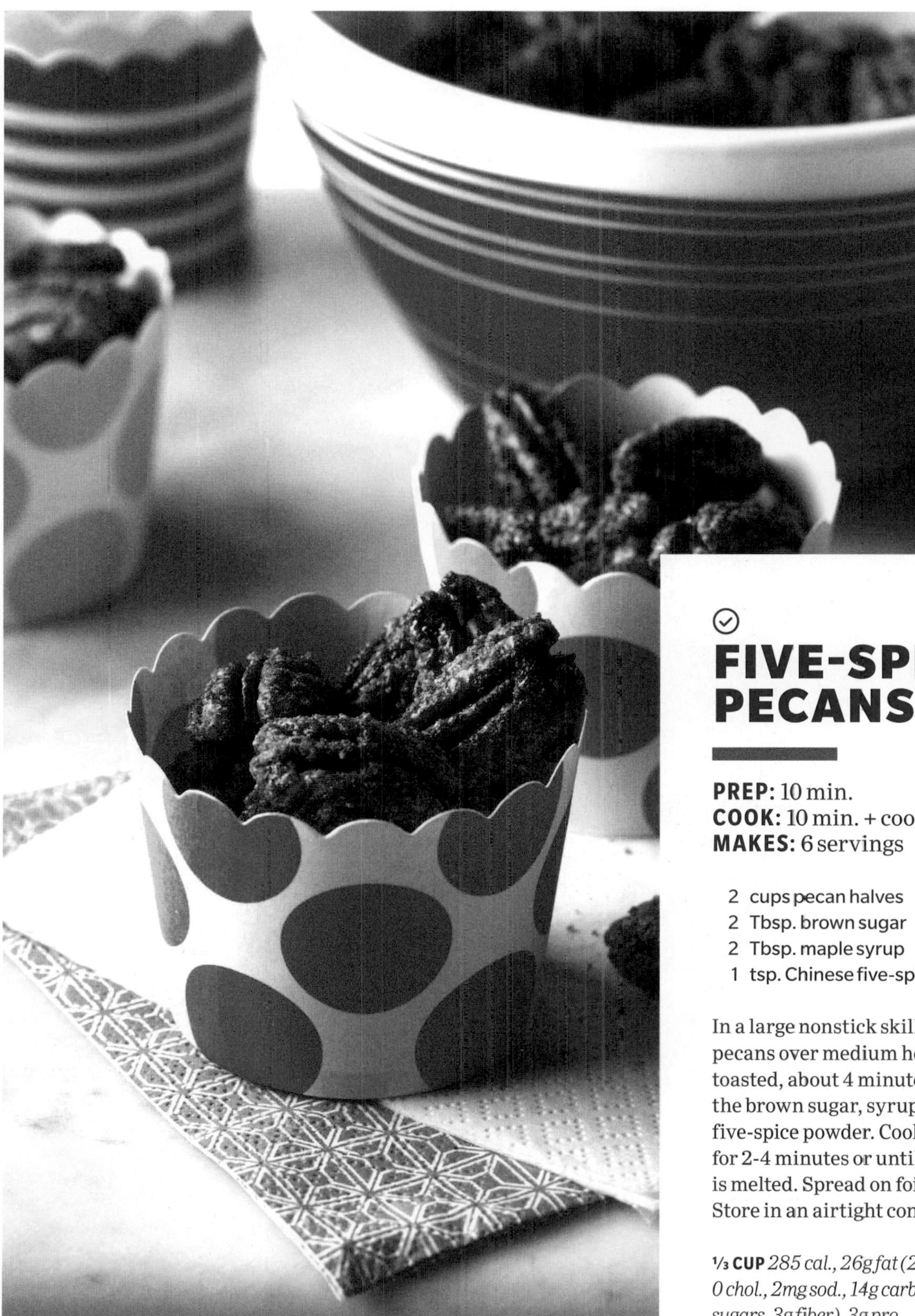

FIVE-SPICE PECANS

PREP: 10 min.
COOK: 10 min. + cooling
MAKES: 6 servings

2 cups pecan halves
2 Tbsp. brown sugar
2 Tbsp. maple syrup
1 tsp. Chinese five-spice powder

In a large nonstick skillet, cook pecans over medium heat until toasted, about 4 minutes. Add the brown sugar, syrup and five-spice powder. Cook and stir for 2-4 minutes or until sugar is melted. Spread on foil to cool. Store in an airtight container.

1/3 CUP *285 cal., 26g fat (2g sat. fat), 0 chol., 2mg sod., 14g carb. (10g sugars, 3g fiber), 3g pro.*

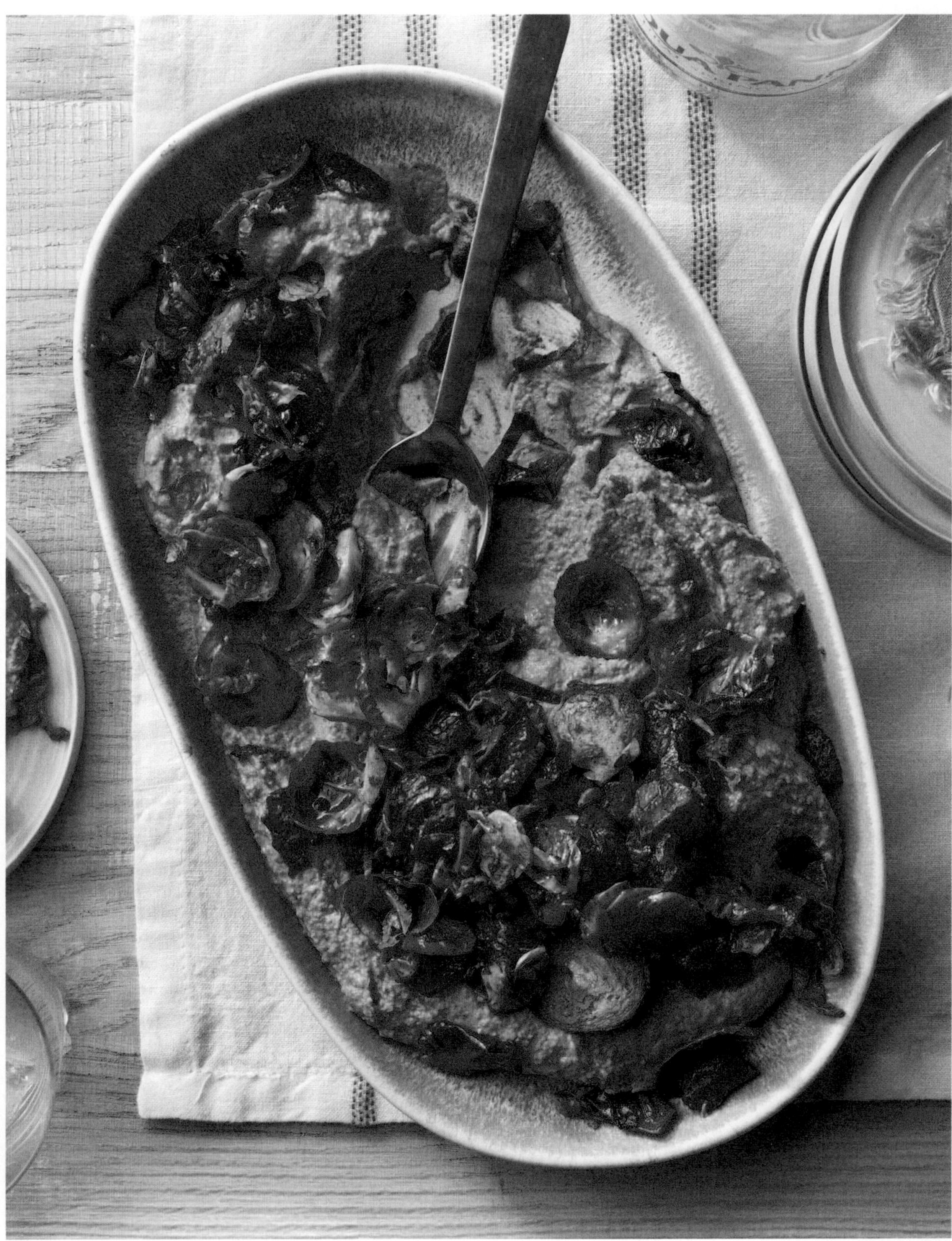

RED LENTIL HUMMUS WITH BRUSSELS SPROUT HASH

PREP: 20 min. **COOK:** 15 min. **MAKES:** 10 servings

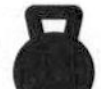

- 1 cup dried red lentils, rinsed
- ¼ cup tahini
- 2 Tbsp. lemon juice
- 1 Tbsp. olive oil
- 3 garlic cloves, halved
- 1 tsp. ground cumin
- 1 tsp. curry powder
- ½ tsp. salt
- ½ tsp. ground ginger
- ⅛ tsp. white pepper
- ⅛ tsp. cayenne pepper

BRUSSELS SPROUT HASH

- 1 Tbsp. olive oil
- 1 shallot, minced
- ½ lb. fresh Brussels sprouts, thinly sliced
- 1 cup canned diced tomatoes
- ¼ tsp. salt
- ¼ tsp. crushed red pepper flakes
- Assorted fresh vegetables

1 Place the lentils in a small saucepan; add water to cover. Bring to a boil; reduce heat. Simmer, covered, until lentils are tender, 12-15 minutes. Drain; cool for 10 minutes. Transfer to a food processor. Add tahini, lemon juice, oil, garlic and seasonings. Process until smooth.

2 For hash, in a large skillet, heat oil over medium heat. Add shallot; cook and stir until tender, 3-4 minutes. Add the Brussels sprouts and tomatoes; cook until sprouts are crisp-tender, 12-15 minutes longer. Remove from heat; stir in salt and red pepper flakes.

3 Spread hummus on a serving plate; top with hash. Serve with vegetables.

1 SERVING *154 cal., 7g fat (1g sat. fat), 0 chol., 226mg sod., 18g carb. (2g sugars, 4g fiber), 7g pro.* ***Diabetic exchanges:*** *1½ fat, 1 starch*

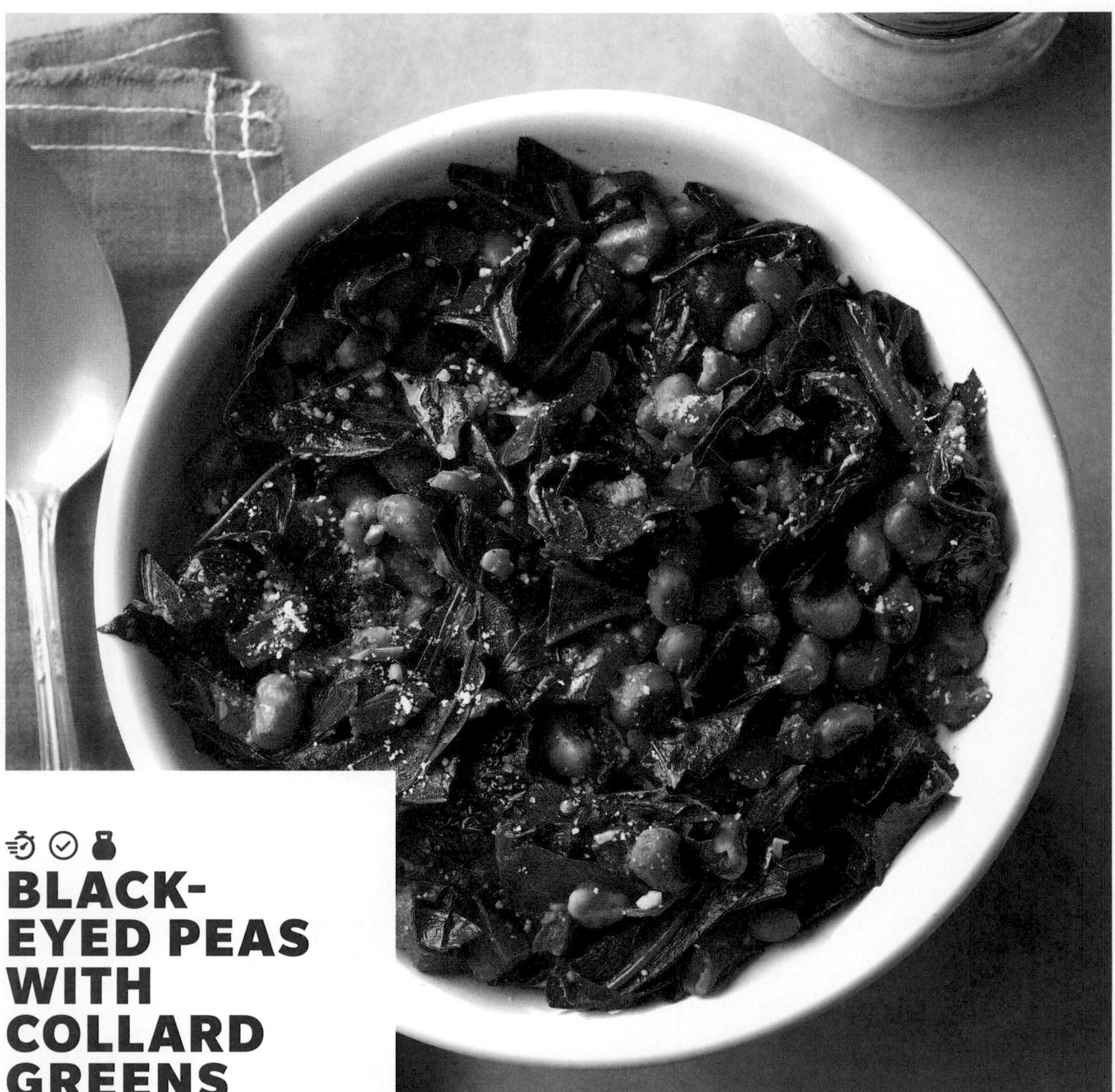

BLACK-EYED PEAS WITH COLLARD GREENS

TAKES: 25 min.
MAKES: 6 servings

- 2 Tbsp. olive oil
- 1 garlic clove, minced
- 8 cups chopped collard greens
- ½ tsp. salt
- ¼ tsp. cayenne pepper
- 2 cans (15½ oz. each) black-eyed peas, rinsed and drained
- 4 plum tomatoes, seeded and chopped
- ¼ cup lemon juice
- 2 Tbsp. grated Parmesan or vegan Parmesan-style cheese

In a Dutch oven, heat oil over medium heat. Add garlic; cook and stir 1 minute. Add collard greens, salt and cayenne; cook and stir 6-8 minutes or until greens are tender. Add peas, tomatoes and lemon juice; heat through. Sprinkle with cheese.

¾ CUP *177 cal., 5g fat (1g sat. fat), 1mg chol., 412mg sod., 24g carb. (3g sugars, 6g fiber), 9g pro.*

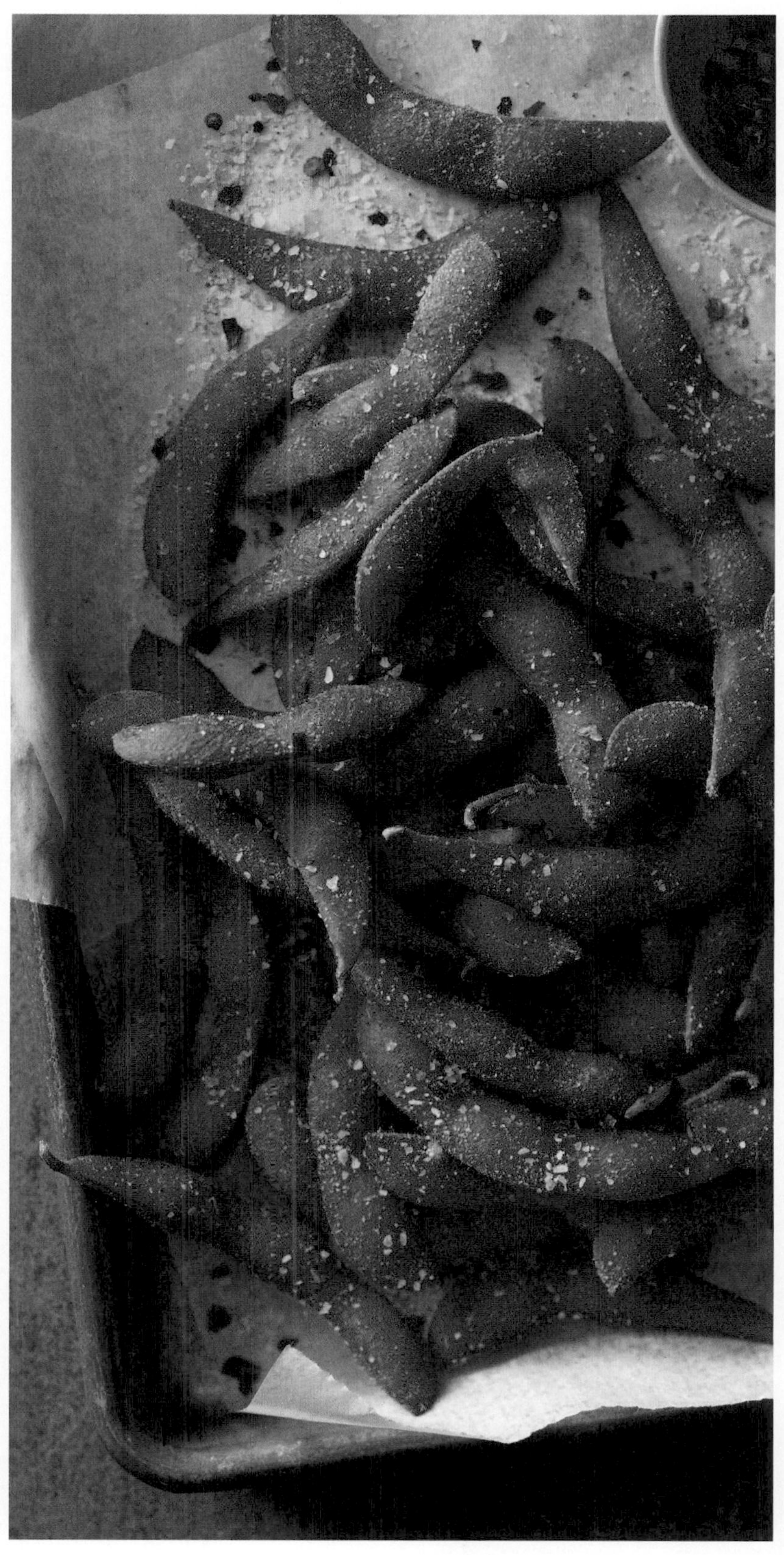

SPICY EDAMAME

TAKES: 20 min.
MAKES: 6 servings

- 1 pkg. (16 oz.) frozen edamame pods
- 2 tsp. kosher salt
- ¾ tsp. ground ginger
- ½ tsp. garlic powder
- ¼ tsp. crushed red pepper flakes

Place the edamame in a large saucepan and cover with water. Bring to a boil. Cover and cook until tender, 4-5 minutes; drain. Transfer to a large bowl. Add the seasonings; toss to coat.

1 SERVING *52 cal., 2g fat (0 sat. fat), 0 chol., 642mg sod., 5g carb. (1g sugars, 2g fiber), 4g pro.*

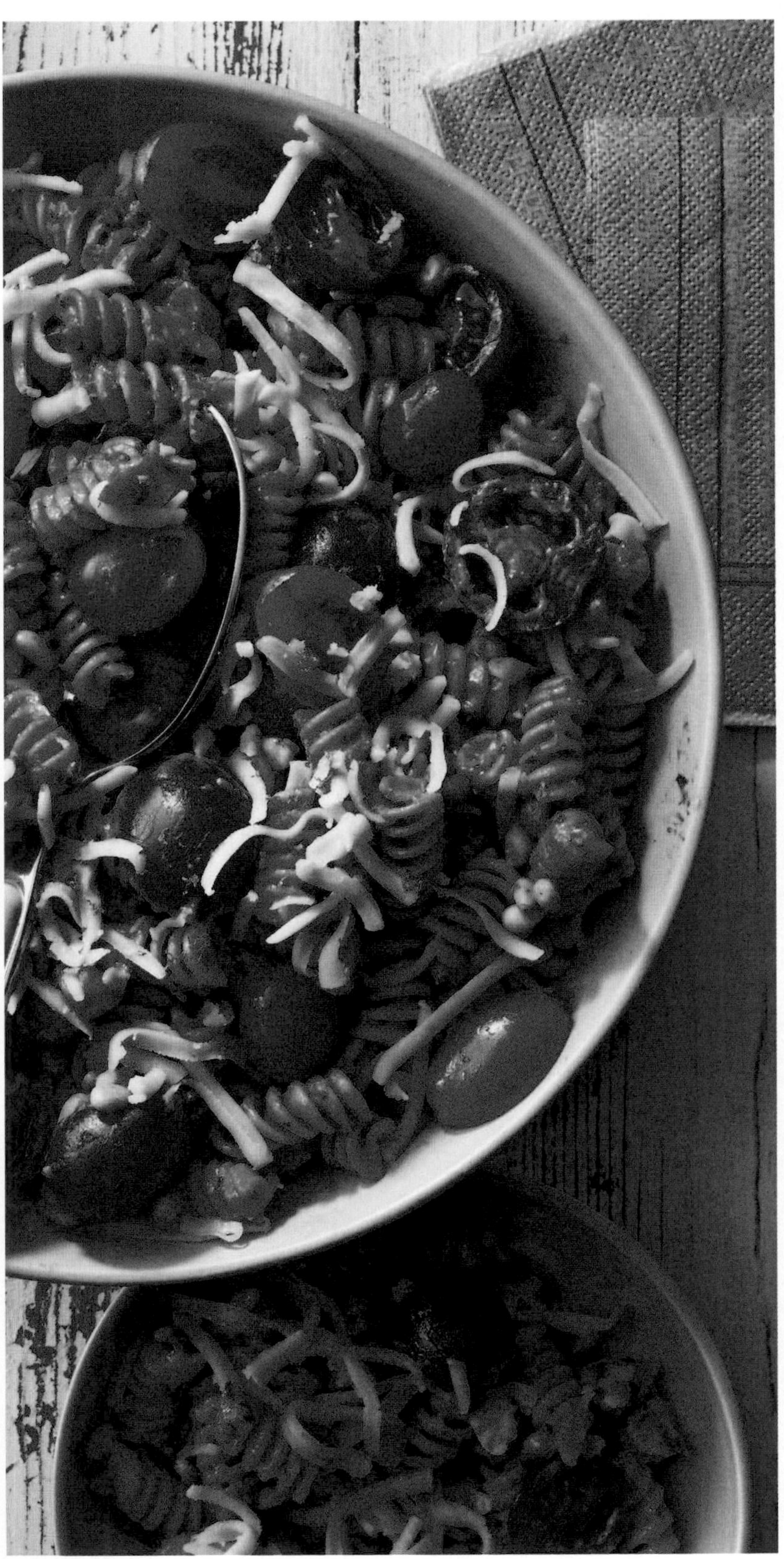

PASTA WITH AVOCADO SAUCE

TAKES: 30 min.
MAKES: 10 servings

- 1 pkg. (14½ oz.) protein-enriched rotini (about 3½ cups uncooked)
- 2 medium ripe avocados, peeled and pitted
- 1 cup fresh spinach
- ¼ cup loosely packed basil leaves
- 2 garlic cloves, halved
- 2 Tbsp. lime juice
- ½ tsp. kosher salt
- ¼ tsp. coarsely ground pepper
- ⅓ cup olive oil
- 1 cup cherry tomatoes, halved
- ½ cup pine nuts
- Optional toppings: Shredded vegan Parmesan-style cheese, shredded vegan mozzarella-style cheese and grated lime zest

1 Cook the rotini according to package directions for al dente. Meanwhile, place avocados, spinach, basil, garlic, lime juice, salt and pepper in a food processor; pulse until chopped. Continue processing while adding oil in a steady stream.

2 Drain the rotini; transfer to a large bowl. Add avocado mixture and tomatoes; toss to coat. Top with pine nuts and toppings of your choice.

¾ CUP *314 cal., 18g fat (2g sat. fat), 0 chol., 125mg sod., 32g carb. (2g sugars, 5g fiber), 9g pro.*

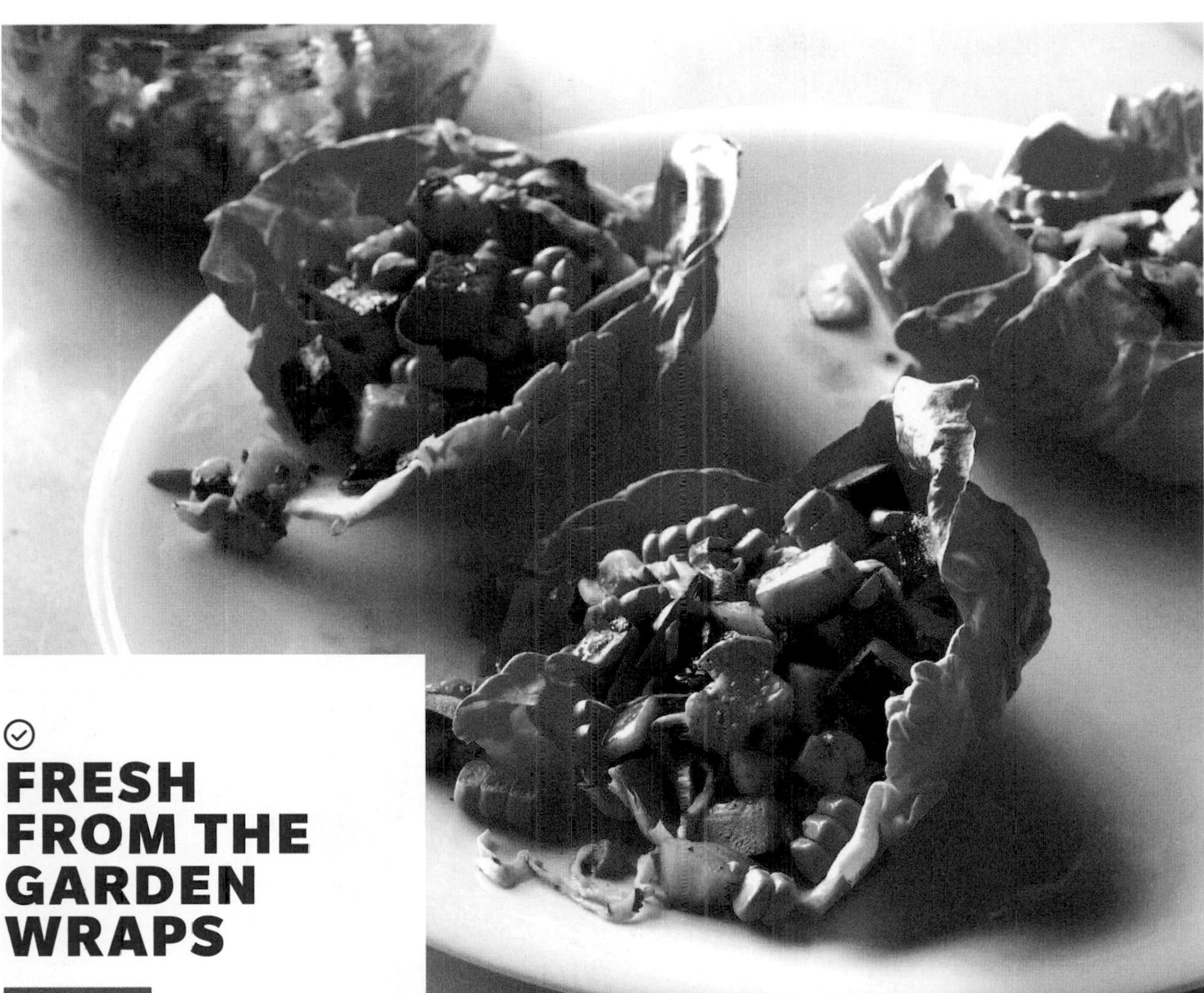

FRESH FROM THE GARDEN WRAPS

PREP: 20 min. + standing
MAKES: 8 servings

- 1 medium ear sweet corn
- 1 medium cucumber, chopped
- 1 cup shredded cabbage
- 1 medium tomato, chopped
- 1 small red onion, chopped
- 1 jalapeno pepper, seeded and minced
- 1 Tbsp. minced fresh basil
- 1 Tbsp. minced fresh cilantro
- 1 Tbsp. minced fresh mint
- ⅓ cup Thai chili sauce
- 3 Tbsp. rice vinegar
- 2 tsp. reduced-sodium soy sauce
- 2 tsp. creamy peanut butter
- 8 Bibb or Boston lettuce leaves

1 Cut corn from cob and place in a large bowl. Add cucumber, cabbage, tomato, onion, jalapeno and herbs.

2 Whisk together chili sauce, vinegar, soy sauce and peanut butter. Pour over vegetable mixture; toss to coat. Let stand 20 minutes.

3 Using a slotted spoon, place ½ cup salad in each lettuce leaf. Fold lettuce over filling.

1 FILLED LETTUCE WRAP *64 cal., 1g fat (0 sat. fat), 0 chol., 319mg sod., 13g carb. (10g sugars, 2g fiber), 2g pro.* ***Diabetic exchanges:*** *1 vegetable, ½ starch.*

NOTE *Wear disposable gloves when cutting hot peppers; the oils can burn skin. Avoid touching your face.*

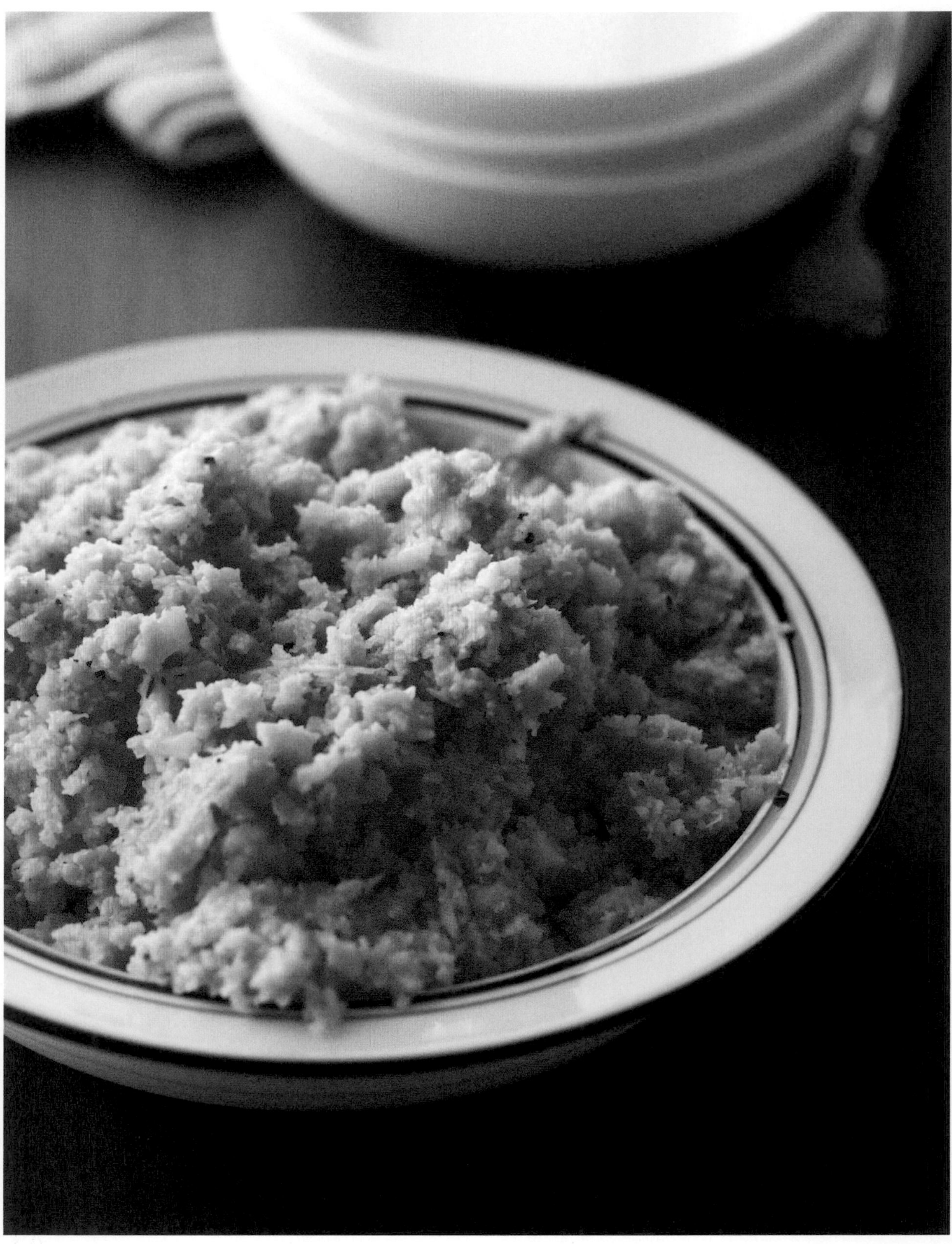

GARLIC ASIAGO CAULIFLOWER RICE

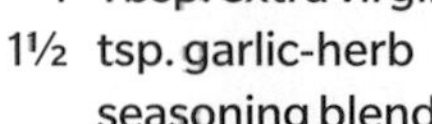

TAKES: 20 min. **MAKES:** 6 servings

- 1 medium head cauliflower
- 2 Tbsp. unsalted dairy or vegan butter
- 1 Tbsp. extra virgin olive oil
- 1½ tsp. garlic-herb seasoning blend
- ½ cup finely grated Asiago or vegan Asiago-style cheese

1 Using a box grater or a food processor fitted with the steel blade, finely shred cauliflower (about 6 cups).

2 In a large cast-iron or other heavy skillet, heat the butter, oil and seasoning blend over medium-high heat. When butter is melted, stir in cauliflower, working in batches if necessary. Cook, uncovered, until tender, 10-15 minutes, stirring occasionally. Stir in cheese.

⅔ CUP *112 cal., 9g fat (4g sat. fat), 18mg chol., 103mg sod., 5g carb. (2g sugars, 2g fiber), 4g pro.* ***Diabetic exchanges:*** *2 fat, 1 vegetable*

STICKY SESAME CAULIFLOWER

PREP: 40 min. **BAKE:** 25 min. **MAKES:** 12 servings

- 1 cup dry bread crumbs
- ½ cup cornmeal
- 2 Tbsp. all-purpose flour
- ½ tsp. salt
- ½ tsp. garlic powder
- ½ tsp. pepper

BATTER

- 1 cup all-purpose flour
- 1 Tbsp. adobo seasoning
- 1 tsp. garlic powder
- ½ tsp. salt
- ½ tsp. pepper
- 1 bottle (12 oz.) beer
- 1 large head cauliflower, broken into florets (about 8 cups)
- 1 Tbsp. peanut oil

SAUCE

- ¼ cup orange juice
- ¼ cup sweet chili sauce
- ¼ cup island teriyaki sauce
- 2 Tbsp. sesame oil
- 1 tsp. soy sauce
- ½ tsp. rice vinegar
- ½ tsp. Sriracha chili sauce
- Optional toppings: Thinly sliced green onions, grated orange zest and sesame seeds

1 Preheat oven to 400°. In a shallow bowl, combine the first 6 ingredients. For batter, in a large bowl, mix flour, adobo seasoning, garlic powder, salt and pepper; whisk in beer until smooth. Dip cauliflower in batter, then in bread crumb mixture. Place on a greased baking sheet. Drizzle with peanut oil; gently toss to coat. Bake until golden brown and cauliflower is just tender, 25-30 minutes.

2 Meanwhile, for sauce, in a small saucepan, combine orange juice, chili sauce, teriyaki sauce, sesame oil, soy sauce, vinegar and Sriracha chili sauce. Cook and stir over low heat just until warmed, about 5 minutes.

3 Transfer cauliflower to a large bowl. Drizzle with sauce; gently toss to coat. Serve with toppings of your choice.

⅔ CUP *140 cal., 4g fat (1g sat. fat), 0 chol., 714mg sod., 23g carb. (8g sugars, 2g fiber), 4g pro.*

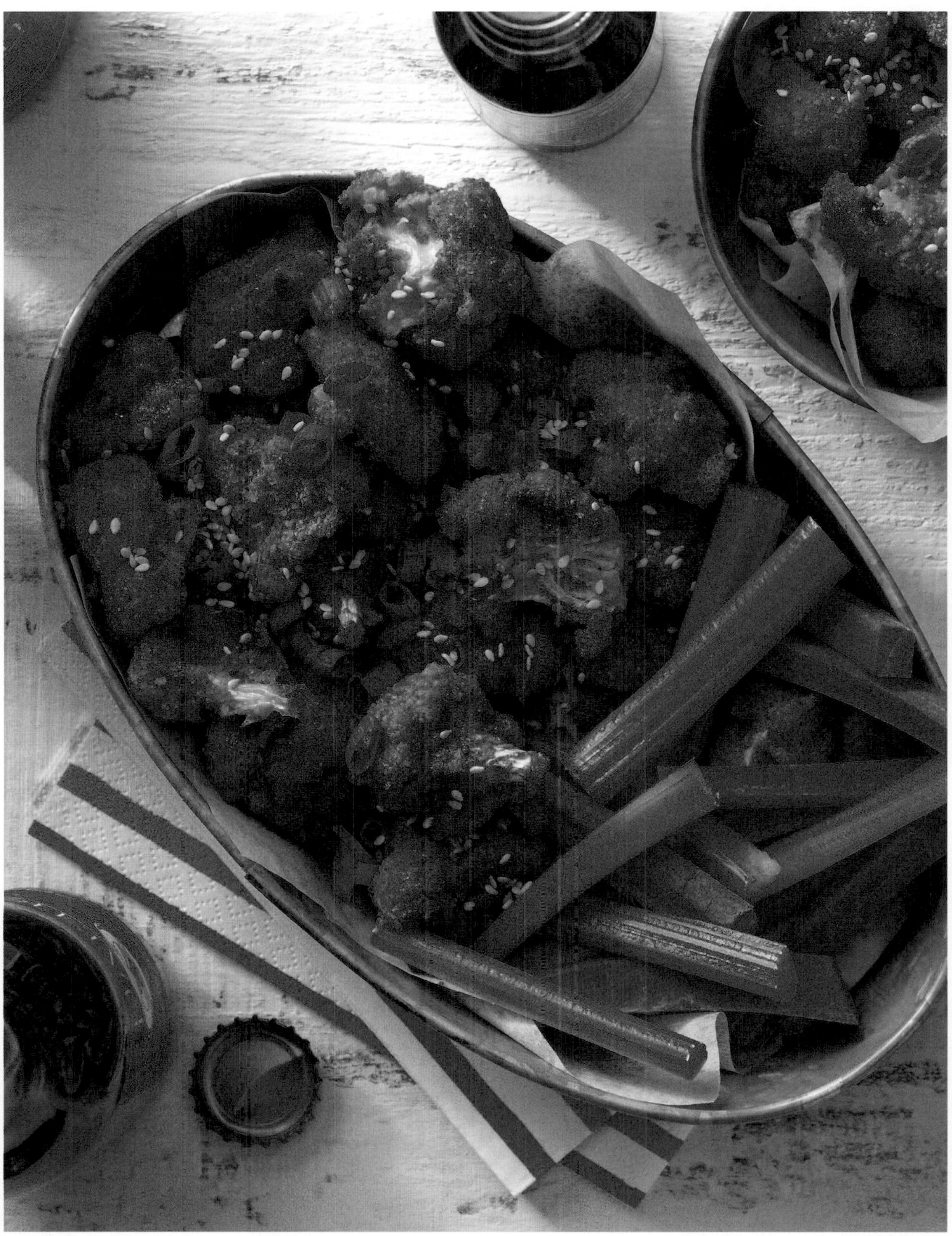

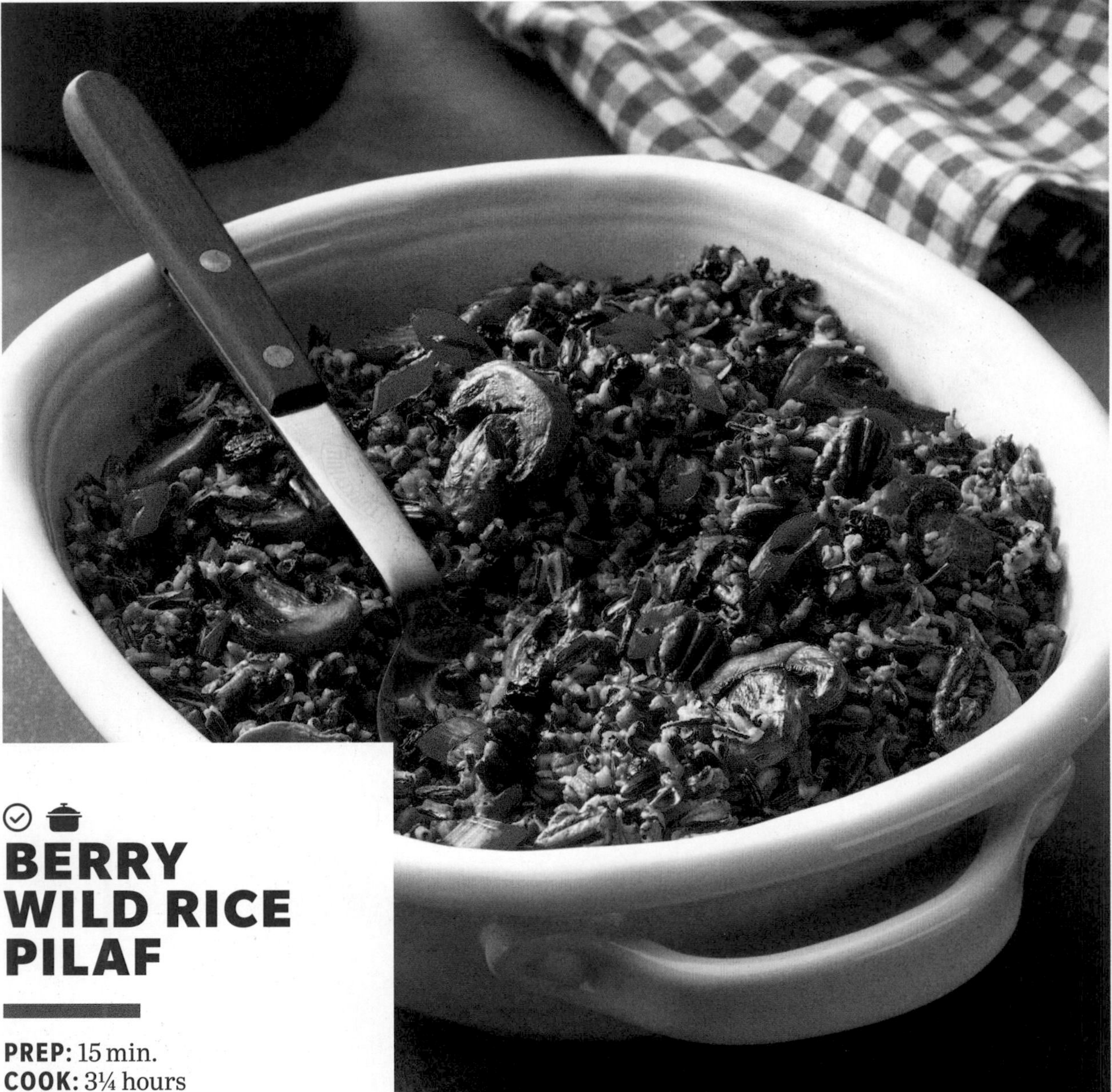

BERRY WILD RICE PILAF

PREP: 15 min.
COOK: 3¼ hours
MAKES: 16 servings

- 2 Tbsp. dairy or vegan butter
- 8 oz. sliced fresh mushrooms
- 3 cups uncooked wild rice
- 8 green onions, sliced
- 1 tsp. salt
- ½ tsp. pepper
- 4 cans (14½ oz. each) vegetable broth
- 1 cup chopped pecans, toasted
- 1 cup dried blueberries

In a large skillet, heat butter over medium heat. Add mushrooms; cook and stir 4-5 minutes or until tender. In a 5-qt. slow cooker, combine rice, mushrooms, onions, salt and pepper. Pour broth over rice mixture. Cook, covered, on low 3-4 hours or until rice is tender. Stir in pecans and blueberries. Cook, covered, 15 minutes longer or until heated through. If desired, top with additional green onions.

¾ CUP *199 cal., 7g fat (1g sat. fat), 4mg chol., 163mg sod., 31g carb. (5g sugars, 4g fiber), 6g pro.* ***Diabetic exchanges:*** *2 starch, 1½ fat*

VEGETABLE BARLEY SAUTE

TAKES: 30 min.
MAKES: 4 servings

- ½ cup quick-cooking barley
- ⅓ cup water
- 3 Tbsp. reduced-sodium soy sauce
- 2 tsp. cornstarch
- 1 garlic clove, minced
- 1 Tbsp. canola oil
- 2 carrots, thinly sliced
- 1 cup cut fresh green beans (2-in. pieces)
- 2 green onions, sliced
- ½ cup unsalted cashews, optional

1 Prepare barley according to package directions. In a small bowl, combine water, soy sauce and cornstarch until smooth; set aside.

2 In a large skillet or wok, saute garlic in oil for 15 seconds. Add carrots and beans; stir-fry for 2 minutes. Add onions; stir-fry 1 minute longer. Stir soy sauce mixture; stir into skillet. Bring to a boil; cook and stir until thickened, about 1 minute. Add barley; heat through. If desired, stir in cashews.

⅔ CUP *148 cal., 4g fat (1g sat. fat), 0 chol., 458mg sod., 24g carb. (3g sugars, 6g fiber), 5g pro.* ***Diabetic exchanges:*** *1½ starch, 1 fat*

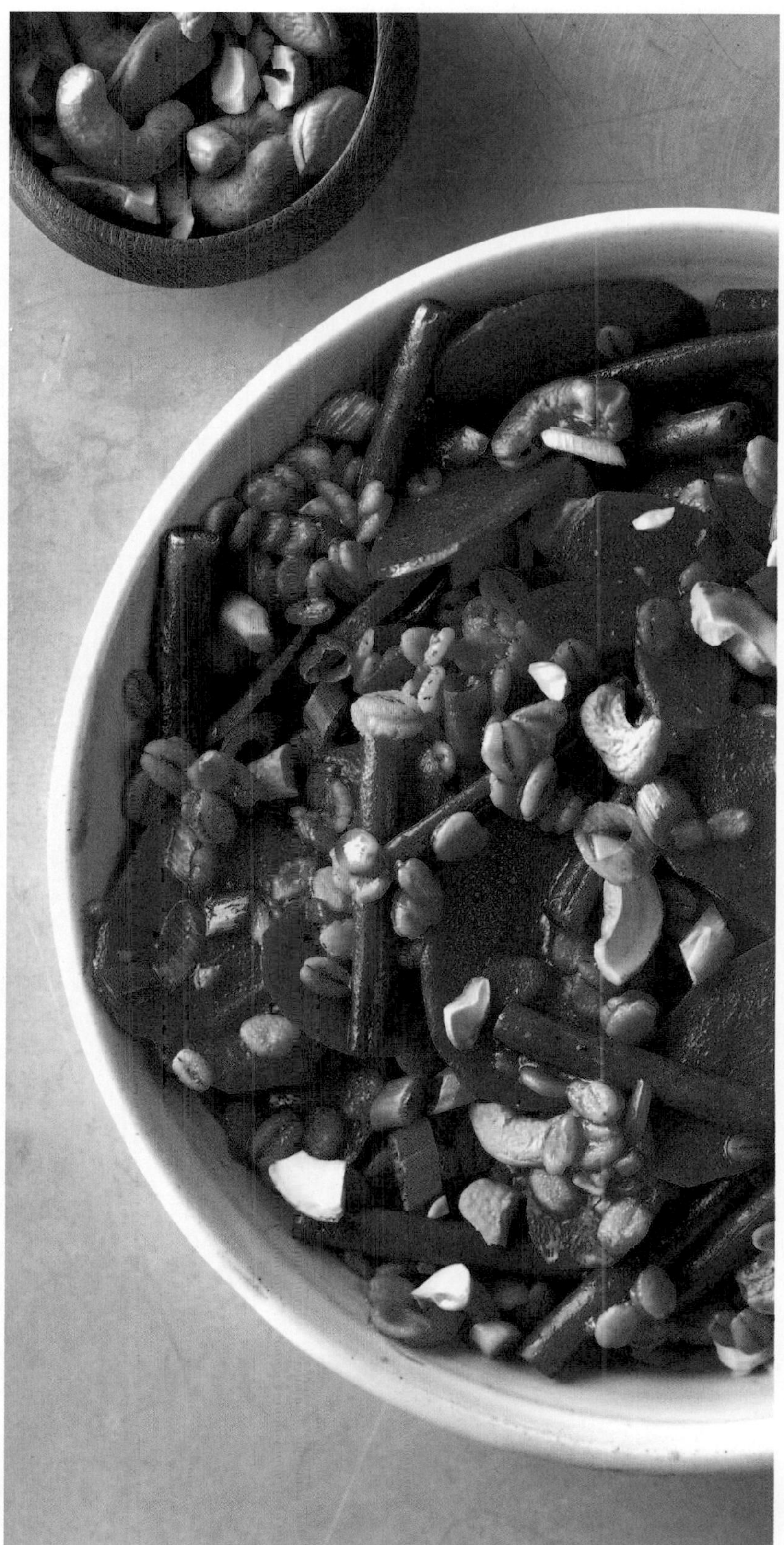

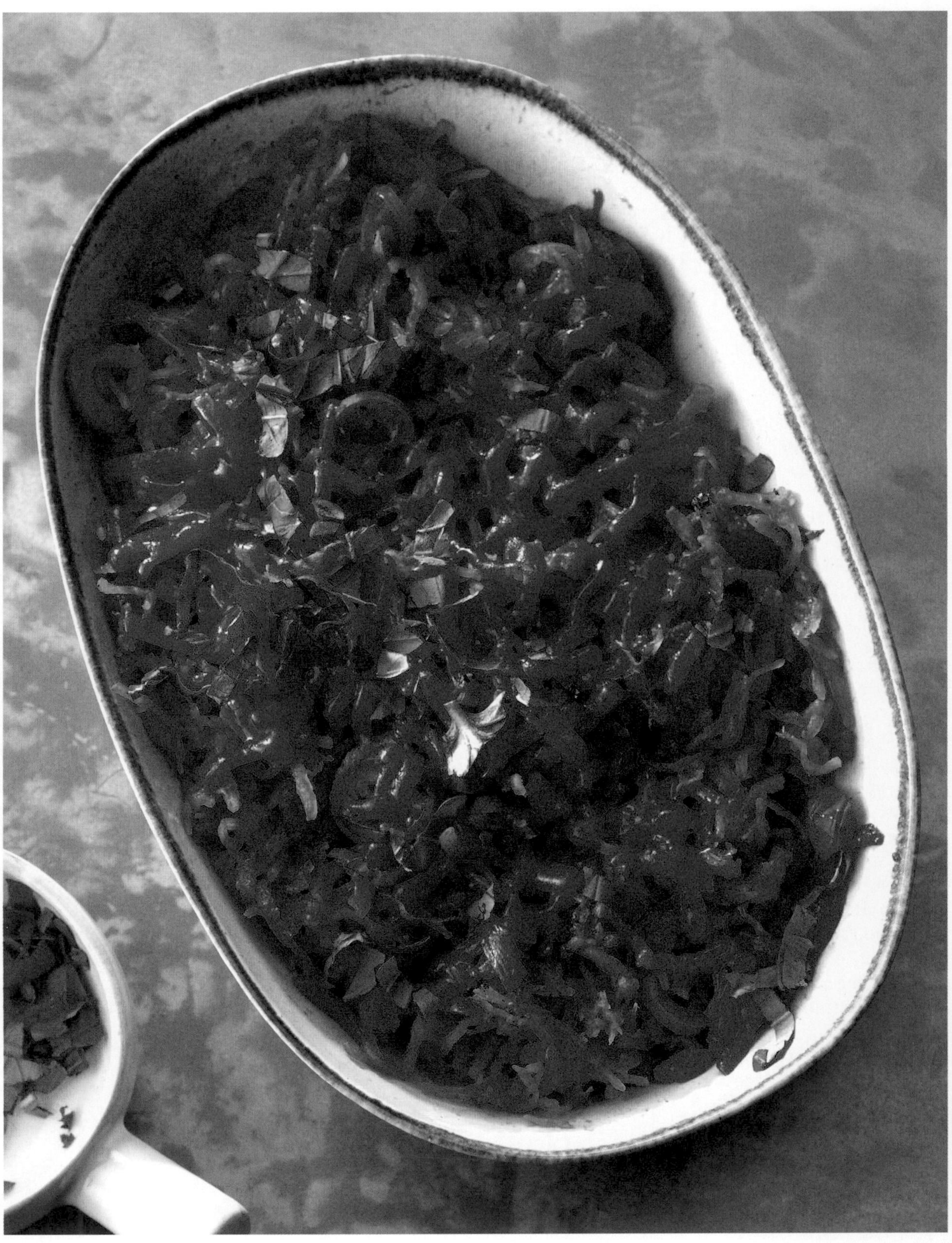

PRESSURE-COOKER SPAGHETTI SQUASH WITH TOMATOES

PREP: 15 min. **COOK:** 10 min. **MAKES:** 10 servings

- 1 medium spaghetti squash, halved lengthwise, seeds removed
- 1 can (14 oz.) diced tomatoes, drained
- ¼ cup sliced green olives with pimientos
- 1 tsp. dried oregano
- ½ tsp. salt
- ½ tsp. pepper
- ½ cup shredded cheddar or vegan cheddar-style cheese
- ¼ cup minced fresh basil

1 Place trivet insert and 1 cup water in a 6-qt. electric pressure cooker. Set the squash on trivet, overlapping as needed to fit. Lock lid; close pressure-release valve. Adjust to pressure-cook on high for 7 minutes. Quick-release the pressure.

2 Remove squash and trivet from pressure cooker; drain cooking liquid from pressure cooker. Using a fork, separate squash into strands resembling spaghetti; discard the skin. Return squash to pressure cooker. Stir in tomatoes, olives, oregano, salt and pepper. Select saute setting and adjust for low heat. Cook and stir until heated through, about 3 minutes. Top with cheese and basil.

¾ CUP *92 cal., 3g fat (1g sat. fat), 6mg chol., 296mg sod., 15g carb. (1g sugars, 4g fiber), 3g pro.* ***Diabetic exchanges:*** *1 starch, ½ fat*

SLOW-COOKER RATATOUILLE

PREP: 20 min. + standing **COOK:** 3 hours **MAKES:** 10 servings

- 1 large eggplant, peeled and cut into 1-in. cubes
- 2 tsp. salt, divided
- 3 medium tomatoes, chopped
- 3 medium zucchini, halved lengthwise and sliced
- 2 medium onions, chopped
- 1 large green pepper, chopped
- 1 large sweet yellow pepper, chopped
- 1 can (6 oz.) pitted ripe olives, drained and chopped
- 1 can (6 oz.) tomato paste
- ½ cup minced fresh basil
- 2 garlic cloves, minced
- ½ tsp. pepper
- 2 Tbsp. olive oil

1 Place eggplant in a colander over a plate; sprinkle with 1 tsp. salt and toss. Let eggplant stand for 30 minutes. Rinse and drain well. Transfer to a 5-qt. slow cooker coated with cooking spray.

2 Stir in tomatoes, zucchini, onions, green and yellow peppers, olives, tomato paste, basil, garlic, pepper and the remaining salt. Drizzle with oil. Cover and cook on high until vegetables are tender, 3-4 hours.

¾ CUP *116 cal., 5g fat (1g sat. fat), 0 chol., 468mg sod., 18g carb. (10g sugars, 6g fiber), 3g pro.* ***Diabetic exchanges:*** *1 starch, 1 fat*

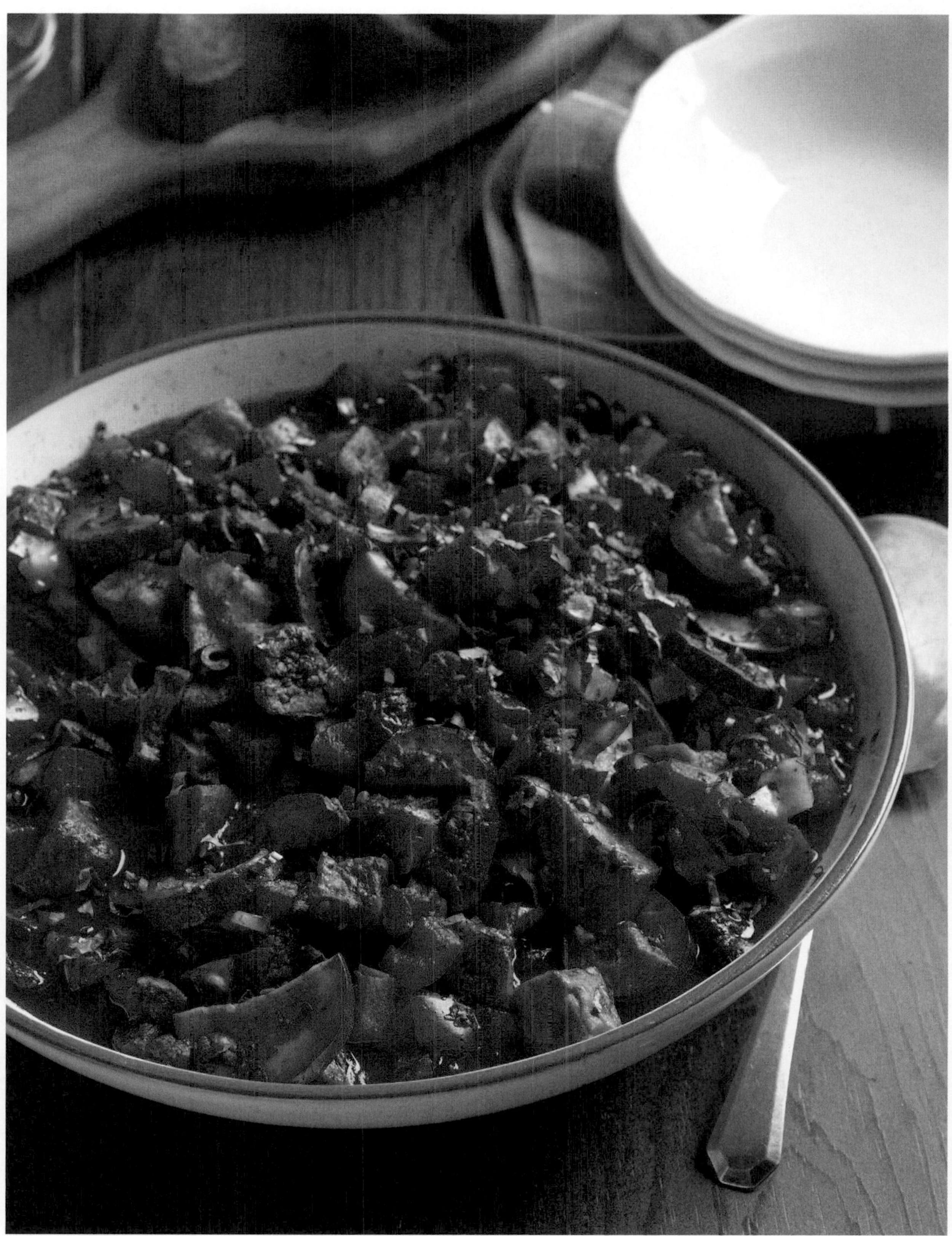

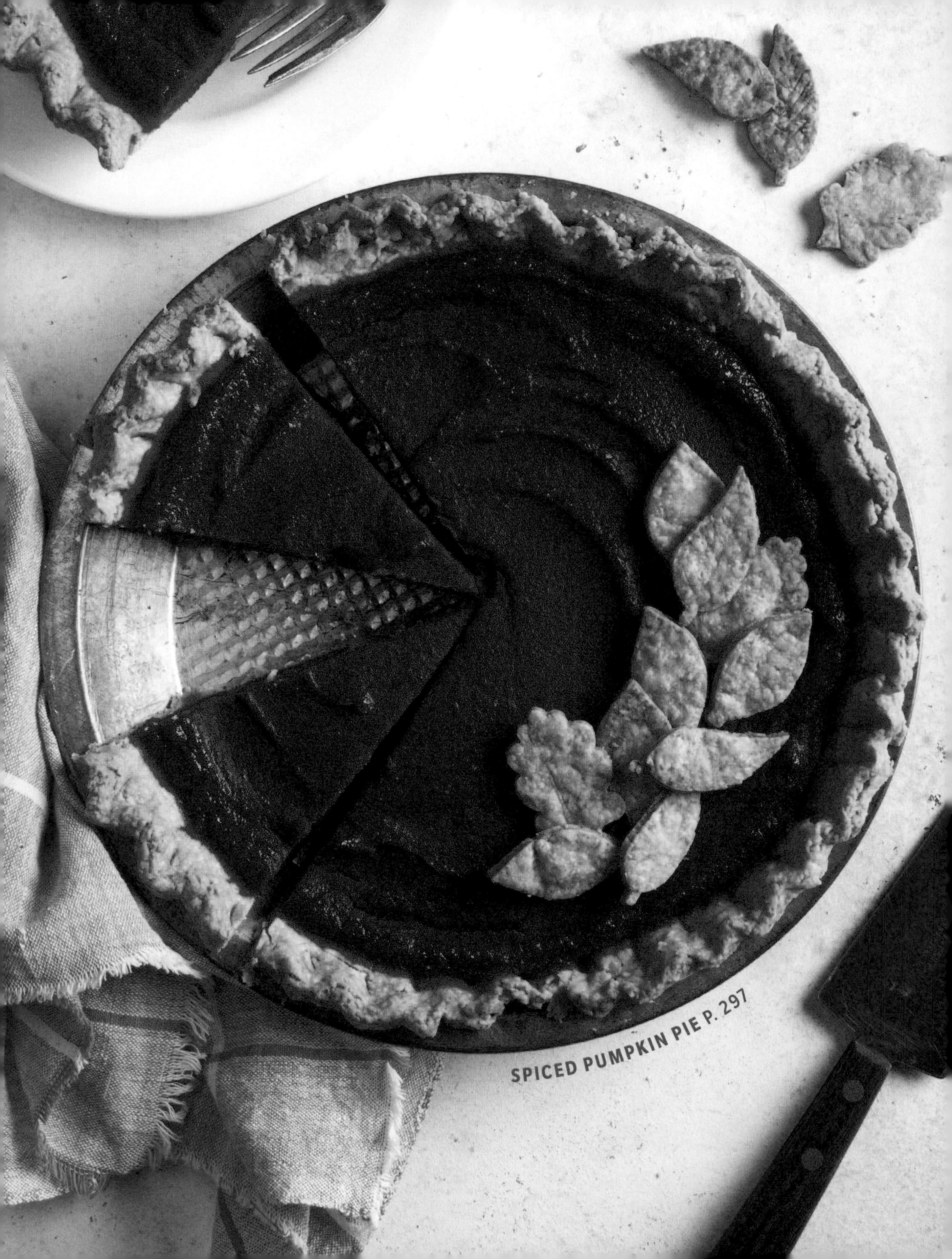

SPICED PUMPKIN PIE P. 297

CHAPTER 13

DESSERTS

ALMOND-PECAN DATE TRUFFLES

PREP: 20 min. + chilling **MAKES:** 1½ dozen

- ⅓ cup apple juice
- 1 pkg. (8 oz.) chopped dates
- 1 cup finely chopped pecans, toasted
- 1¼ tsp. ground cinnamon
- ¼ tsp. ground nutmeg
- 1 cup ground almonds, toasted

1 In a microwave, warm apple juice. Stir in dates; let stand 5 minutes to soften, stirring occasionally. Remove dates from apple juice; discard liquid. Transfer dates to the bowl of a food processor fitted with the blade attachment; process until smooth. Add pecans and spices; pulse just until combined (mixture will be thick).

2 Shape the mixture into 1-in. balls; place on a waxed paper-lined baking sheet. Refrigerate, covered, 30-60 minutes.

3 Roll date balls in almonds.

1 DATE BALL *109 cal., 7g fat (1g sat. fat), 0 chol., 0 sod., 12g carb. (9g sugars, 2g fiber), 2g pro.*

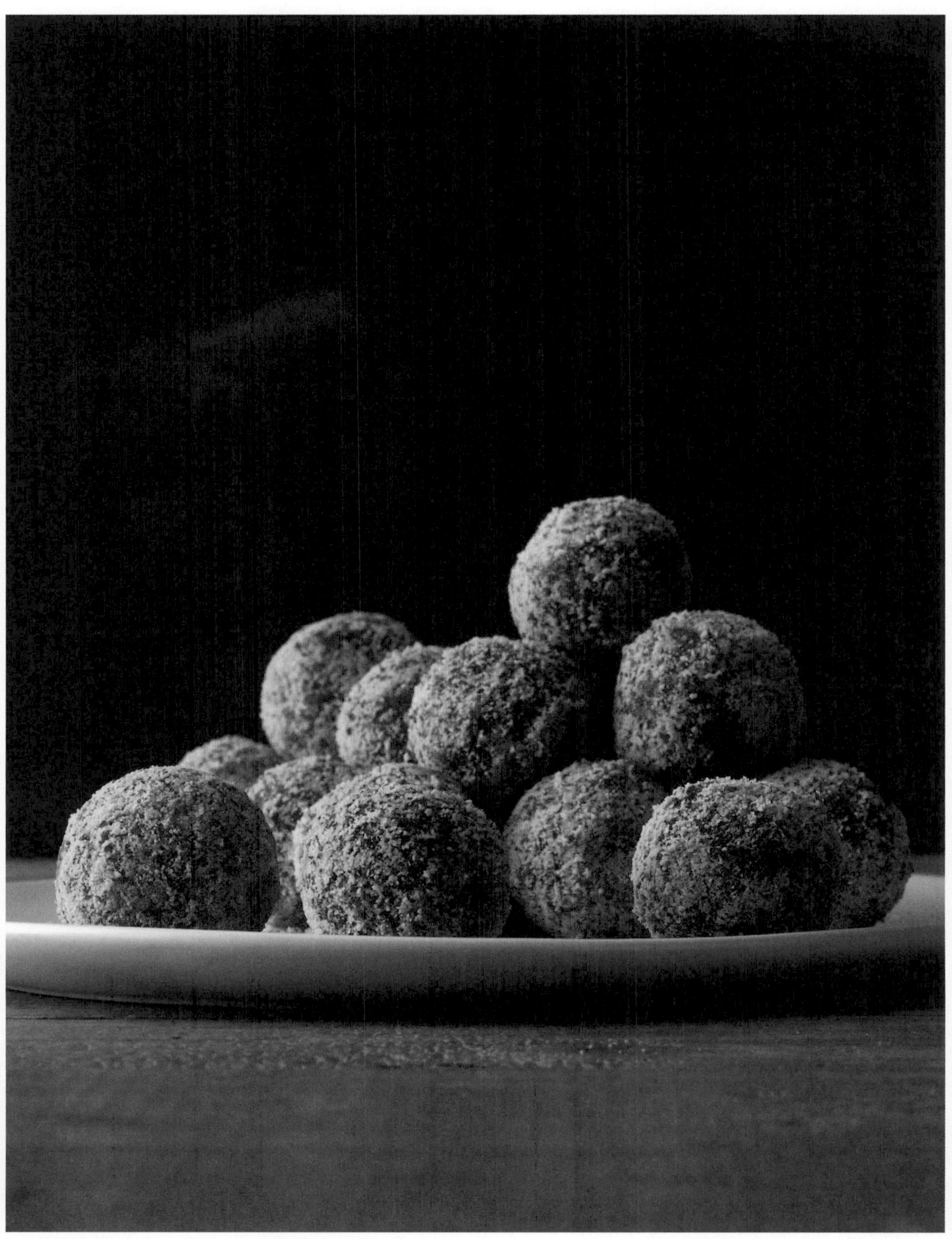

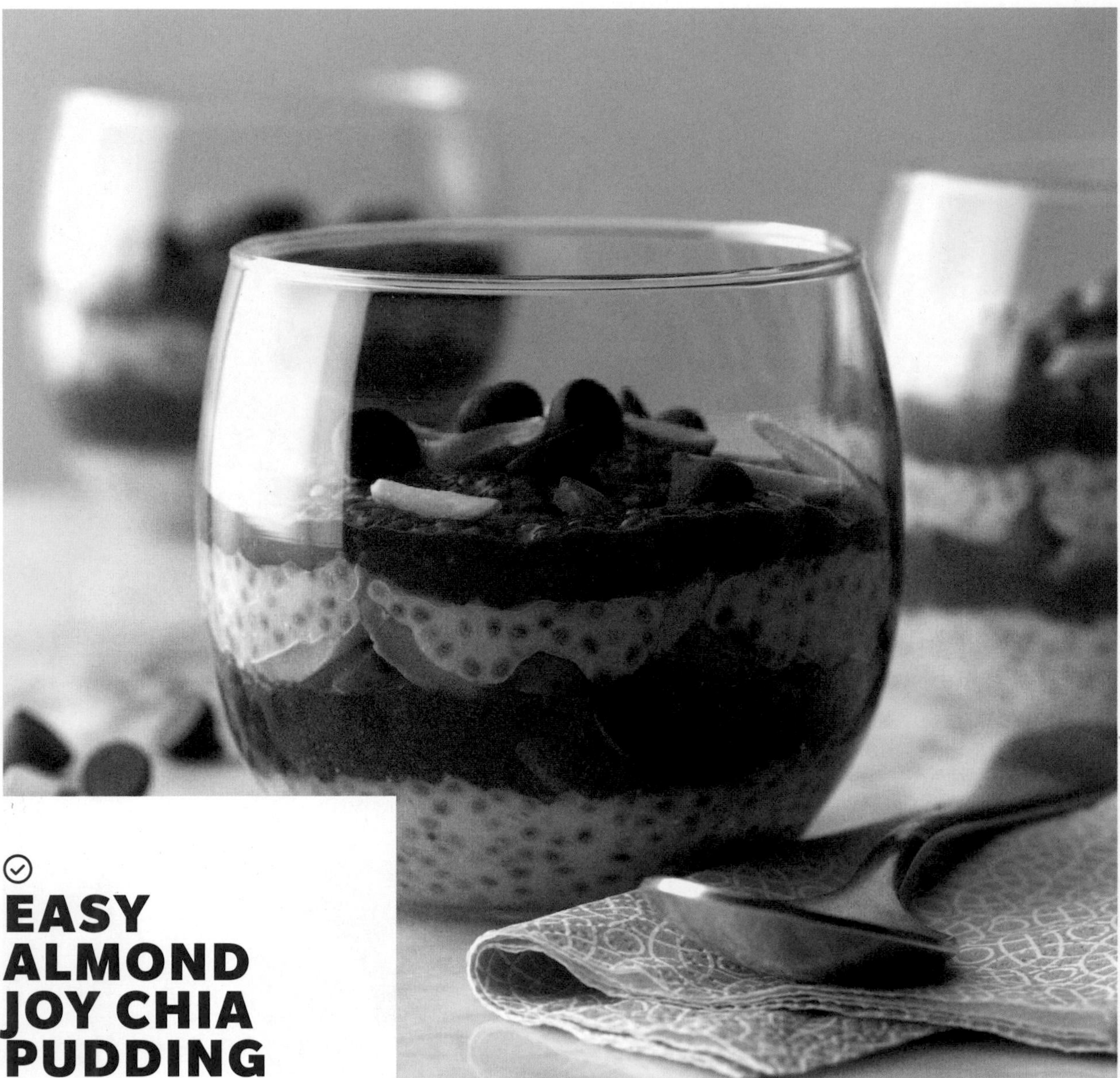

EASY ALMOND JOY CHIA PUDDING

PREP: 15 min. + chilling
MAKES: 2 servings

- 1 cup refrigerated unsweetened coconut milk
- 4 Tbsp. chia seeds
- 3 Tbsp. maple syrup
- 2 Tbsp. baking cocoa
- ¼ cup dairy-free semisweet chocolate chips
- ¼ cup slivered almonds

In a small bowl, mix coconut milk, chia seeds and maple syrup. Remove half the mixture to a small bowl; stir in cocoa until blended. Refrigerate both plain and chocolate mixtures, covered, until thickened, at least 6 hours. In dessert dishes, layer ¼ each of the white pudding, chocolate pudding, chocolate chips and almonds. Repeat layers. Serve immediately or store in the refrigerator up to 3 days.

1 SERVING *414 cal., 24g fat (8g sat. fat), 0 chol., 7mg sod., 50g carb. (30g sugars, 12g fiber), 9g pro.*

GLUTEN-FREE ALMOND CRISPIES

PREP: 20 min.
BAKE: 10 min./batch
MAKES: 3 dozen

- ⅓ cup maple syrup
- ¼ cup canola oil
- 1 Tbsp. water
- 1 tsp. almond extract
- 1 cup brown rice flour
- ½ cup almond flour
- ¼ cup sugar
- 1 tsp. baking powder
- 1 tsp. ground cinnamon
- ⅛ tsp. salt
- ½ cup finely chopped almonds

1 In a small bowl, beat syrup, oil, water and extract until well blended. Combine flours, sugar, baking powder, cinnamon and salt; gradually beat into syrup mixture until blended. Stir in the almonds.

2 Drop by rounded teaspoonfuls onto parchment-lined baking sheets; flatten slightly. Bake at 350° for 10-12 minutes or until the bottoms are lightly browned. Cool for 1 minute before removing from pans to wire racks.

1 COOKIE *54 cal., 3g fat (0 sat. fat), 0 chol., 18mg sod., 6g carb. (3g sugars, 1g fiber), 1g pro.* ***Diabetic exchanges:*** *½ starch, ½ fat*

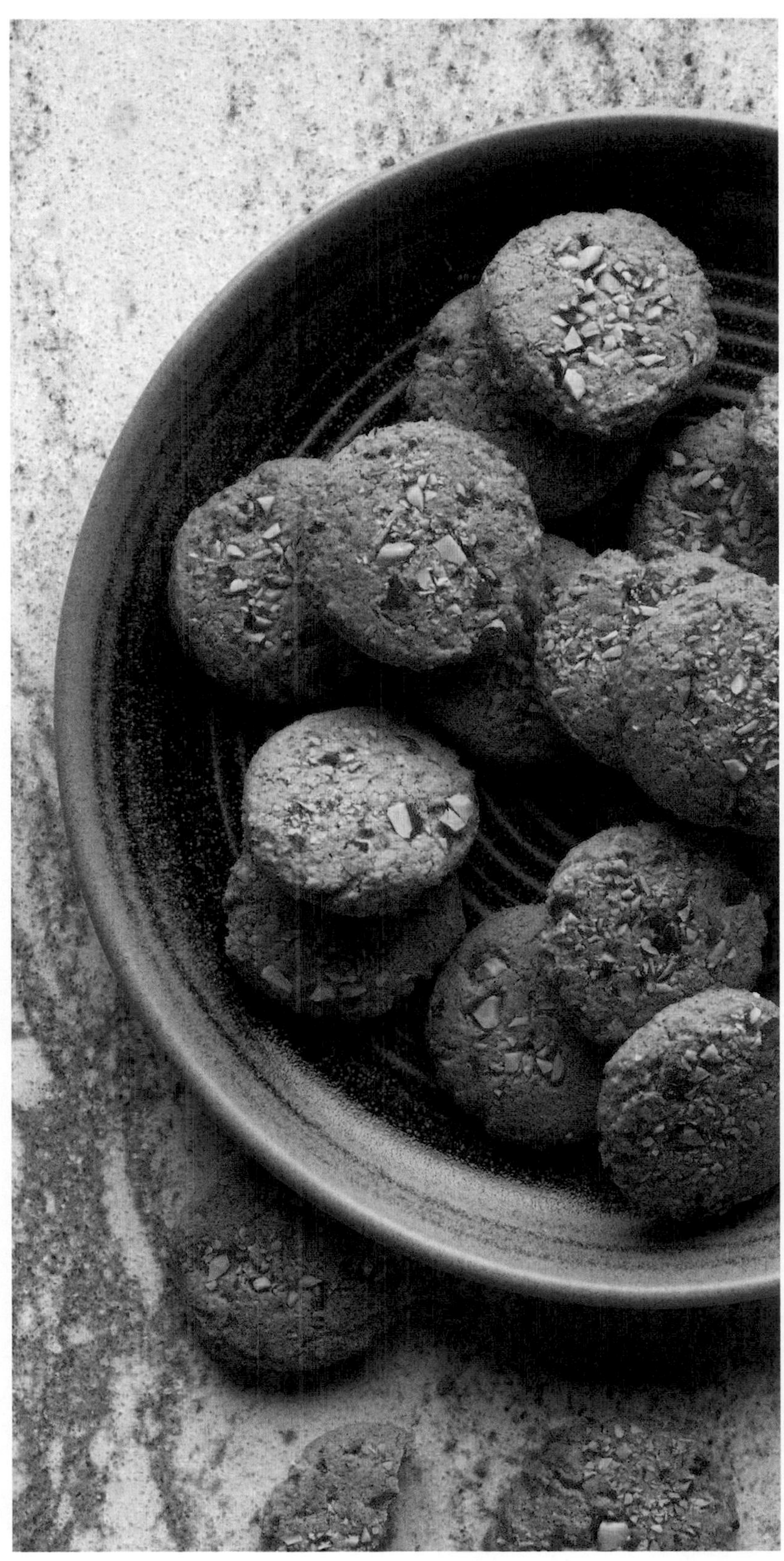

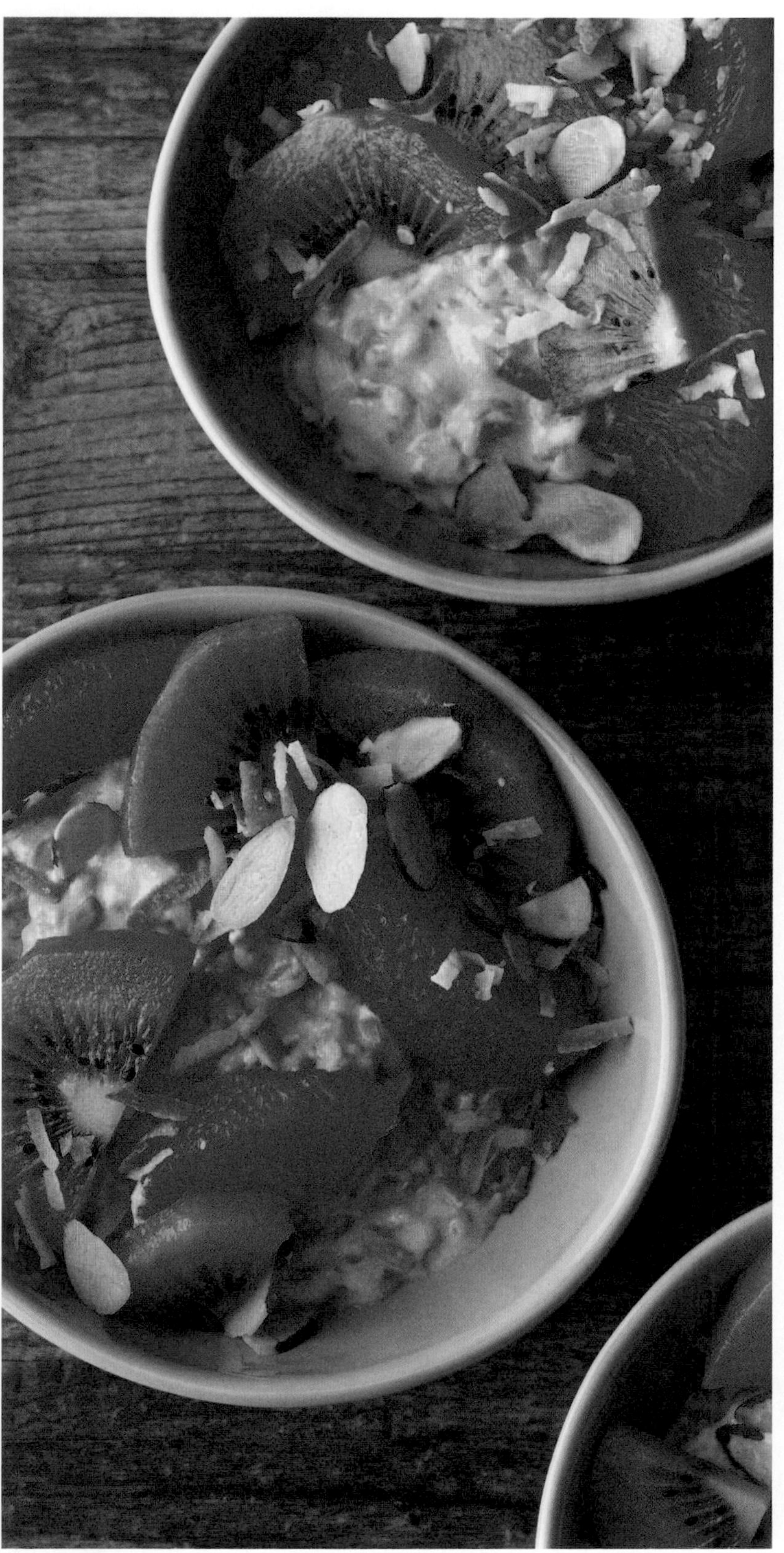

CREAMY COCONUT RICE PUDDING PARFAITS

PREP: 15 min. **COOK:** 45 min.
MAKES: 6 servings

- 2 cups 2% milk or milk alternative
- 1½ cups coconut milk
- 1½ cups cold cooked brown rice
- ¼ cup maple syrup
- ¼ tsp. salt
- 2 tsp. vanilla extract
- ¼ tsp. almond extract
- 2 medium oranges, peeled and sectioned
- 2 medium kiwifruit, peeled and sliced
- ¼ cup sliced almonds, toasted
- Toasted sweetened shredded coconut

1 In a large heavy saucepan, combine the first 5 ingredients; bring to a boil over medium heat. Reduce heat to maintain a low simmer. Cook, uncovered, 35-45 minutes or until rice is soft and milk is almost absorbed, stirring occasionally.

2 Remove from heat; stir in extracts. Cool slightly. Serve warm, or refrigerate, covered, and serve cold. To serve, spoon pudding into dishes. Top with fruit; sprinkle with almonds and coconut.

1 SERVING *291 cal., 13g fat (10g sat. fat), 7mg chol., 157mg sod., 37g carb. (19g sugars, 3g fiber), 7g pro.*

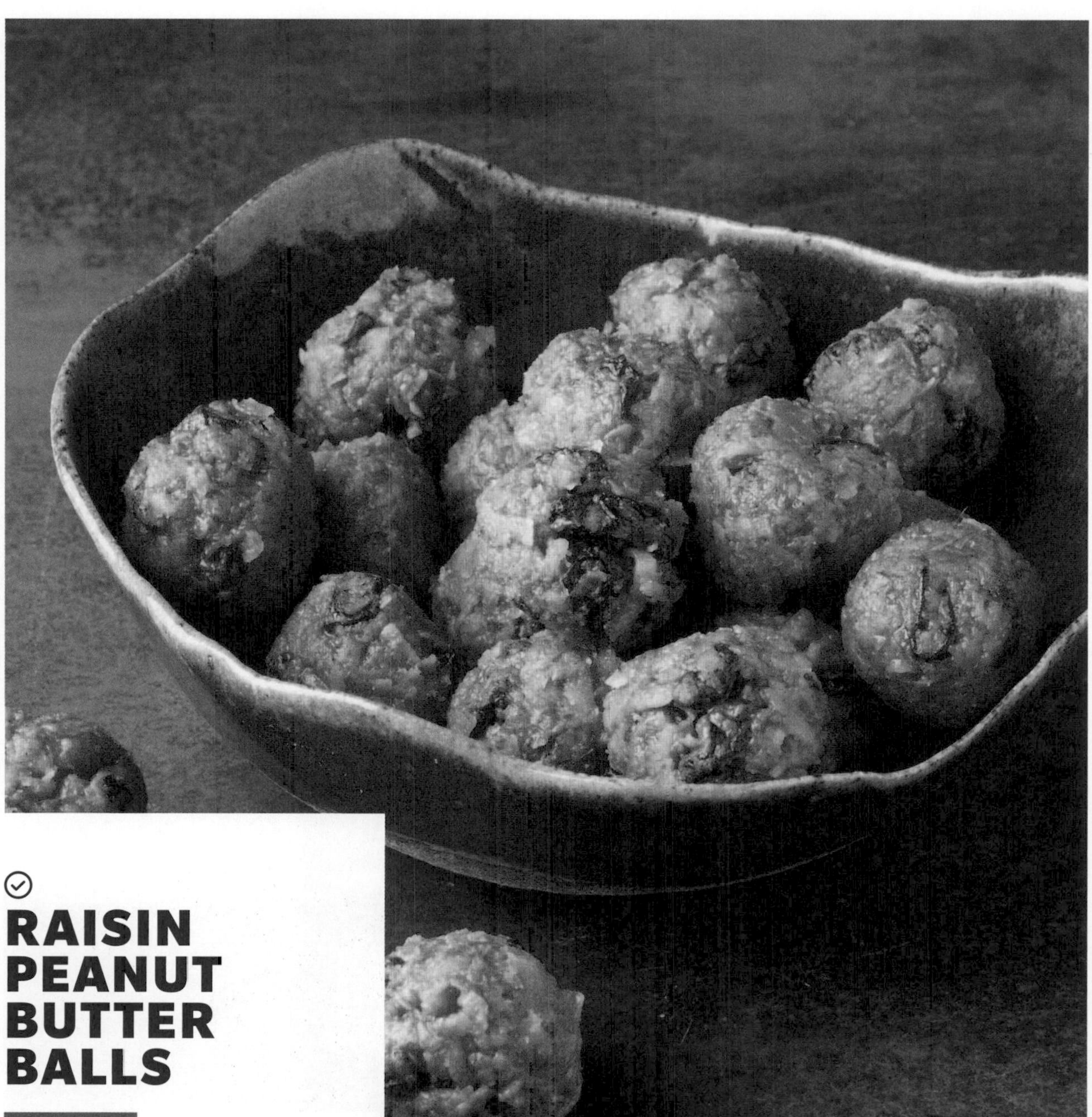

RAISIN PEANUT BUTTER BALLS

PREP: 10 min. + chilling
MAKES: 2 dozen

- ½ cup sweetened shredded coconut
- ½ cup raisins
- 4 tsp. sugar or 2 tsp. agave nectar
- 2 Tbsp. finely chopped walnuts
- ⅓ cup creamy peanut butter
- ¼ tsp. coconut extract

In a bowl, combine the first 4 ingredients; beat well. Add peanut butter and extract. Refrigerate for 30 minutes or until easy to handle. Shape into ¾-in. balls.

1 PIECE *47 cal., 3g fat (1g sat. fat), 0 chol., 21mg sod., 5g carb. (4g sugars, 0 fiber), 1g pro.*

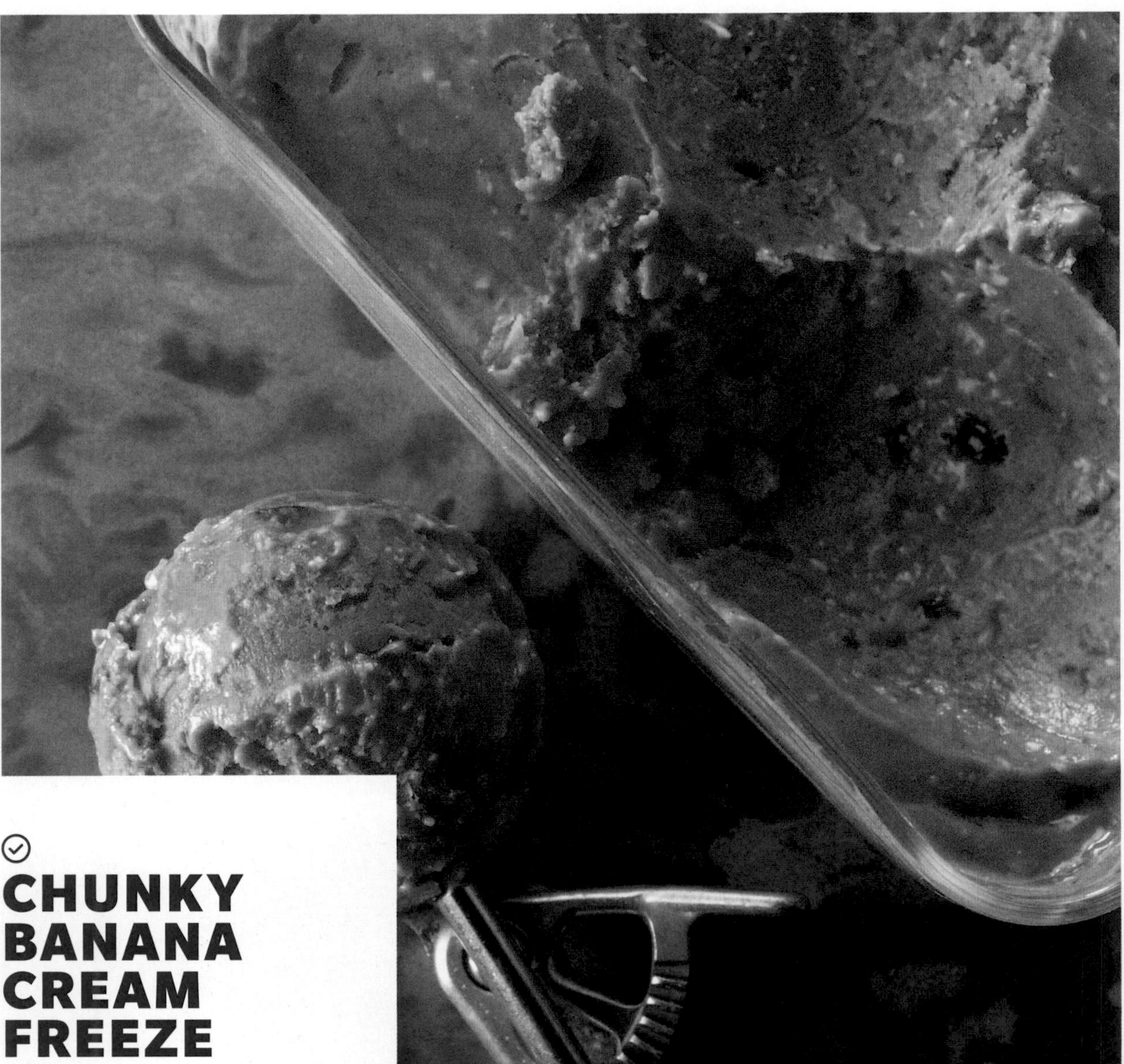

CHUNKY BANANA CREAM FREEZE

PREP: 15 min. + freezing
MAKES: 3 cups

- 5 medium bananas, peeled and frozen
- ⅓ cup almond milk
- 2 Tbsp. unsweetened finely shredded coconut
- 2 Tbsp. creamy peanut butter
- 1 tsp. vanilla extract
- ¼ cup chopped walnuts
- 3 Tbsp. raisins

1 Place bananas, milk, coconut, peanut butter and vanilla in a food processor; cover and process until blended.

2 Transfer to a freezer container; stir in the walnuts and raisins. Freeze mixture for 2-4 hours before serving.

½ CUP *181 cal., 7g fat (2g sat. fat), 0 chol., 35mg sod., 29g carb. (16g sugars, 4g fiber), 3g pro.* ***Diabetic exchanges:*** *1 fruit, 1 fat, ½ starch*

COCONUT MILK BERRY-BANANA POPS

PREP: 10 min. + freezing
MAKES: 12 servings

- 1 can (13.66 oz.) coconut milk
- 1 pint fresh strawberries, chopped, divided
- 1 medium banana, sliced
- 2 Tbsp. maple syrup
- 12 freezer pop molds or 12 paper cups (3 oz. each) and wooden pop sticks

Place coconut milk, 1½ cups strawberries, banana and syrup in a blender; cover and process until smooth. Divide remaining strawberries among 12 molds or paper cups. Pour pureed mixture into molds or cups, filling ¾ full. Top molds with holders. If using cups, top with foil and insert sticks through foil. Freeze until firm, at least 4 hours.

1 POP *51 cal., 3g fat (3g sat. fat), 0 chol., 5mg sod., 7g carb. (5g sugars, 1g fiber), 1g pro.*

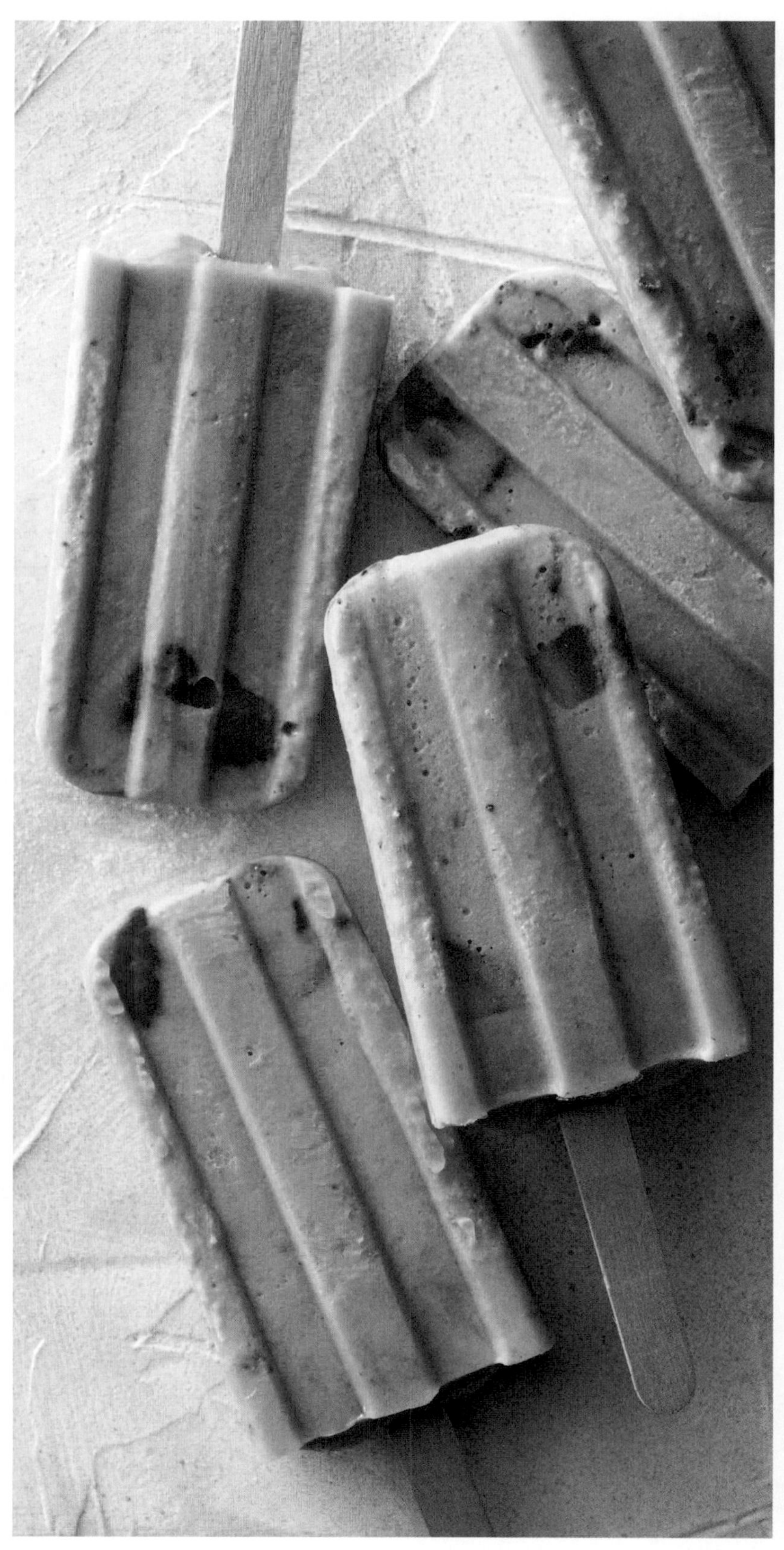

FROSTY WATERMELON ICE

PREP: 20 min. + freezing **MAKES:** 4 servings

- 1 tsp. unflavored gelatin
- 2 Tbsp. water
- 2 Tbsp. lime juice
- 2 Tbsp. honey or agave nectar
- 4 cups cubed seedless watermelon, divided

1 In a microwave-safe bowl, sprinkle gelatin over water; let stand 1 minute. Microwave on high for 40 seconds. Stir and let stand until gelatin is completely dissolved, 1-2 minutes.

2 Place lime juice, honey and gelatin mixture in a blender. Add 1 cup watermelon; cover and process until blended. Add remaining watermelon, 1 cup at a time, processing until smooth after each addition.

3 Transfer to a shallow dish; freeze until almost firm. In a chilled bowl, beat with an electric mixer until the mixture is bright pink. Divide among 4 serving dishes; freeze, covered, until firm. Remove from the freezer 15-20 minutes before serving.

¾ CUP *81 cal., 0 fat (0 sat. fat), 0 chol., 3mg sod., 21g carb. (18g sugars, 1g fiber), 1g pro.* ***Diabetic exchanges:*** *1 fruit, ½ starch*

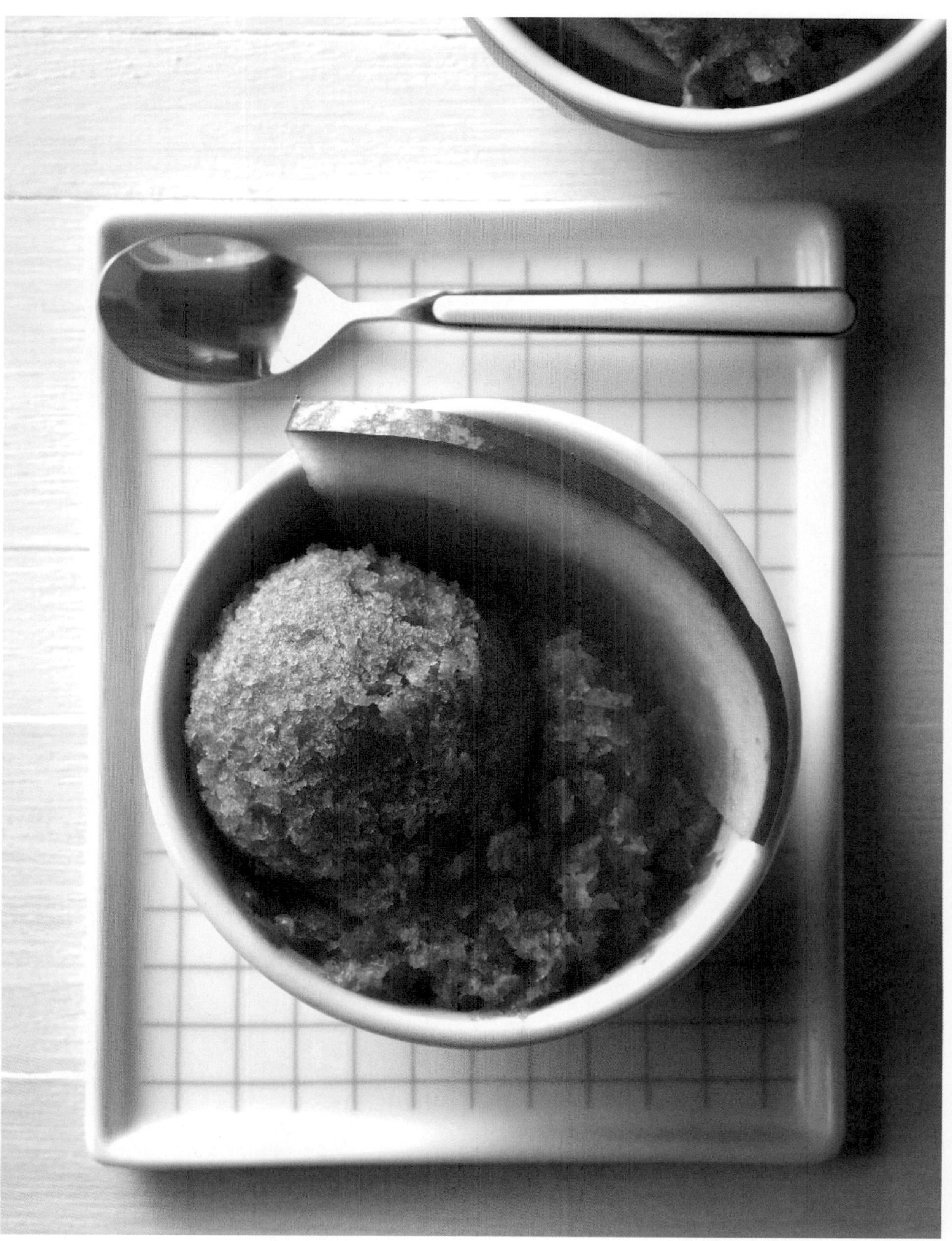

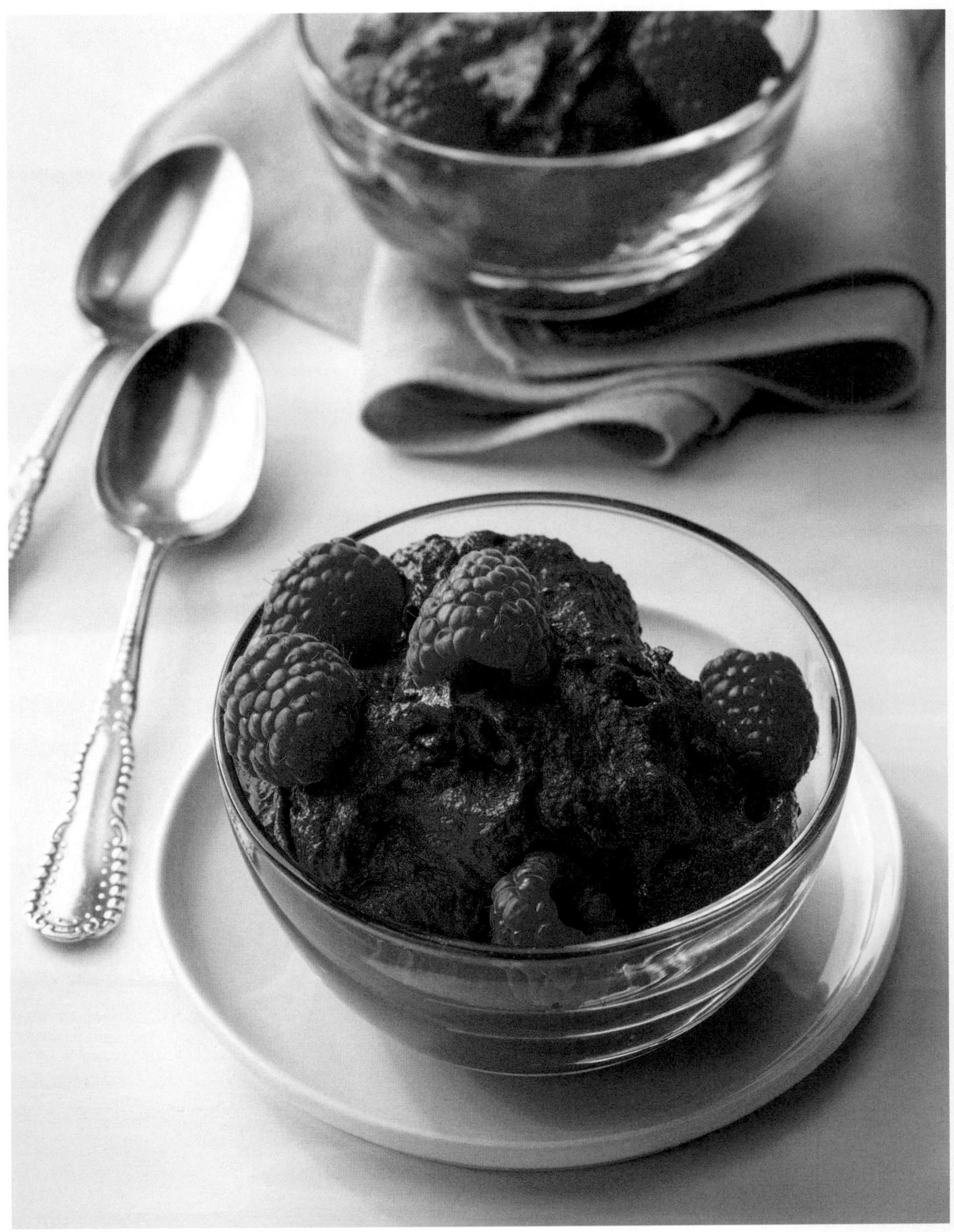

FIG & AVOCADO CHOCOLATE MOUSSE

PREP: 25 min. + chilling **MAKES:** 6 servings

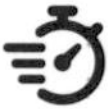

- 1/3 cup boiling water
- 3/4 cup dried mission figs, stemmed and halved lengthwise
- 1 cup dairy-free dark chocolate chips
- 2 medium ripe avocados, peeled and pitted
- 1/3 cup baking cocoa
- 2 Tbsp. unsweetened almond milk
- 1 Tbsp. maple syrup
- 1 tsp. vanilla extract
- 1/8 tsp. sea salt
- 1 can (15 oz.) garbanzo beans or chickpeas, undrained
- 1/4 tsp. cream of tartar
- Fresh raspberries, optional

1 Pour boiling water over figs in a small bowl; let stand 45 minutes. In a microwave, melt chocolate chips; stir until smooth. Cool to room temperature. Place figs and liquid in a food processor. Pulse until a paste forms. Add avocados, cooled chocolate, cocoa, almond milk, syrup, vanilla and sea salt; pulse until pureed. Transfer to a large bowl.

2 To make aquafaba, drain the garbanzo beans, reserving liquid (save beans for another use). Add the drained liquid and cream of tartar to bowl of a stand mixer. Beat on high speed until stiff peaks form, 2-3 minutes. Gently fold aquafaba into fig mixture. Spoon into dessert dishes. Refrigerate at least 2 hours or overnight before serving. If desired, serve with fresh raspberries.

2/3 CUP *310 cal., 18g fat (7g sat. fat), 0 chol., 149mg sod., 41g carb. (26g sugars, 8g fiber), 5g pro.*

GRILLED STONE FRUITS WITH BALSAMIC SYRUP

TAKES: 20 min. **MAKES:** 4 servings

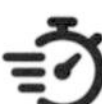

- ½ cup balsamic vinegar
- 2 Tbsp. brown sugar
- 2 medium peaches, peeled and halved
- 2 medium nectarines, peeled and halved
- 2 medium plums, peeled and halved

1 In a small saucepan, combine vinegar and brown sugar. Bring to a boil; cook until liquid is reduced by half.

2 On a lightly oiled grill rack, grill peaches, nectarines and plums, covered, over medium heat or broil 4 in. from the heat until tender, 3-4 minutes on each side.

3 Slice the fruit; arrange on a serving plate. Drizzle with sauce.

1 SERVING *114 cal., 1g fat (0 sat. fat), 0 chol., 10mg sod., 28g carb. (24g sugars, 2g fiber), 2g pro.* ***Diabetic exchanges:*** *1 starch, 1 fruit*

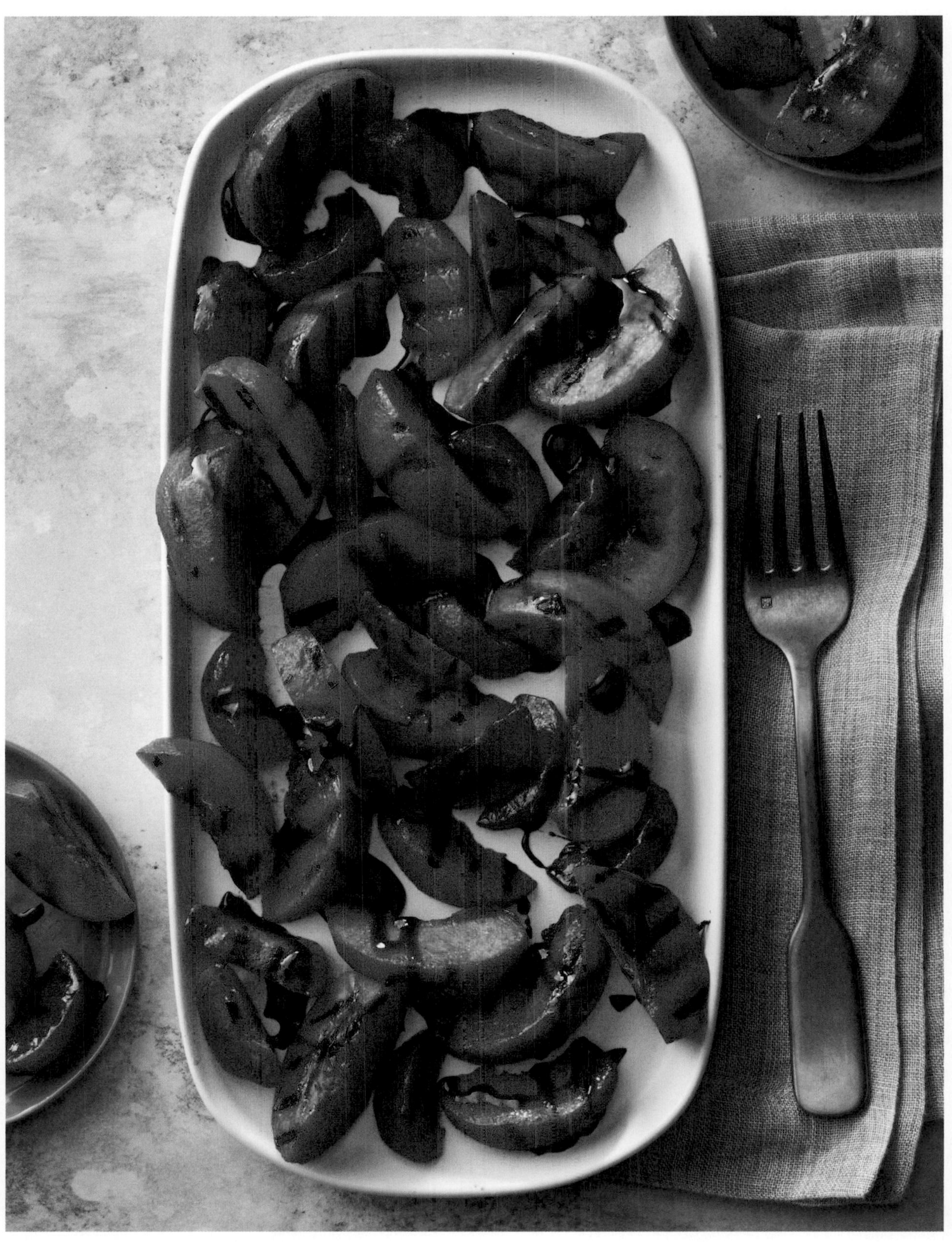

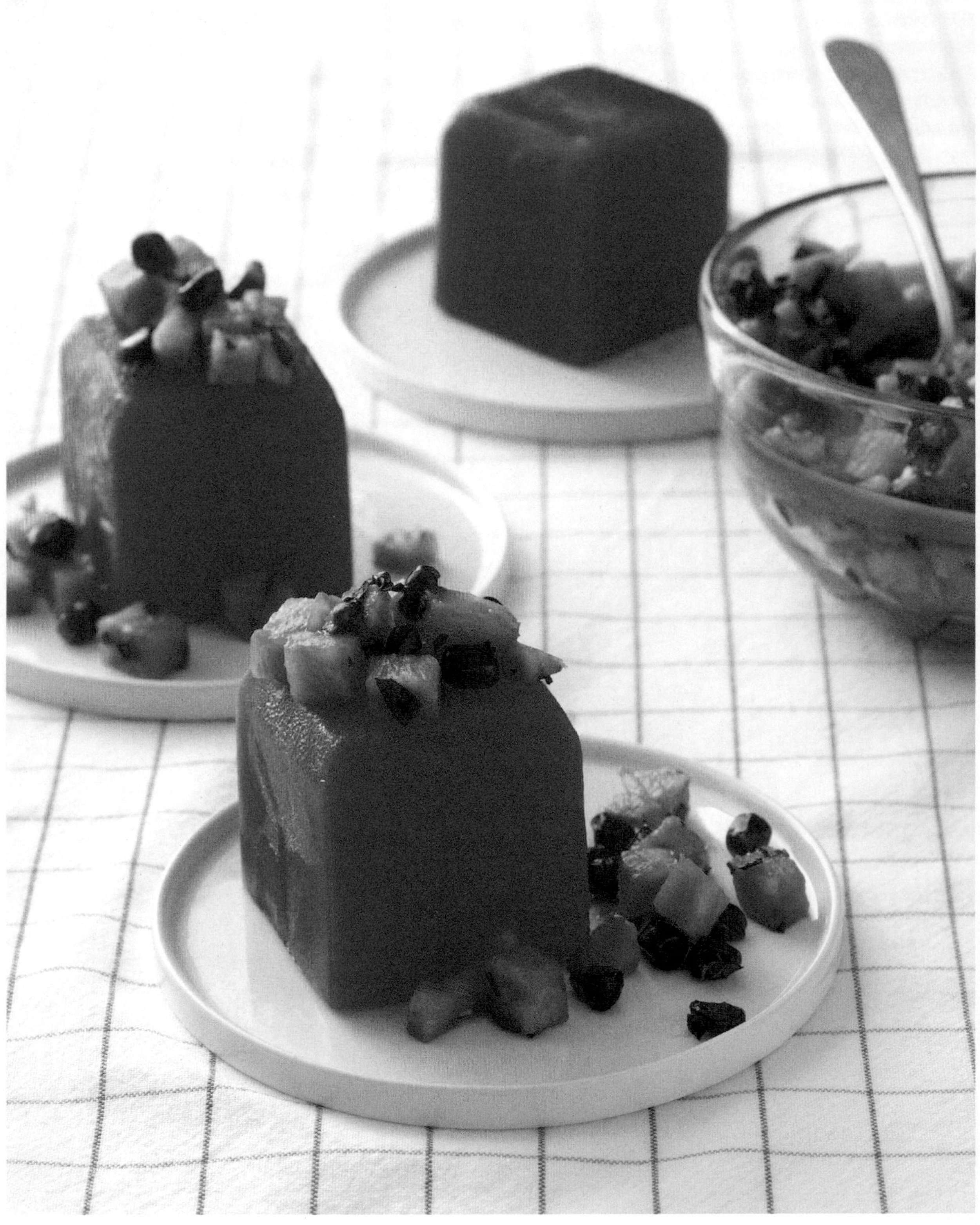

MANGO GLACE WITH PINEAPPLE POMEGRANATE SALSA

PREP: 45 min. + freezing **MAKES:** 1 dozen

4 medium ripe mangoes, peeled and chopped
1 fresh ripe pineapple, peeled and cut into ½-in. pieces
2 Tbsp. lime juice

SALSA

1 cup finely chopped fresh pineapple
2 Tbsp. pomegranate seeds
1 Tbsp. minced fresh mint

1 Combine mangoes, pineapple and lime juice in a blender. Cover and process until smooth. Strain through a fine-mesh strainer into a large bowl. Pour into 1¾-in. silicone ice cube trays. Freeze until firm, 8 hours or overnight.

2 Combine salsa ingredients; cover and refrigerate overnight.

3 Take the cubes out of freezer 10 minutes before serving. Run a small spatula around the edge of each fruit cube to loosen; remove from trays. Serve with salsa.

1 CUBE WITH 4 TSP. SALSA *114 cal., 1g fat (0 sat. fat), 0 chol., 2mg sod., 29g carb. (24g sugars, 3g fiber), 1g pro.*

QUINOA, FRESH FIG & HONEY-BALSAMIC PARFAITS

TAKES: 30 min. **MAKES:** 4 servings

- 1 cup water
- ½ cup quinoa, rinsed
- ¼ cup balsamic vinegar
- 1 tsp. vanilla extract
- ¼ tsp. ground cinnamon
- ⅛ tsp. salt
- ¼ cup honey or agave nectar
- 8 fresh figs, quartered
- 1 cup (8 oz.) vanilla dairy or vegan yogurt

1 In a small saucepan, bring water to a boil. Add the quinoa. Reduce heat; simmer, covered, until the liquid is absorbed, 12-15 minutes. Remove from heat; fluff with a fork.

2 Meanwhile, place vinegar in a small saucepan. Bring to a boil; cook 1-2 minutes or until liquid is reduced by half.

3 In a small bowl, mix cooked quinoa, vanilla, cinnamon and salt. Layer half the quinoa mixture, half the honey, the balsamic vinegar, half the figs and half the yogurt into 4 parfait glasses. Top with the remaining quinoa mixture, honey, yogurt and figs.

1 PARFAIT *272 cal., 2g fat (1g sat. fat), 3mg chol., 117mg sod., 59g carb. (43g sugars, 4g fiber), 7g pro.*

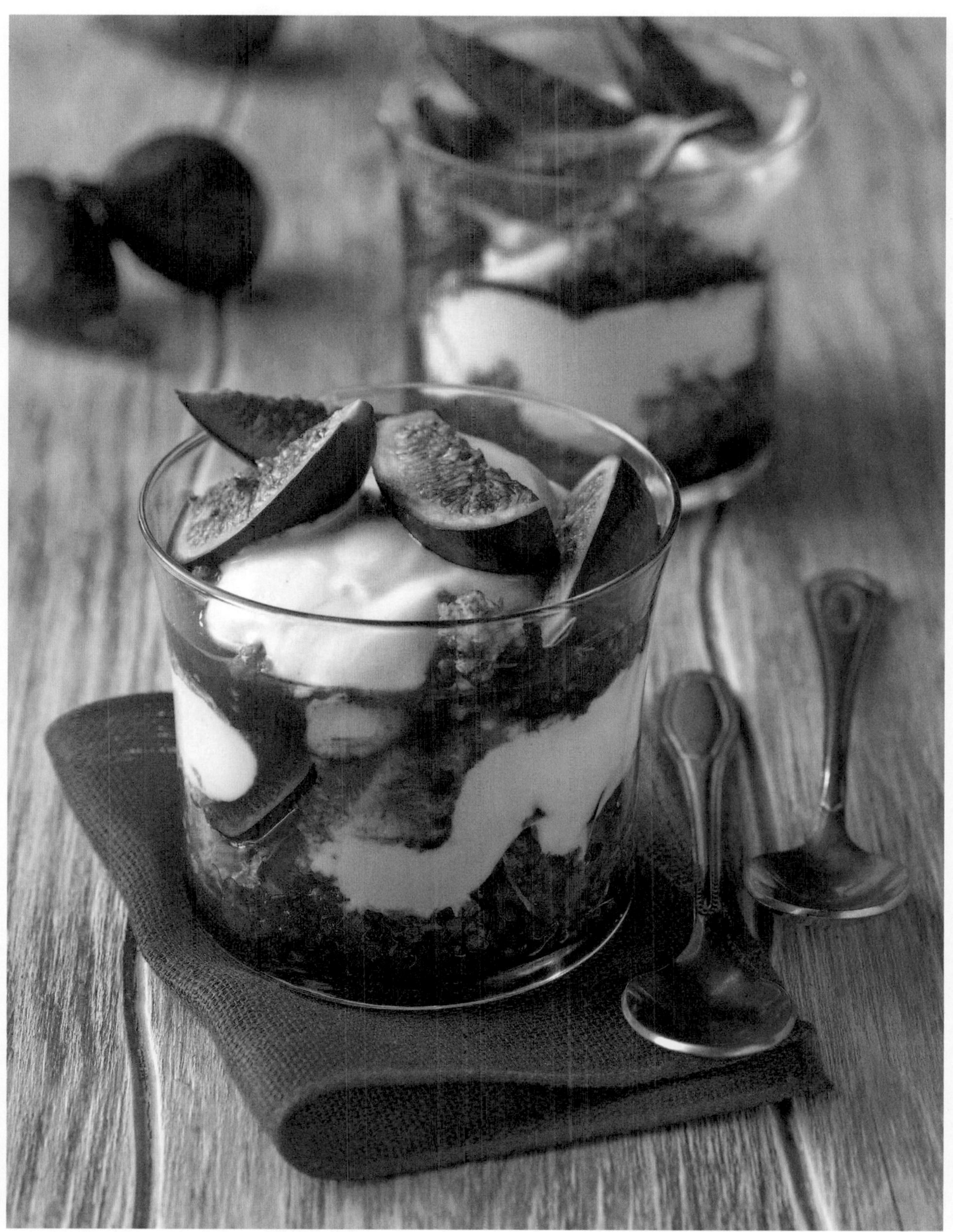

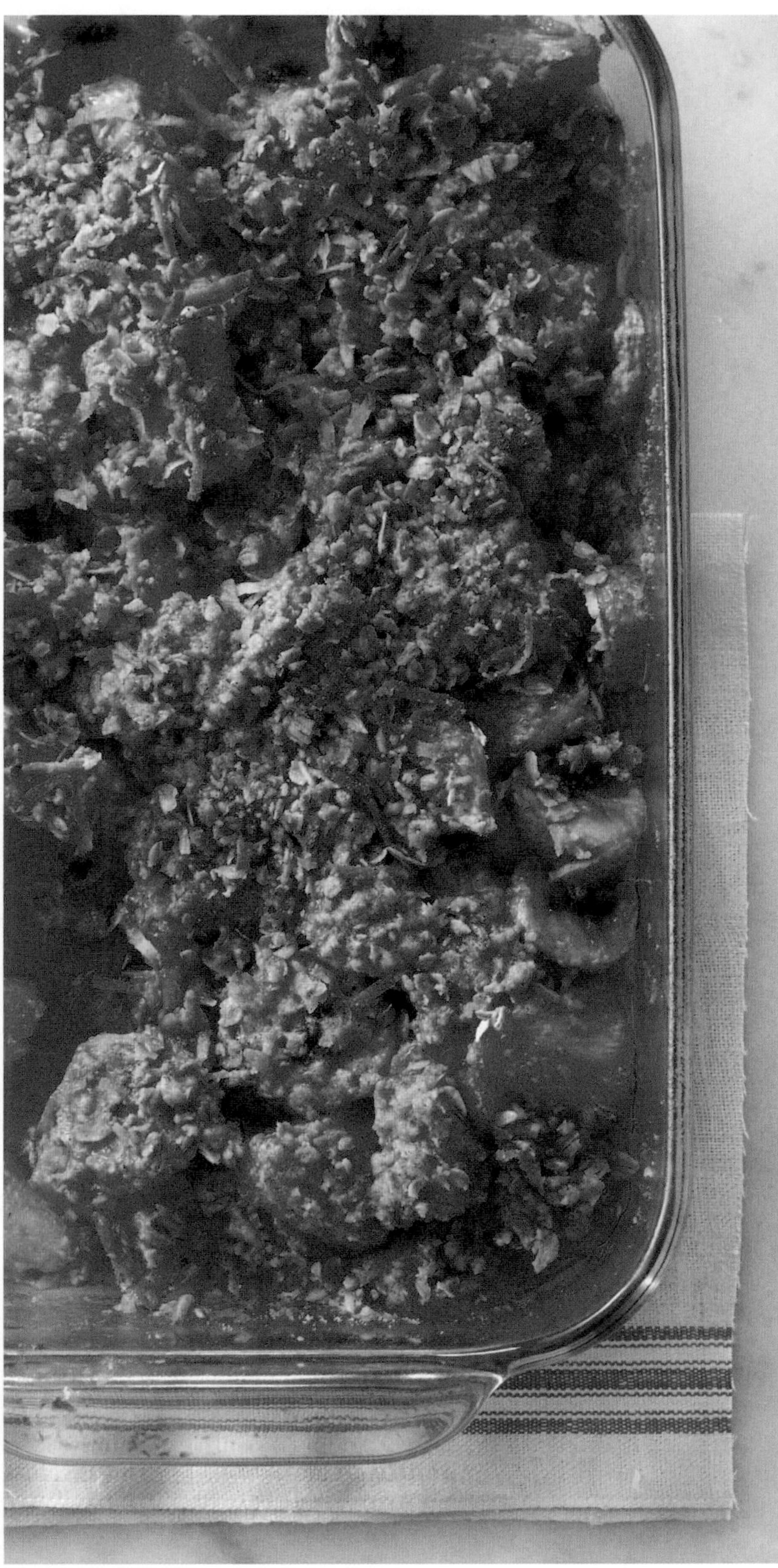

TROPICAL CRISP

PREP: 20 min.
BAKE: 30 min.
MAKES: 9 servings

- 1 fresh pineapple, peeled and cubed
- 4 medium bananas, sliced
- ¼ cup packed brown sugar
- 2 Tbsp. all-purpose flour

TOPPING

- ⅓ cup old-fashioned oats
- ¼ cup all-purpose flour
- 2 Tbsp. sweetened shredded coconut, toasted
- 2 Tbsp. brown sugar
- ¼ tsp. ground nutmeg
- ¼ cup cold dairy or vegan butter, cubed

1 Preheat oven to 350°. In a large bowl, combine pineapple and bananas. Sprinkle with brown sugar and flour; toss to coat. Transfer to an 11x7-in. baking dish coated with cooking spray.

2 In a small bowl, mix the first 5 topping ingredients; cut in butter until crumbly. Sprinkle over pineapple mixture.

3 Bake 30-35 minutes or until filling is bubbly and topping is golden brown. Serve warm.

1 SERVING *188 cal., 6g fat (4g sat. fat), 13mg chol., 44mg sod., 34g carb. (21g sugars, 3g fiber), 2g pro.* ***Diabetic exchanges:*** *1 starch, 1 fruit, 1 fat*

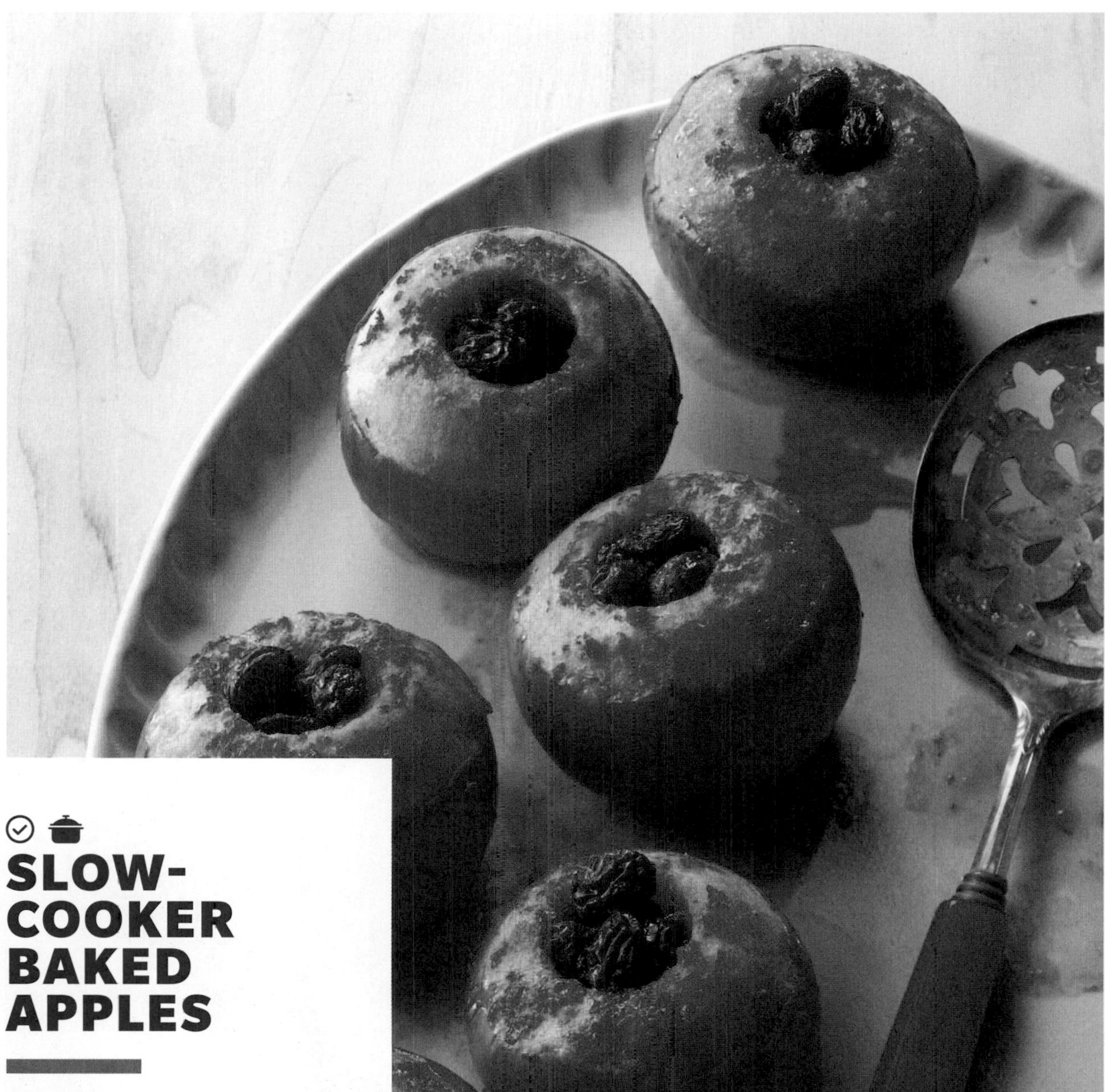

SLOW-COOKER BAKED APPLES

PREP: 25 min.
COOK: 4 hours
MAKES: 6 servings

- 6 medium tart apples
- ½ cup raisins
- ⅓ cup packed brown sugar
- 1 Tbsp. grated orange zest
- 1 cup water
- 3 Tbsp. thawed orange juice concentrate
- 2 Tbsp. dairy or vegan butter

1 Core apples and peel the top third of each if desired. Combine the raisins, brown sugar and orange zest; spoon into apples. Place in a 5-qt. slow cooker.

2 Pour water around apples. Drizzle with the orange juice concentrate. Dot with butter. Cover and cook on low until apples are tender, 4-5 hours.

1 STUFFED APPLE *203 cal., 4g fat (2g sat. fat), 10mg chol., 35mg sod., 44g carb. (37g sugars, 4g fiber), 1g pro.*

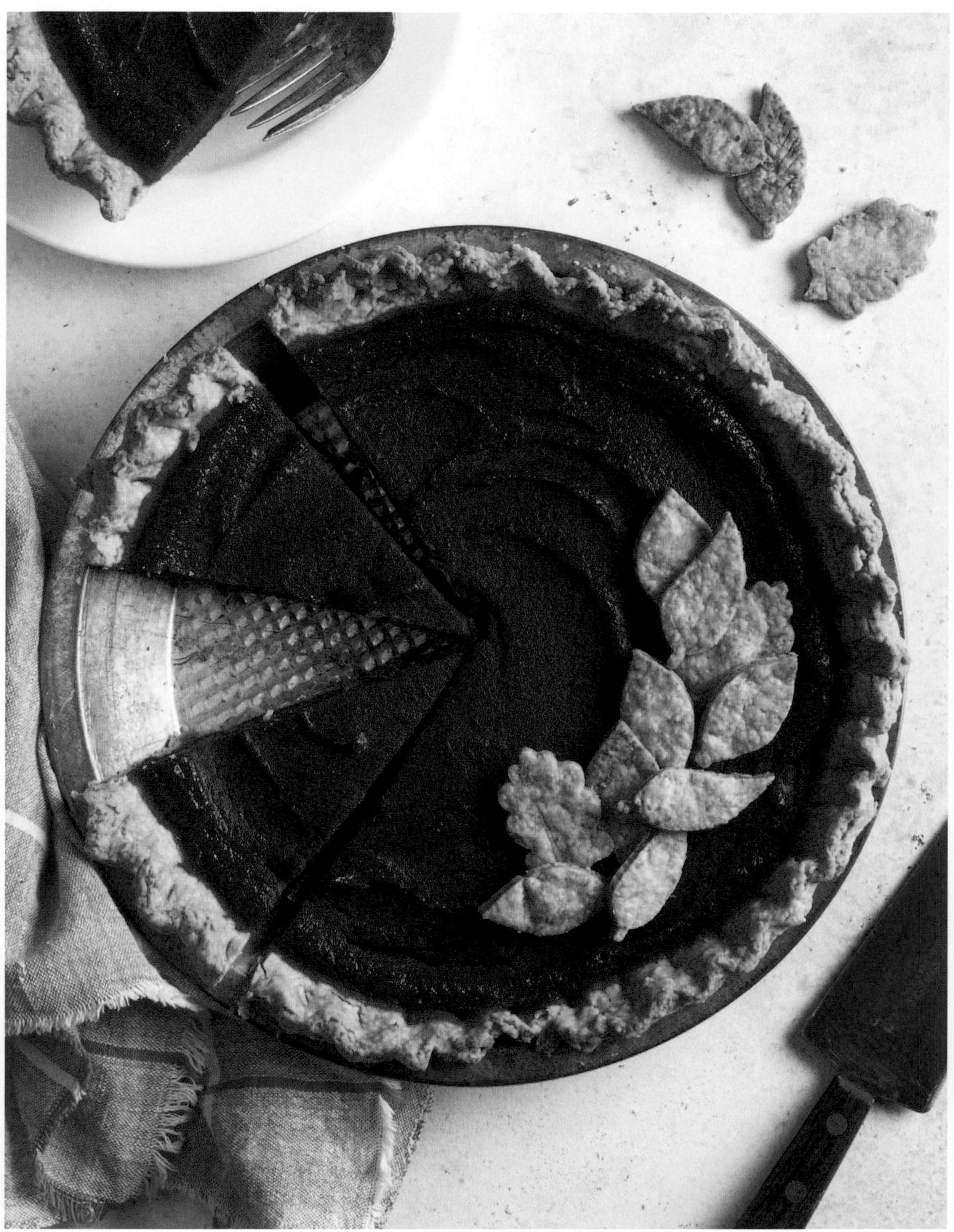

SPICED PUMPKIN PIE

PREP: 20 min. + chilling **BAKE:** 1 hour + cooling **MAKES:** 8 servings

- 1¼ cups all-purpose flour
- 2 tsp. sugar
- ¼ tsp. salt
- ½ cup coconut oil or shortening, cold
- 3 to 4 Tbsp. ice water

FILLING

- 2½ cups canned pumpkin
- ¼ cup packed brown sugar
- ¼ cup maple or agave syrup
- ¾ cup oat milk
- 1 tsp. vanilla extract
- 2 tsp. pumpkin pie spice
- ½ tsp. ground cinnamon
- ½ tsp. salt
- 3 Tbsp. tapioca flour or arrowroot flour

1 In a food processor, mix flour, sugar and salt; pulse in coconut oil until crumbly. Gradually add ice water, pulsing until dough holds together when pressed. Shape into a disk. Cover and refrigerate 30 minutes or up to 2 hours.

2 On a lightly floured surface, roll dough into a ⅛-in.-thick circle; transfer to 9-in. pie plate. Trim crust to ½ in. beyond rim of plate; flute edge by positioning your index finger of one hand at the edge of the crust pointing outward. Use your index finger and the thumb of your other hand to press the crust around your index finger in the shape of a V. Continue around entire edge. Refrigerate 30 minutes. Preheat oven to 425°.

3 Line the crust with a double thickness of foil. Fill with pie weights, dried beans or uncooked rice. Bake on a lower oven rack until crust is set, about 5 minutes. Remove foil and weights; bake until crust just starts to brown, about 10 minutes. Reduce oven temperature to 350°.

4 In a blender, combine filling ingredients. Puree until smooth. Pour filling into crust. Bake 45-50 minutes or until center is set and filling is beginning to crack (cover edges with foil during the last 15 minutes to prevent overbrowning if necessary). Cool on a wire rack for 1 hour. Refrigerate overnight or until set.

1 PIECE *298 cal., 15g fat (12g sat. fat), 0 chol., 239mg sod., 41g carb. (18g sugars, 3g fiber), 3g pro.*

CHOCOLATE CUPCAKES

PREP: 20 min. **BAKE:** 15 min. + cooling **MAKES:** 24 servings

- 2½ cups all-purpose flour
- ⅔ cup baking cocoa
- 2 tsp. baking soda
- 2 cups refrigerated unsweetened coconut milk
- 1½ cups sugar
- ⅓ cup canola oil
- 2 Tbsp. cider vinegar
- 1 tsp. vanilla extract

FROSTING

- 1 cup vegan margarine, softened
- 3 cups confectioners' sugar
- ⅓ cup baking cocoa
- 2 tsp. vanilla extract

1 Preheat oven to 350°. In a large bowl, whisk the flour, cocoa and baking soda. In a small bowl, whisk coconut milk, sugar, oil, vinegar and vanilla. Stir into dry ingredients just until moistened.

2 Fill paper-lined muffin cups half full. Bake until a toothpick inserted in the center comes out clean, 15-20 minutes. Cool 10 minutes before removing from pans to wire racks to cool completely.

3 For frosting, in a large bowl, beat margarine until light and fluffy. Beat in confectioners' sugar, cocoa and vanilla. Frost the cupcakes.

1 CUPCAKE *265 cal., 12g fat (2g sat. fat), 0 chol., 194mg sod., 40g carb. (27g sugars, 1g fiber), 2g pro.*

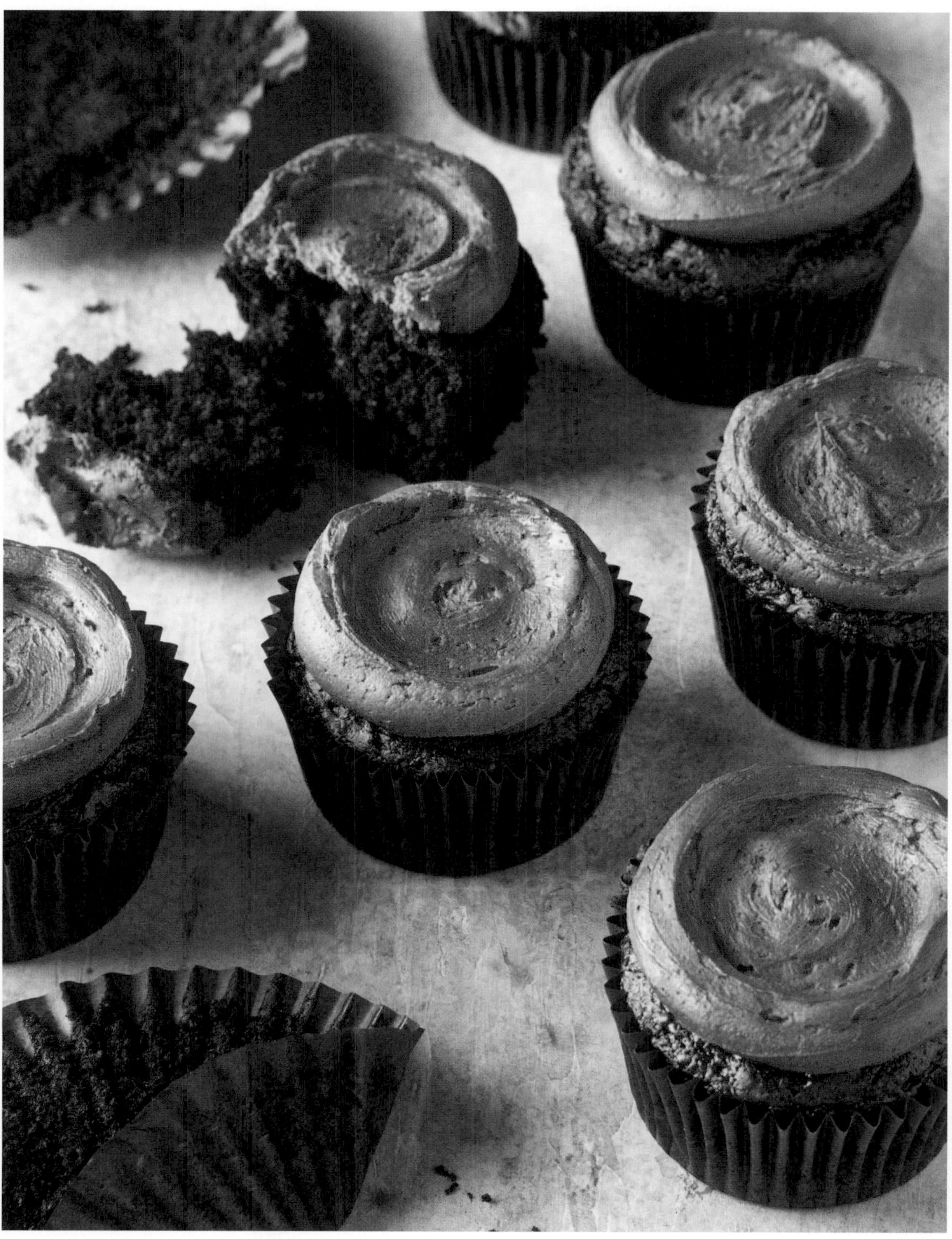

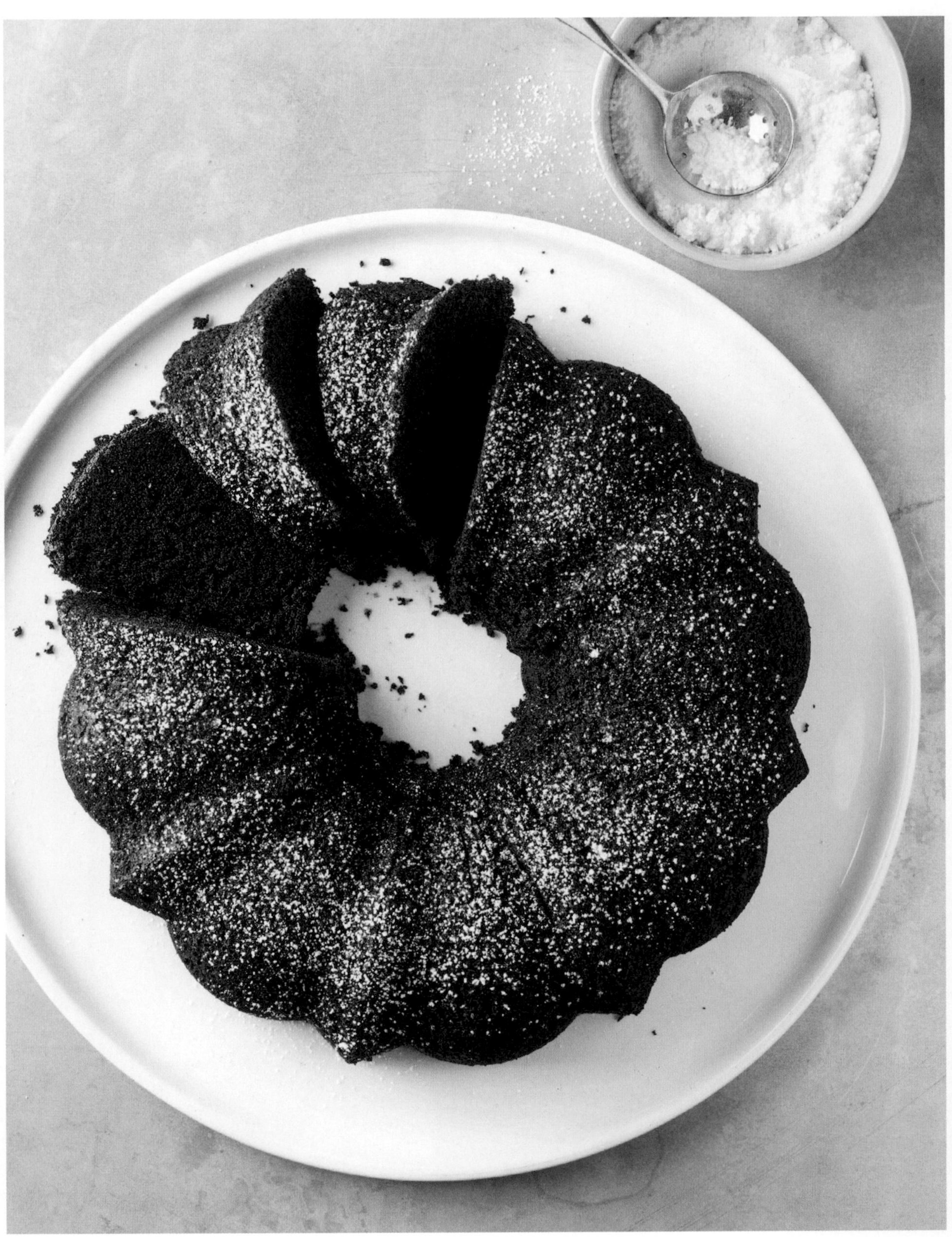

BEST GLUTEN-FREE CHOCOLATE CAKE

PREP: 20 min. **BAKE:** 50 min. + cooling **MAKES:** 16 servings

- 3 Tbsp. plus 2 cups gluten-free all-purpose baking flour, divided
- 2 cups sugar
- ¾ cup baking cocoa
- ¼ cup ground flaxseed
- ¼ cup chia seeds
- 2 tsp. baking powder
- 1½ tsp. baking soda
- 1 tsp. salt
- 1 to 2 tsp. instant espresso powder
- ½ tsp. xanthan gum
- 1 cup boiling water
- 1 cup unsweetened almond milk
- 1 cup canola oil
- 4 tsp. vanilla extract
- Confectioners' sugar

1 Preheat oven to 350°. Grease and flour a 10-in. fluted tube pan using 3 Tbsp. gluten-free flour.

2 In a large bowl, whisk the remaining 2 cups flour and the next 9 ingredients. In another bowl, combine water, almond milk, oil and vanilla until well blended. Gradually beat flour mixture into milk mixture.

3 Transfer to prepared pan. Bake until a toothpick inserted in the center comes out clean, 50-55 minutes. Cool in pan 15 minutes before removing to wire rack to cool completely. Dust with confectioners' sugar before serving.

1 PIECE *310 cal., 17g fat (1g sat. fat), 0 chol., 339mg sod., 41g carb. (26g sugars, 4g fiber), 3g pro.*

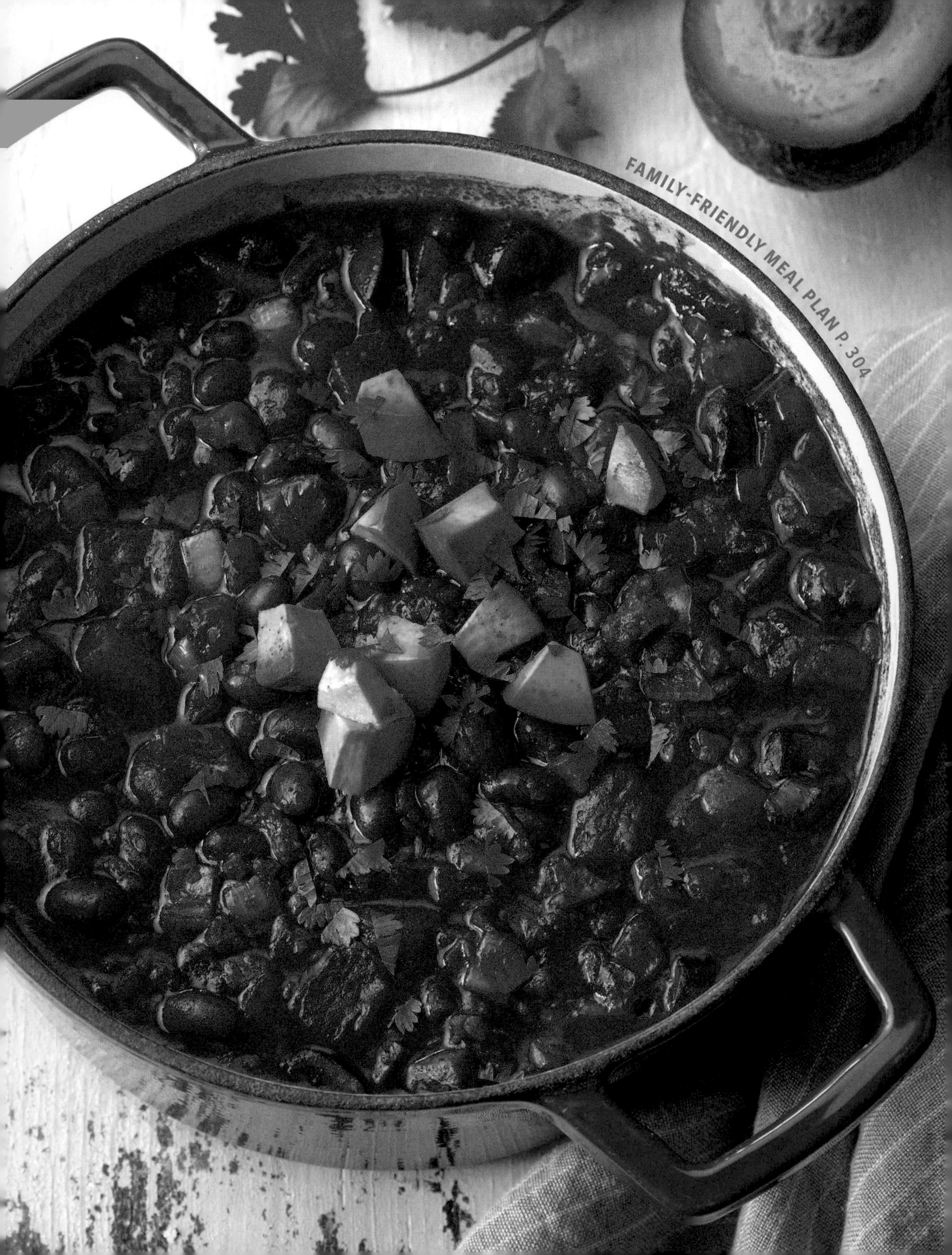
FAMILY-FRIENDLY MEAL PLAN P. 304

CHAPTER 14

MEAL PLANS

The recipes in this book can be mixed and matched to meet many different goals and needs. Use the nutrition information listed with each recipe to help choose the ones that are right for you and your family. We've included two-day sample menus for ten common diets to get you started. Round them out with your favorite sides, snacks and beverages.

FAMILY-FRIENDLY MEAL PLAN

Casual classics such as tacos, sloppy joes and chili are sure to please both kids and adults.

DAY 1

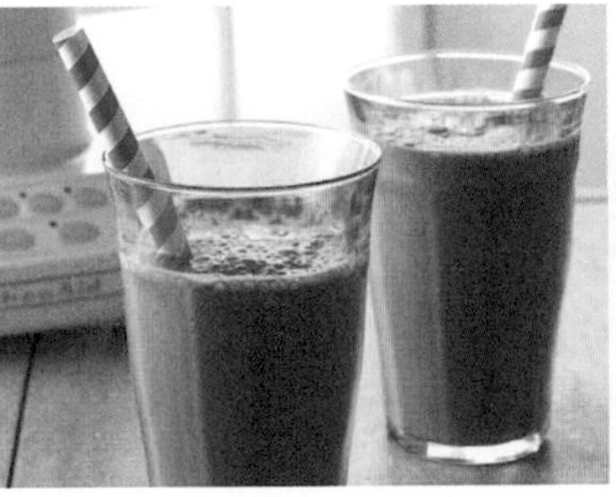

BREAKFAST
Berry-Carrot Smoothie, *p. 59*

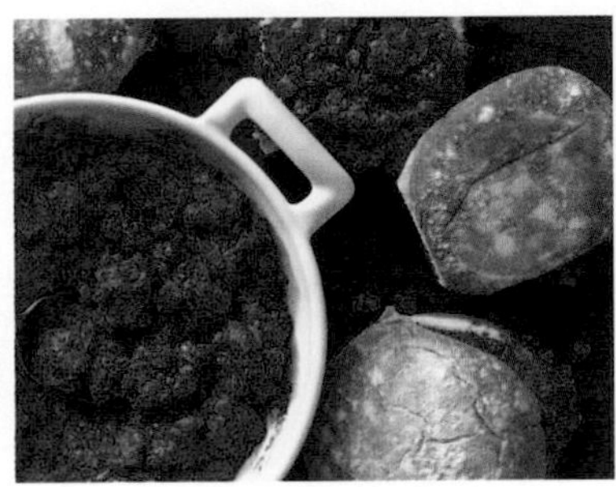

LUNCH
Saucy Tempeh Sloppy Joes, *p. 98*

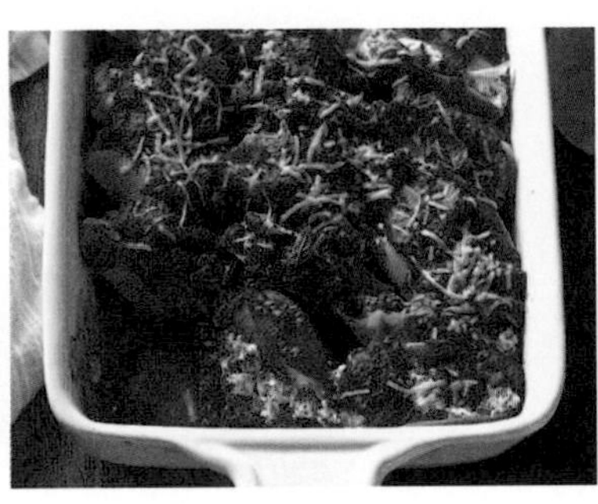

DINNER
Stuffed Shells with Broccoli, *p. 212*

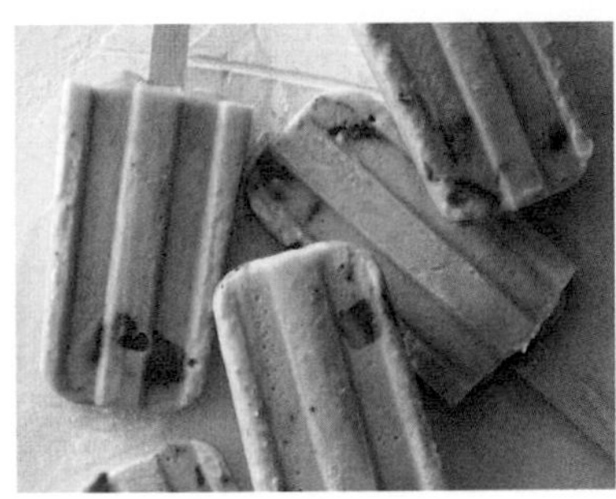

DESSERT
Coconut Milk Berry-Banana Pops, *p. 283*

DAY 2

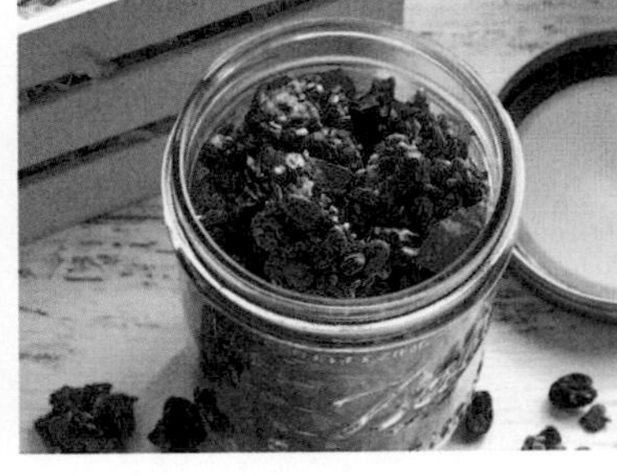

BREAKFAST
Great Granola, *p. 42*

LUNCH
Mushroom Chili, *p. 83*

DINNER
Jackfruit Carnitas Tacos, *p. 134*

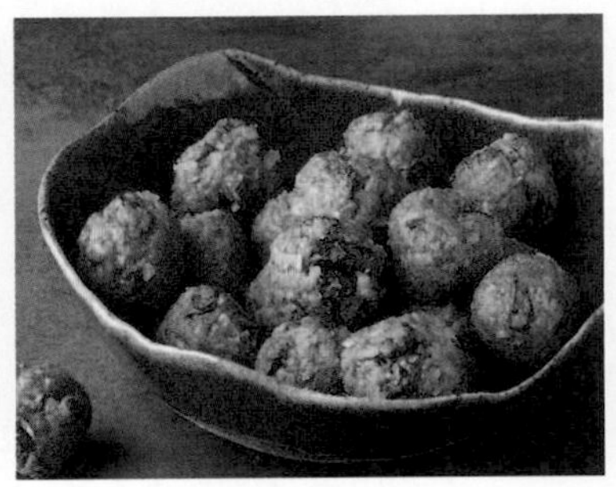

SNACK
Raisin Peanut Butter Balls, *p. 281*

ON-A-BUDGET MEAL PLAN

Low-cost staples, such as garbanzo beans, black beans and chicken thighs help keep menus on budget.

DAY 1

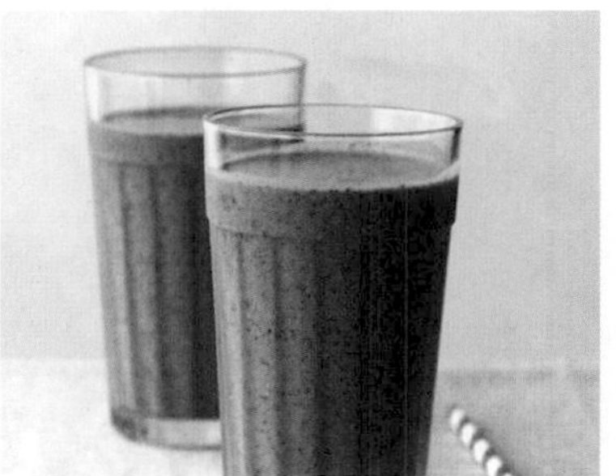

BREAKFAST
Blueberry Pancake Smoothie, *p. 61*

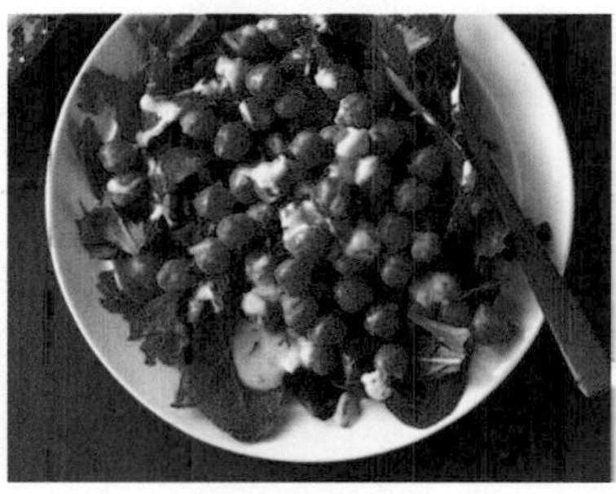

LUNCH
Lemony Garbanzo Salad, *p. 107*

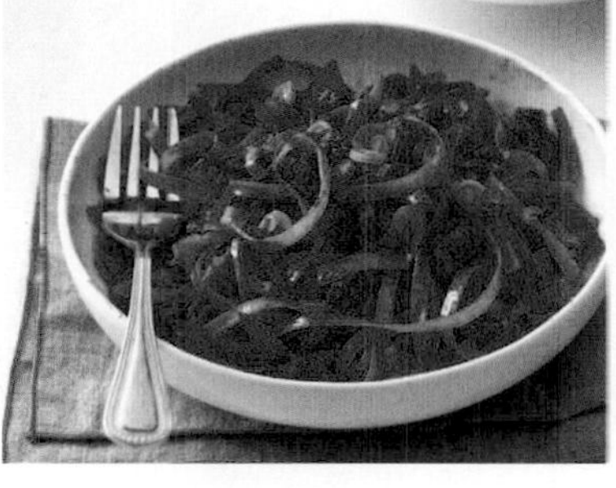

DINNER
Egg Roll Noodles, *p. 207*

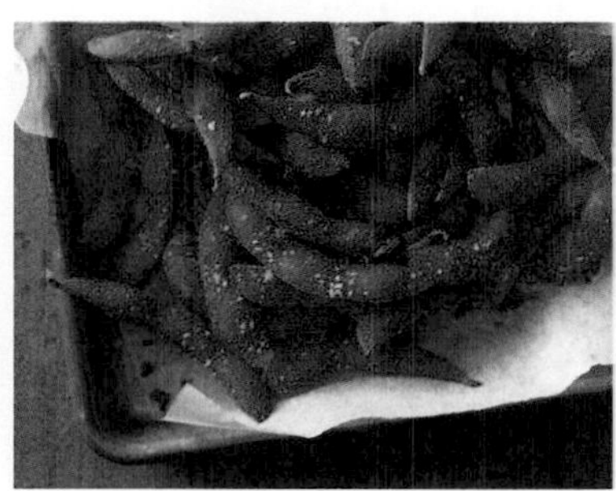

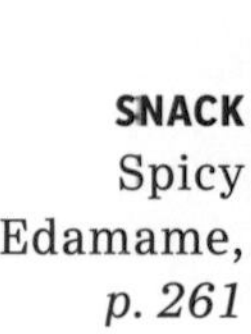

SNACK
Spicy Edamame, *p. 261*

DAY 2

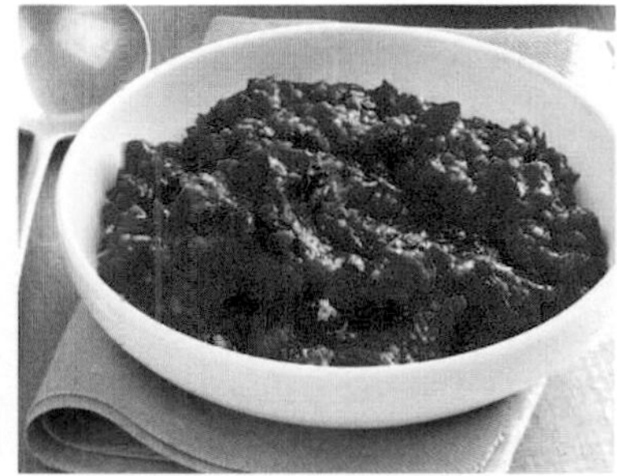

BREAKFAST
Carrot Cake Oatmeal, *p. 45*

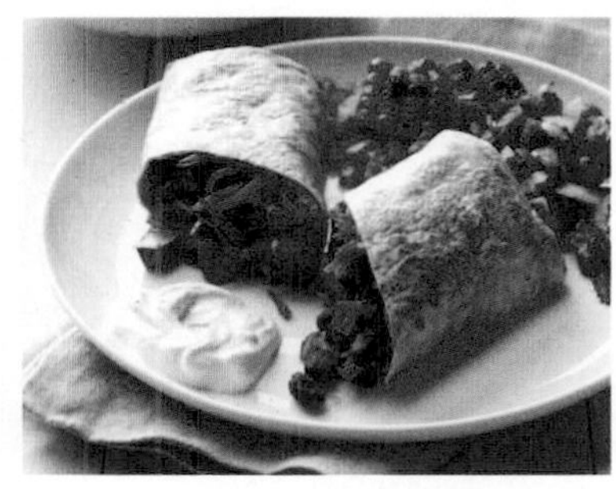

LUNCH
Black Bean Burritos, *p. 165*

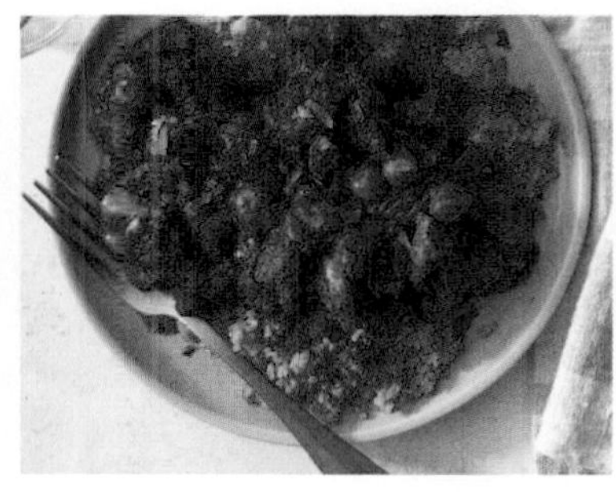

DINNER
Slow-Cooker Pumpkin Chicken Tagine, *p. 190*

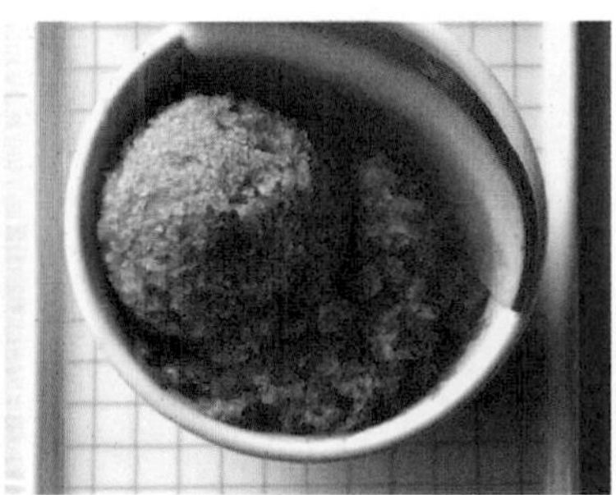

DESSERT
Frosty Watermelon Ice, *p. 284*

IN-A-HURRY MEAL PLAN

Busy families will appreciate recipes that are table-ready in 30 minutes or less or can be made ahead with little prep.

DAY 1

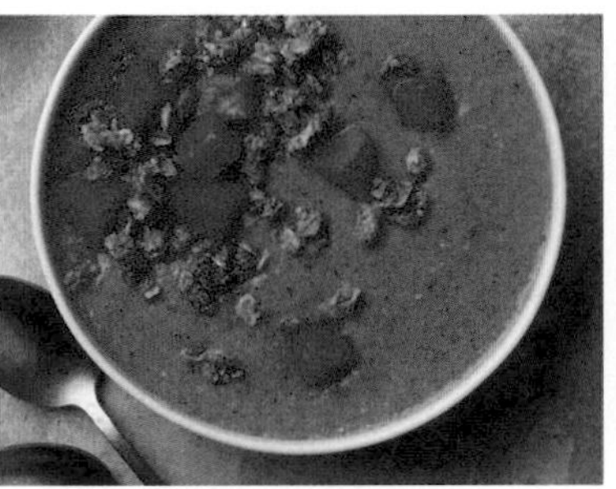

BREAKFAST
Tropical Smoothie Bowls, *p. 57*

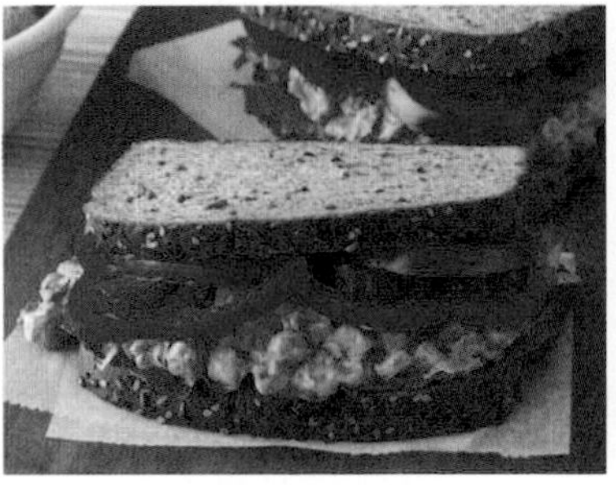

LUNCH
Dilly Chickpea Salad, *p. 89*

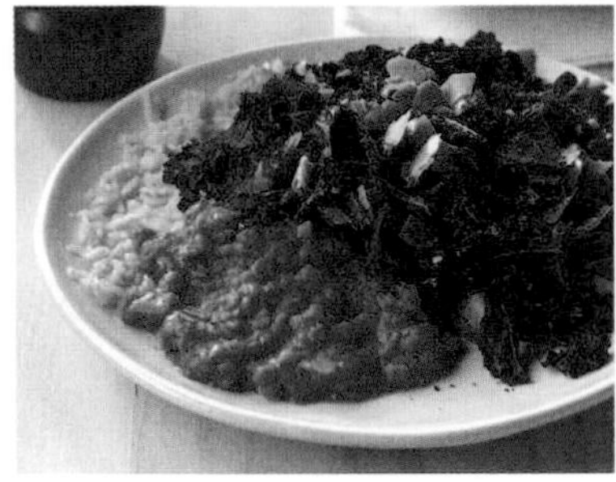

DINNER
Creamy Lentils with Kale Artichoke Saute, *p. 170*

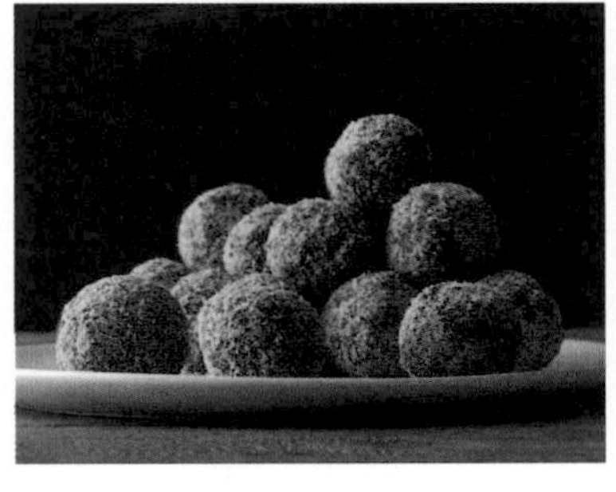

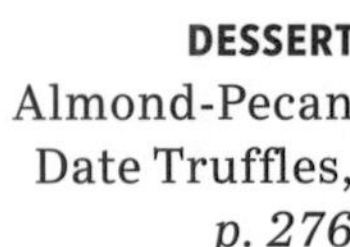

DESSERT
Almond-Pecan Date Truffles, *p. 276*

DAY 2

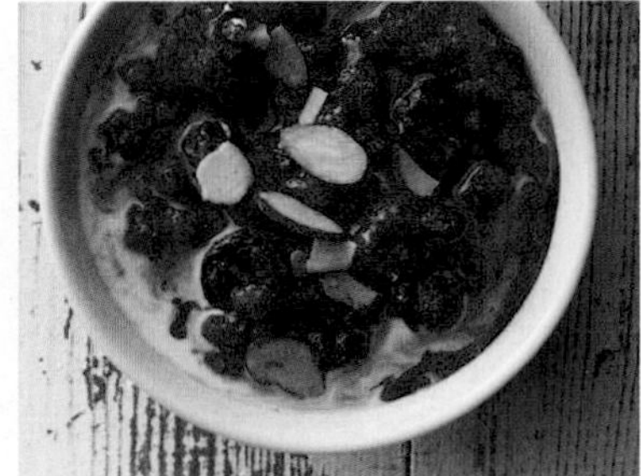

BREAKFAST
Overnight Flax Oatmeal, *p. 43*

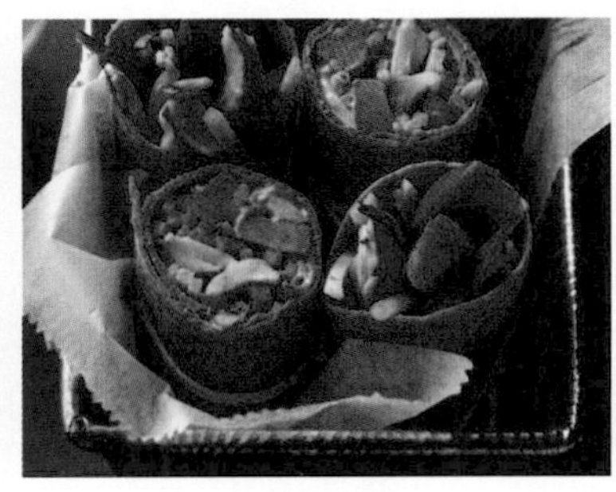

LUNCH
California Roll Wraps, *p. 95*

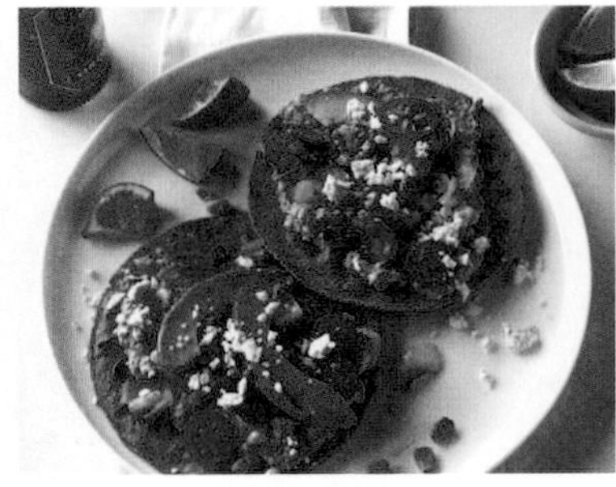

DINNER
Grilled Corn Hummus Tostadas, *p. 141*

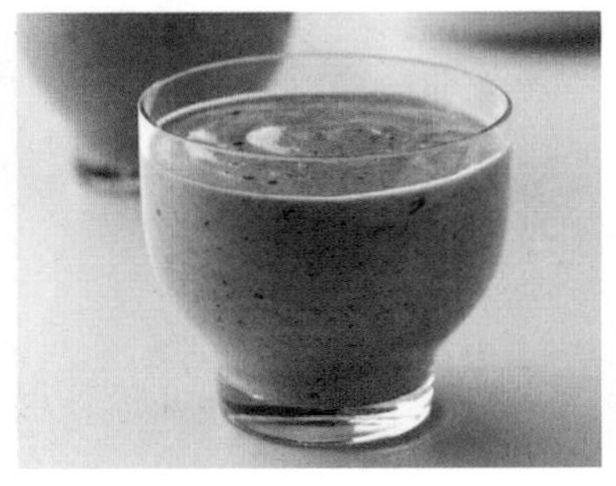

SNACK
Brain Food Smoothie, *p. 60*

HEART-HEALTHY MEAL PLAN

Eat heart smart with recipes that are lower in sodium and unhealthy fats, higher in fiber and include cardio-protective ingredients such as salmon and edamame.

DAY 1

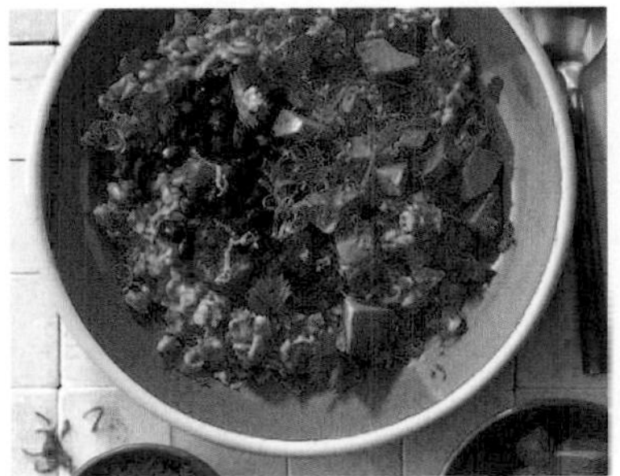

BREAKFAST
Tex-Mex Grain Bowls, *p. 44*

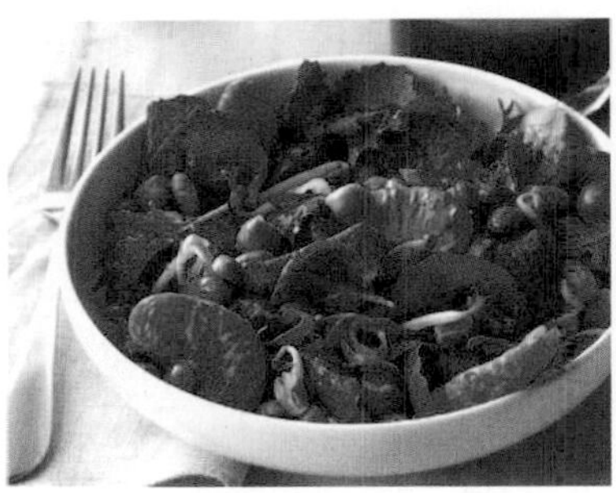

LUNCH
Edamame Salad with Sesame Ginger Dressing, *p. 109*

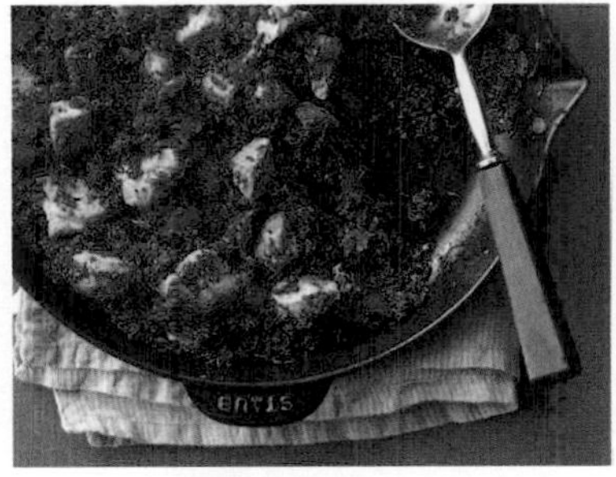

DINNER
Chicken Bulgur Skillet, *p. 236*

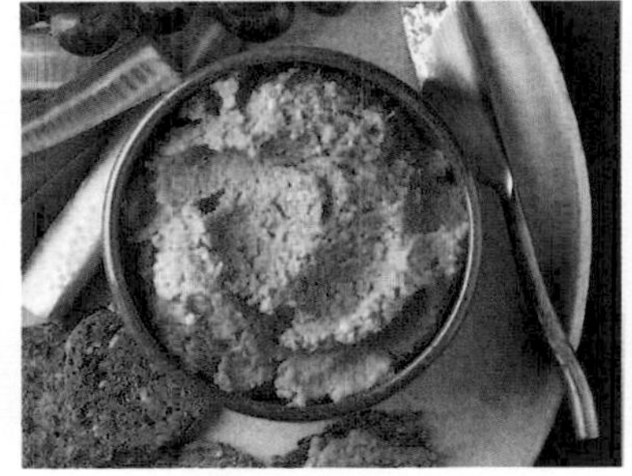

SNACK
Cashew Cheese, *p. 254*

DAY 2

BREAKFAST
Kale Smoothie, *p. 58*

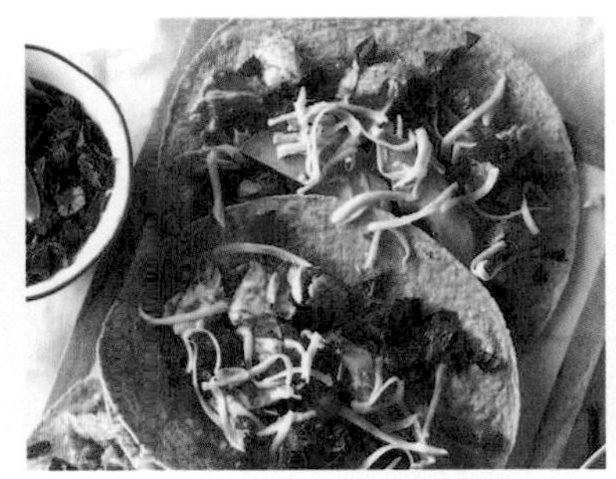

LUNCH
Grilled Salmon Wraps, *p. 94*

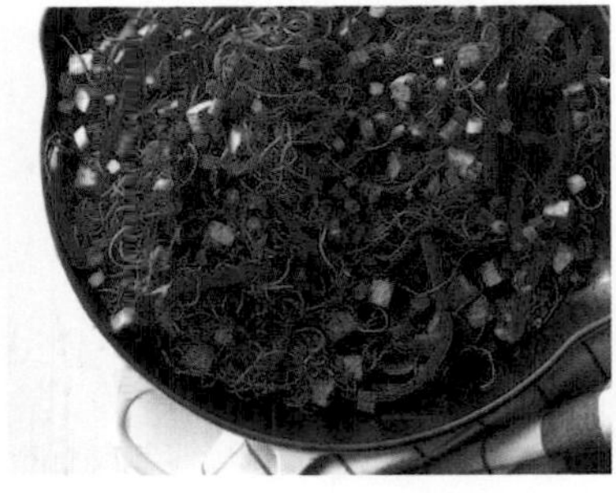

DINNER
Tofu Chow Mein, *p. 216*

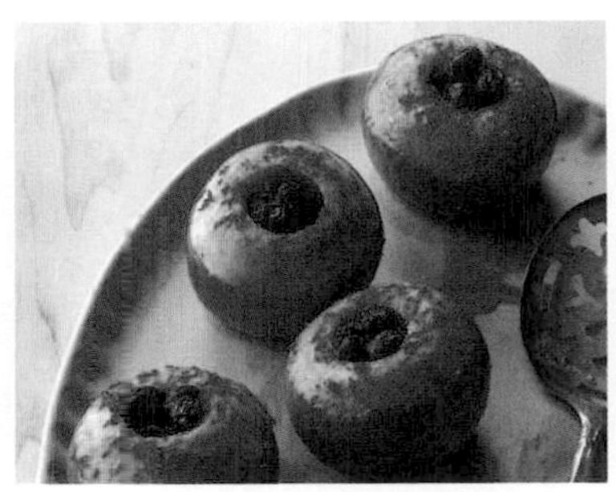

DESSERT
Slow-Cooker Baked Apples, *p. 295*

DIABETES-FRIENDLY MEAL PLAN

These recipes include diabetic exchanges (only those with low enough amounts of sodium, saturated fat and carbohydrates qualify). The plans include a modest amount of carbohydrates spread throughout the day.

DAY 1

BREAKFAST
Slow-Cooker Frittata Provencal, *p. 49*

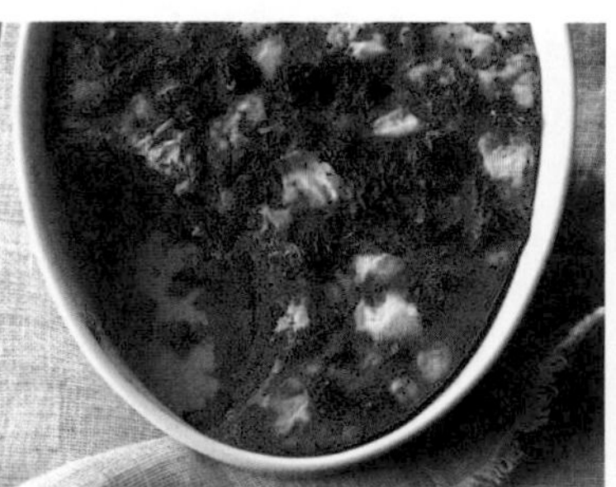

LUNCH
Tomato Basil Tortellini Soup, *p. 69*

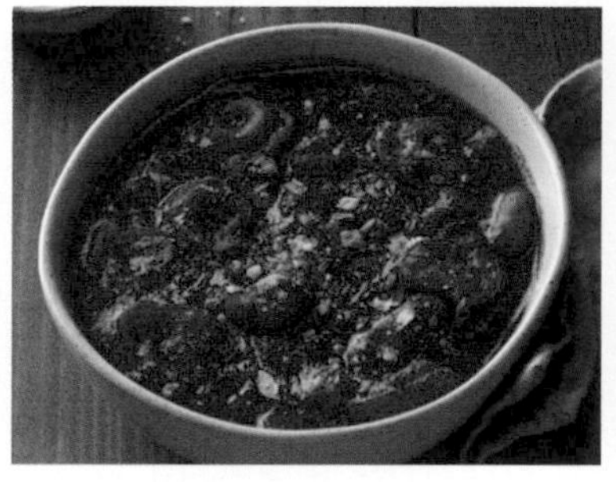

DINNER
Pressure-Cooker Indian-Style Chicken and Vegetables, *p. 153*

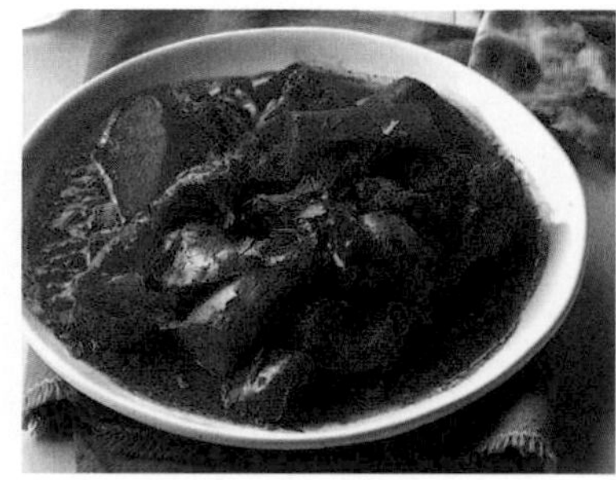

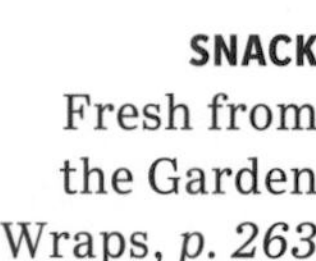

SNACK
Fresh from the Garden Wraps, *p. 263*

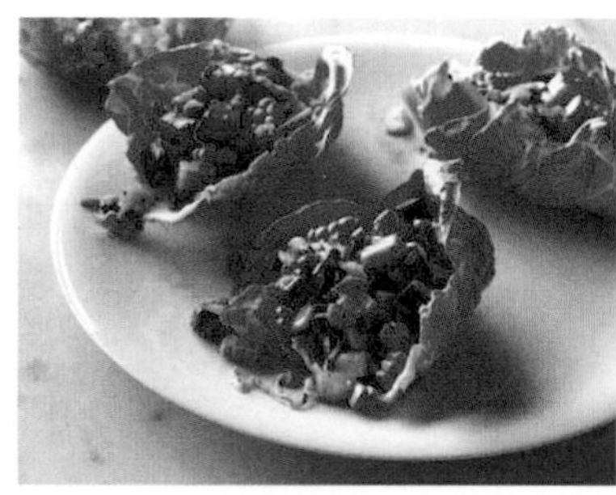

DAY 2

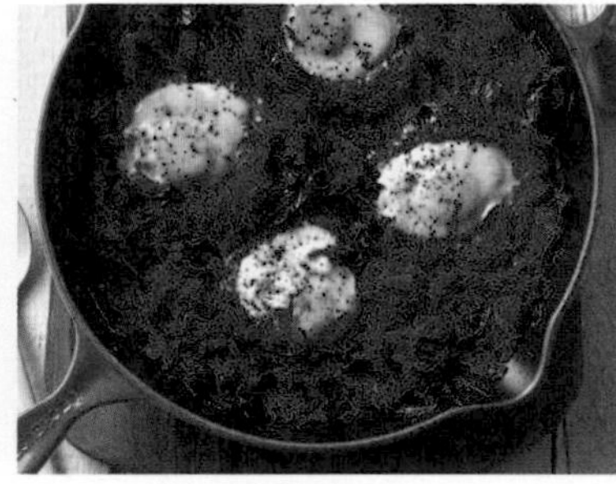

BREAKFAST
Sweet Potato & Egg Skillet, *p. 52*

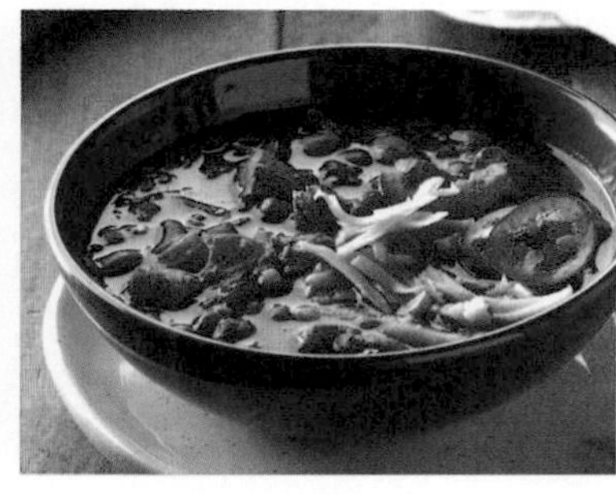

LUNCH
White Chicken Chili, *p. 84*

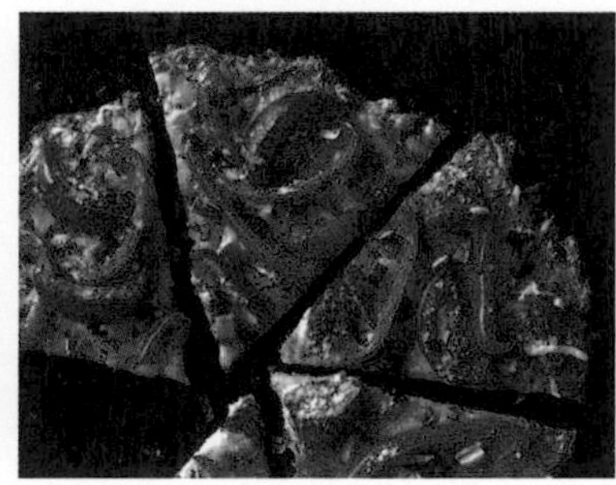

DINNER
Zucchini Crust Pizza, *p. 150*

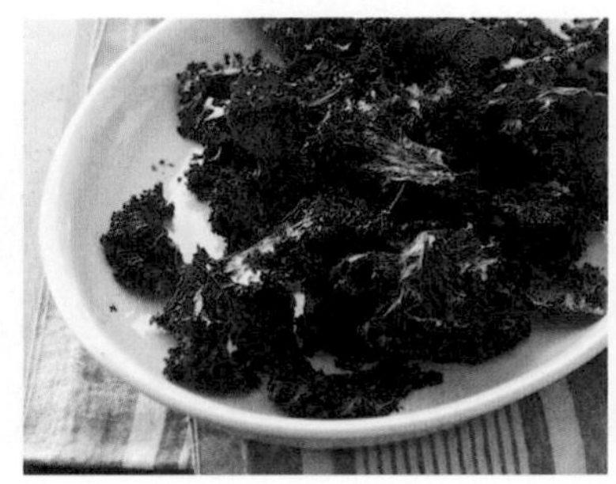

SNACK
Old Bay Crispy Kale Chips, *p. 256*

LOWER-SODIUM MEAL PLAN

Eating a plant-forward diet makes cutting salt easy. These flavorful menus contribute less than 950 milligrams of total sodium per day.

DAY 1

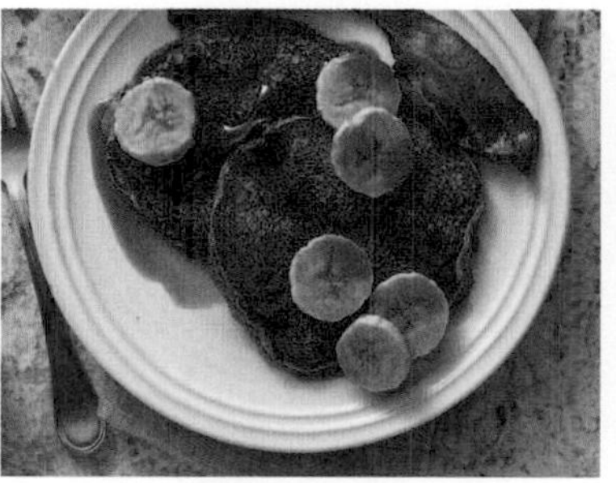

BREAKFAST
Banana Blueberry Pancakes, *p. 55*

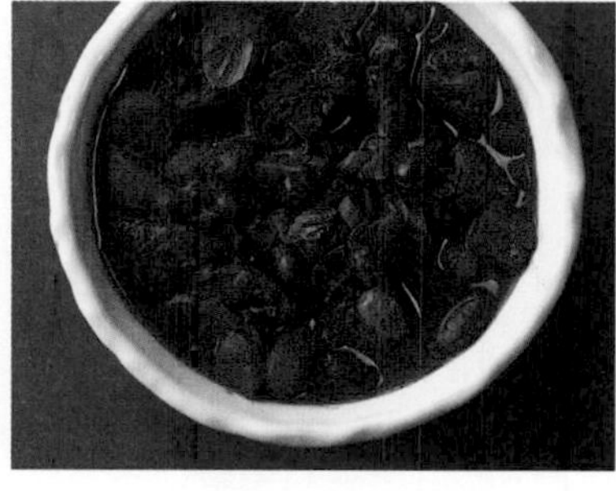

LUNCH
Pressure-Cooker Manchester Stew, *p. 79*

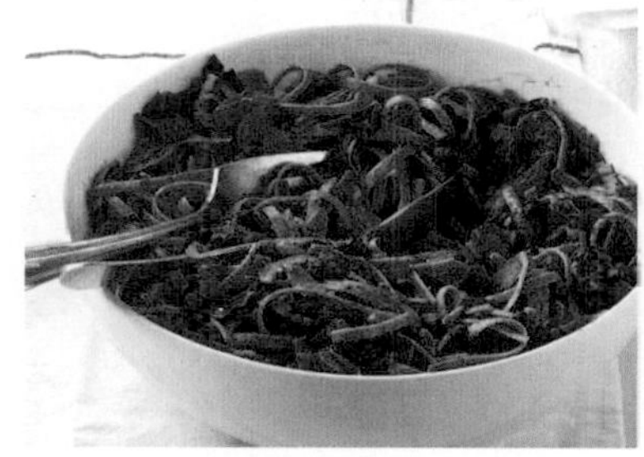

DINNER
Black Bean Pasta, *p. 219*

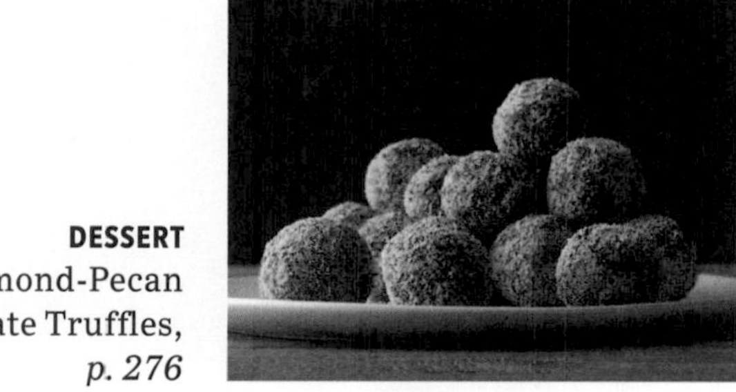

DESSERT
Almond-Pecan Date Truffles, *p. 276*

DAY 2

BREAKFAST
Overnight Flax Oatmeal, *p. 43*

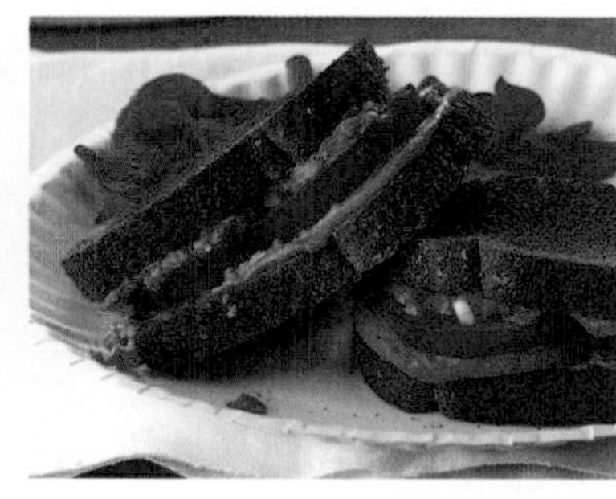

LUNCH
Tomato & Avocado Sandwiches, *p. 93*

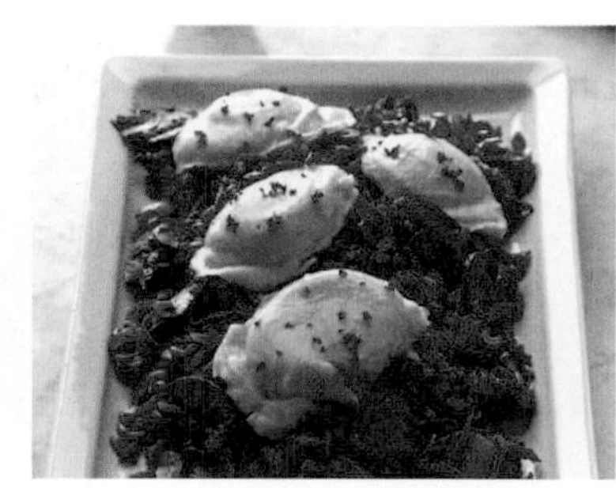

DINNER
Mushroom & Brown Rice Hash with Poached Eggs, *p. 246*

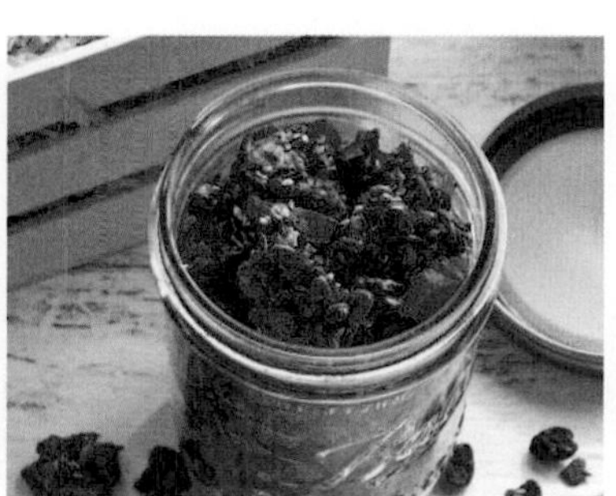

SNACK
Great Granola, *p. 42*

LOWER-FAT MEAL PLAN

If you're cutting fat from your diet, look to these menus for 16 grams of total fat and 5 grams of saturated fat or less per day.

DAY 1

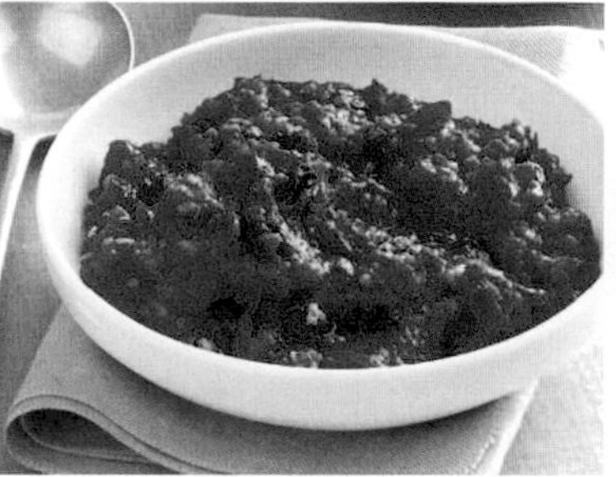

BREAKFAST
Carrot Cake Oatmeal, *p. 45*

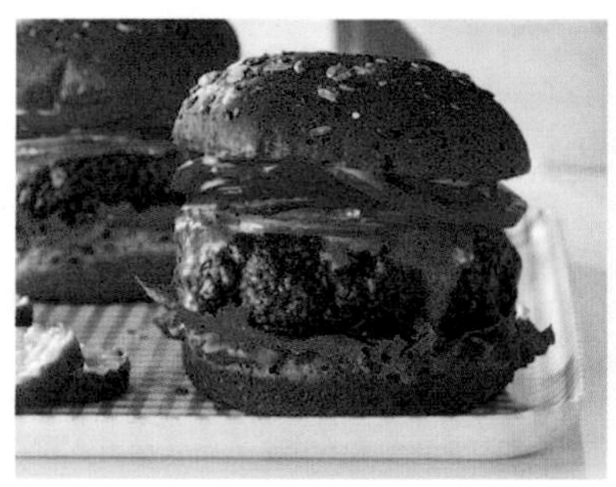

LUNCH
Salsa Black Bean Burgers, *p. 103*

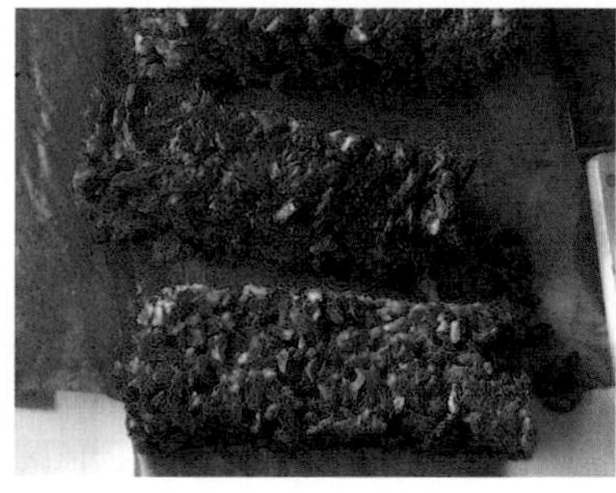

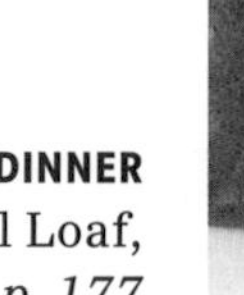

DINNER
Lentil Loaf, *p. 177*

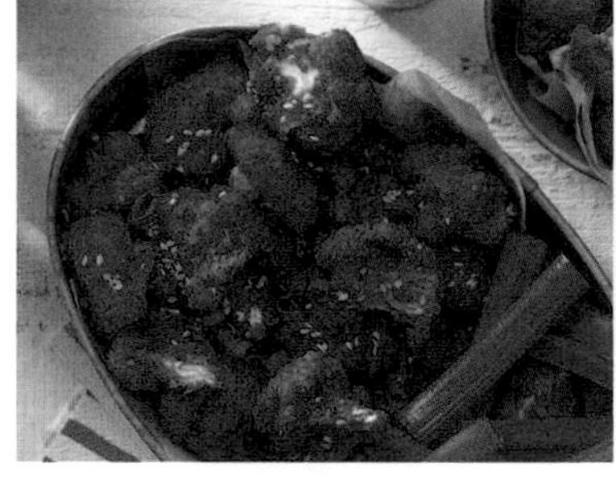

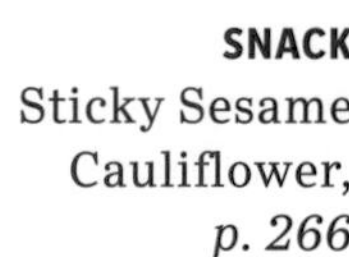

SNACK
Sticky Sesame Cauliflower, *p. 266*

DAY 2

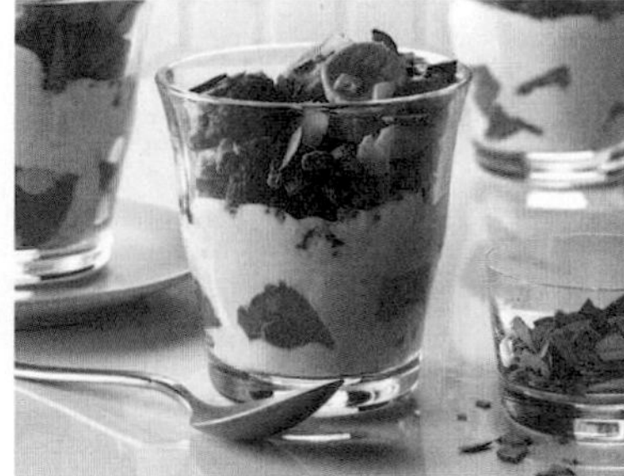

BREAKFAST
Breakfast Parfaits, *p. 56*

LUNCH
Carrot Split Pea Soup, *p. 74*

DINNER
Pressure-Cooker Tomato-Poached Halibut, *p. 151*

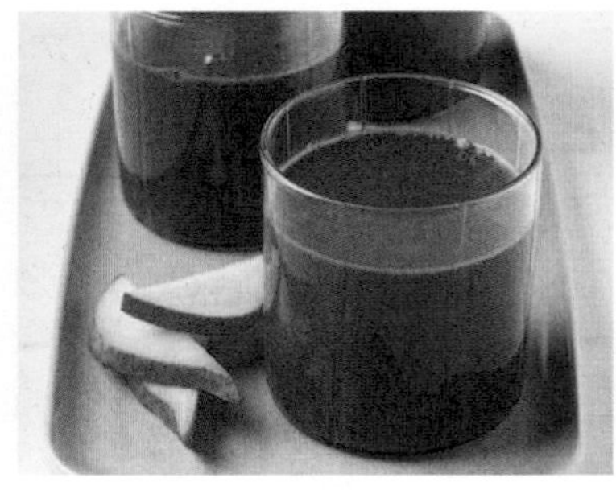

SNACK
Kale Smoothie, *p. 58*

BRAIN-HEALTHY MEAL PLAN

These recipes help support brain health and keep your mind and memory sharp with ingredients such as fatty fish, berries, nuts, seeds, eggs, broccoli and more.

DAY 1

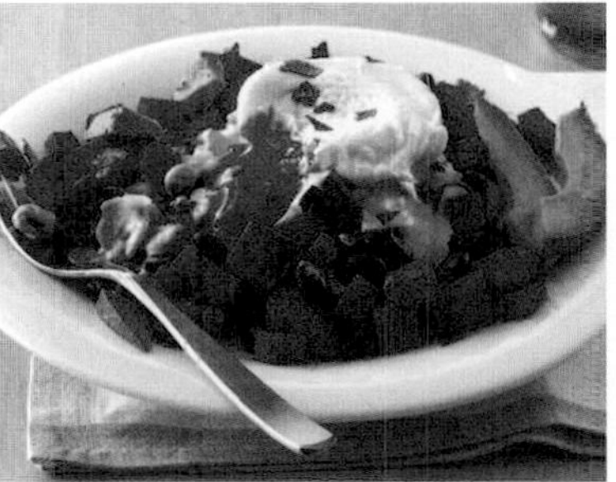

BREAKFAST
Southwest Hash with Adobo-Lime Crema, *p. 50*

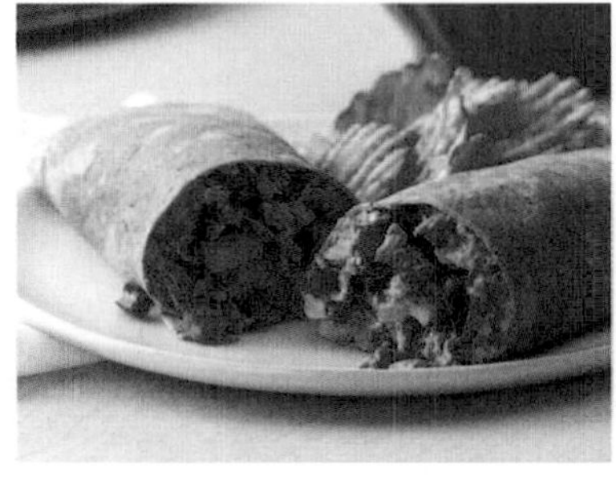

LUNCH
Crunchy Tuna Wraps, *p. 96*

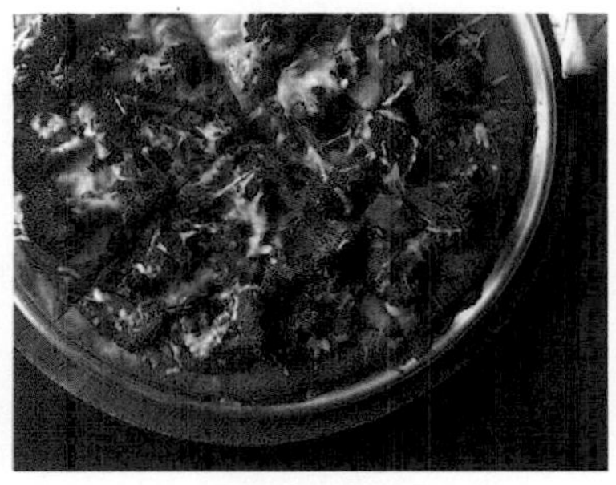

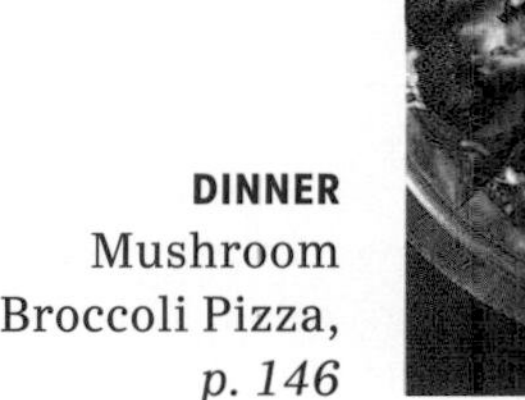

DINNER
Mushroom Broccoli Pizza, *p. 146*

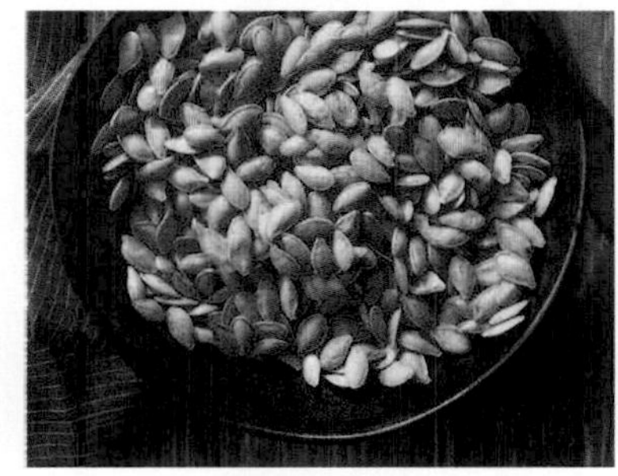

SNACK
Garlic Pumpkin Seeds, *p. 255*

DAY 2

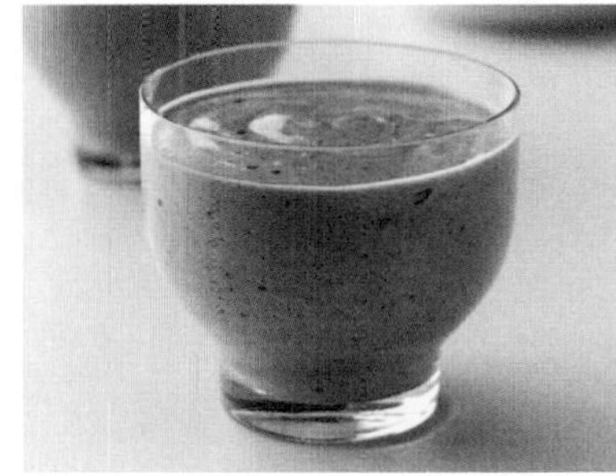

BREAKFAST
Brain Food Smoothie, *p. 60*

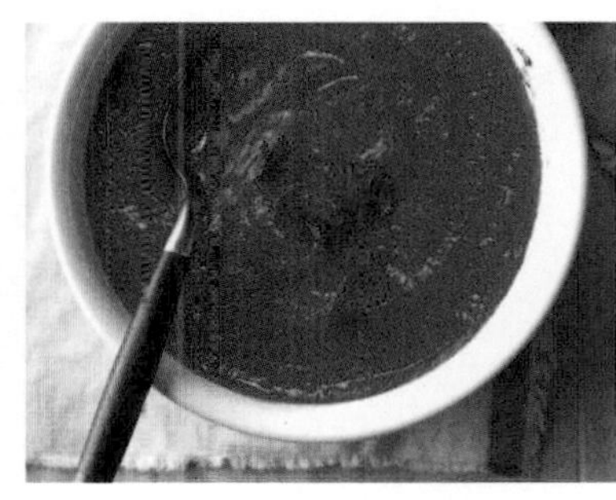

LUNCH
Creamy Cauliflower Pakora Soup, *p. 70*

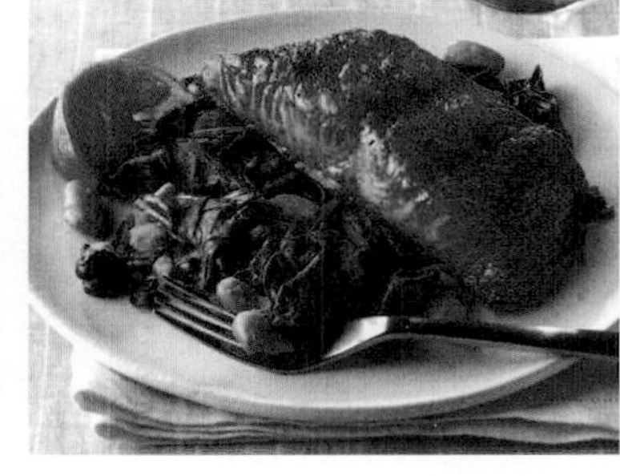

DINNER
Salmon with Spinach & White Beans, *p. 189*

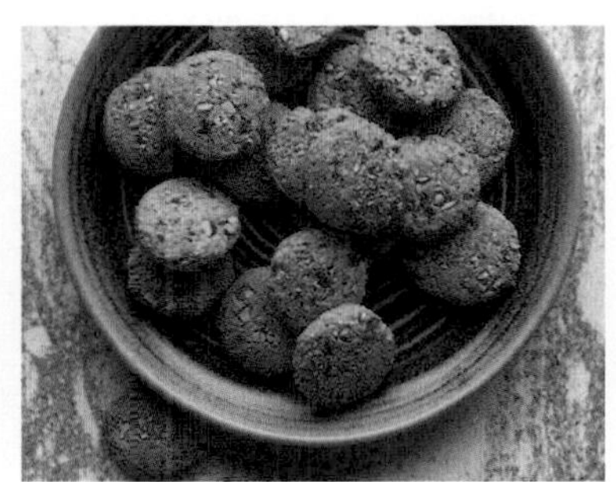

DESSERT
Gluten-Free Almond Crispies, *p. 279*

GUT-FRIENDLY MEAL PLAN

Ingredients rich in prebiotics, probiotics or fiber—such as leeks, yogurt and barley—can help maintain a healthy digestive system.

DAY 1

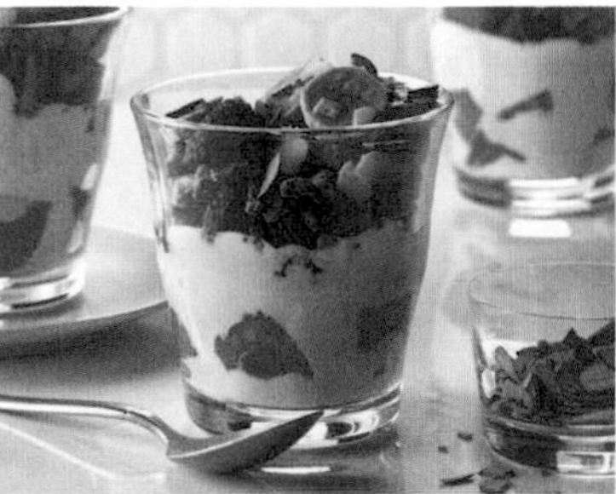

BREAKFAST
Breakfast Parfaits, *p. 56*

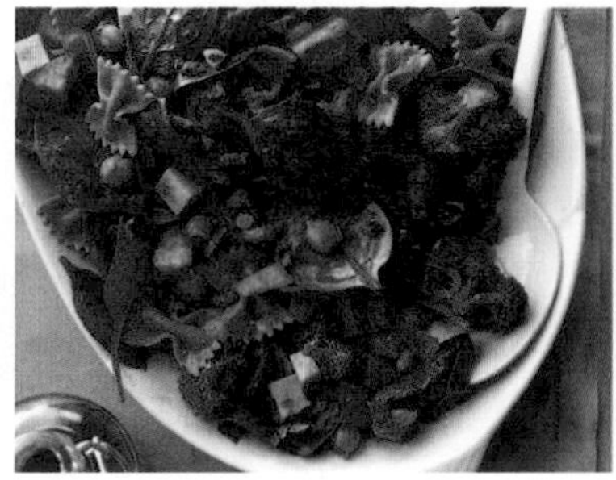

LUNCH
Bow Tie & Spinach Salad, *p. 120*

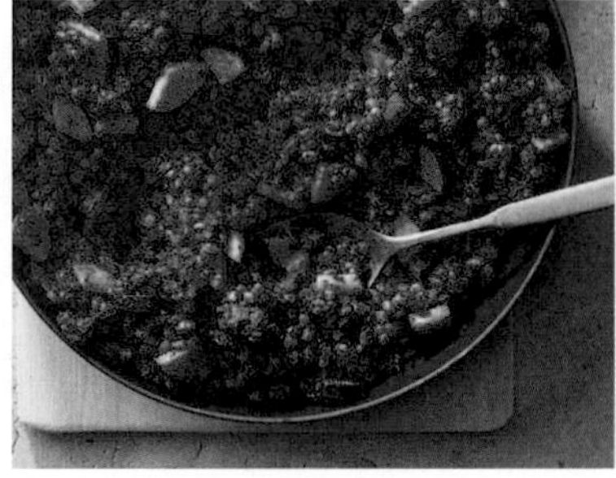

DINNER
Barley Beef Skillet, *p. 235*

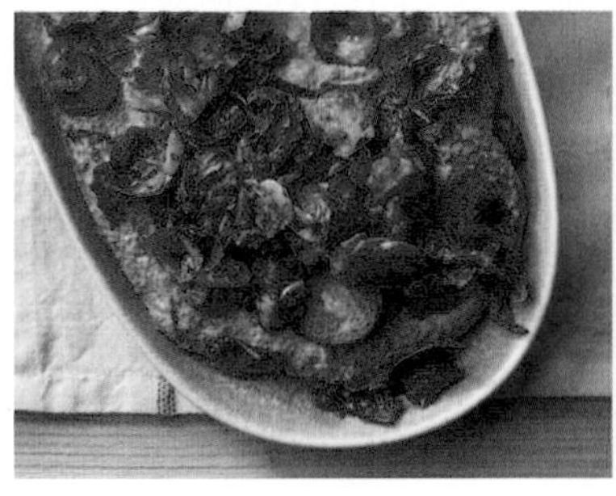

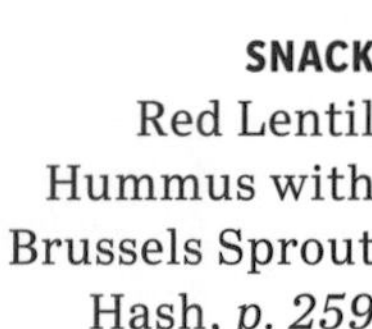

SNACK
Red Lentil Hummus with Brussels Sprout Hash, *p. 259*

DAY 2

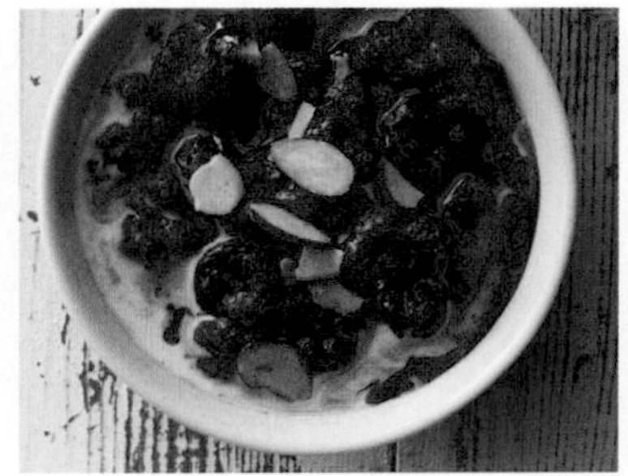

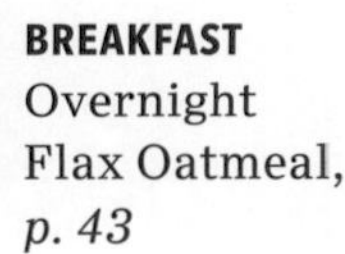

BREAKFAST
Overnight Flax Oatmeal, *p. 43*

LUNCH
Bean & Bulgur Chili, *p. 82*

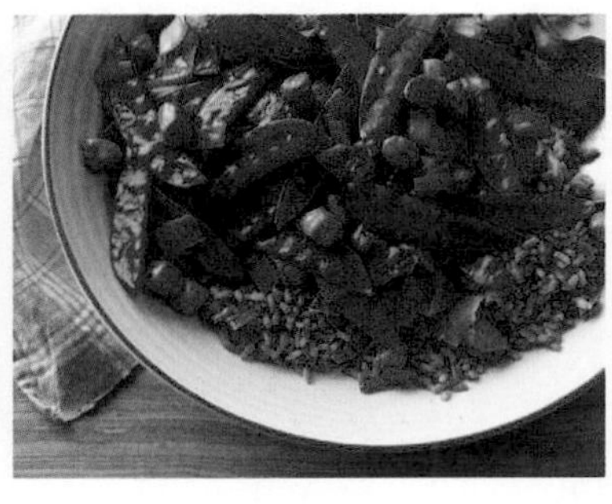

DINNER
Scallops with Snow Peas, *p. 249*

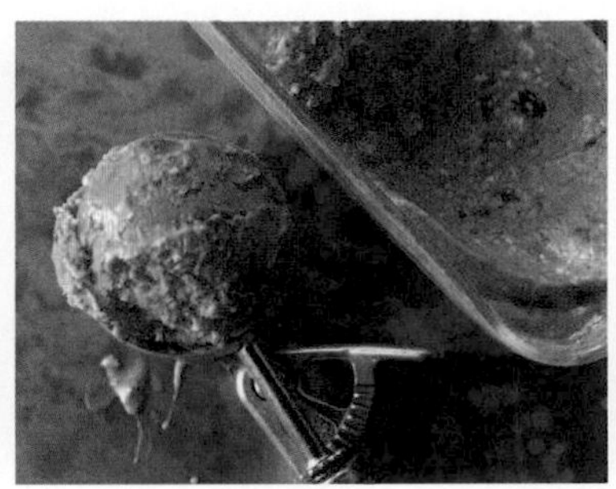

SNACK
Chunky Banana Cream Freeze, *p. 282*

GLUTEN-FREE MEAL PLAN

Skip recipes that include wheat, rye and barley or ingredients made from those grains. Be sure to read package labels to ensure items are truly gluten free.

DAY 1

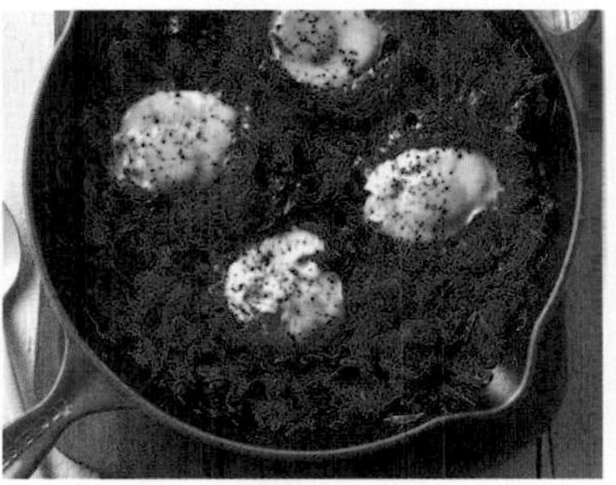

BREAKFAST
Sweet Potato & Egg Skillet, *p. 52*

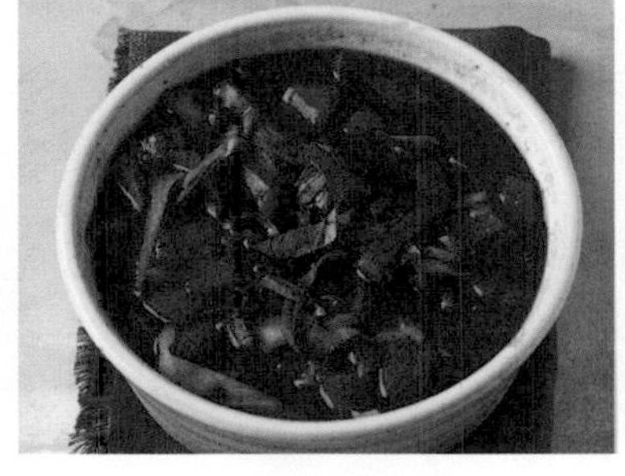

LUNCH
Italian Cabbage Soup, *p. 65*

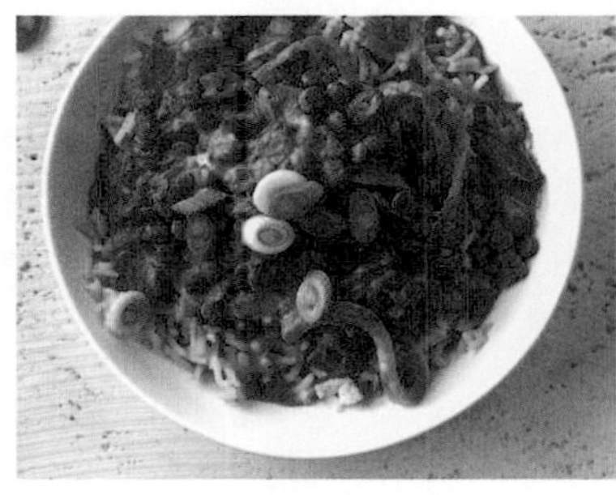

DINNER
Pressure-Cooker Lentil Stew, *p. 76*

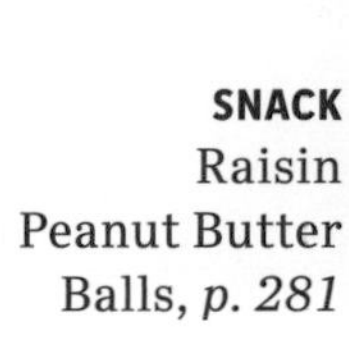

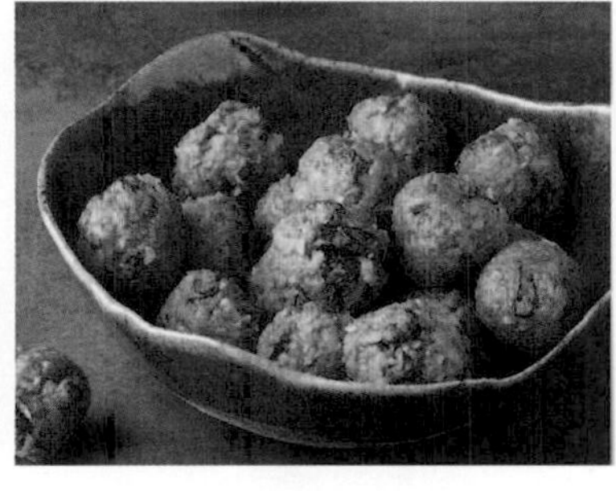

SNACK
Raisin Peanut Butter Balls, *p. 281*

DAY 2

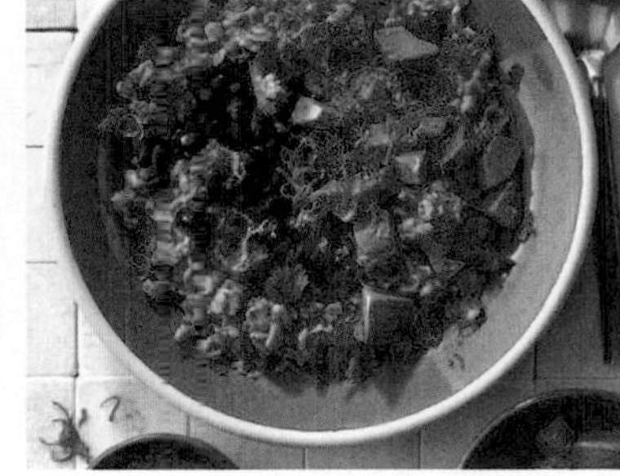

BREAKFAST
Tex Mex Grain Bowls, *p. 44*

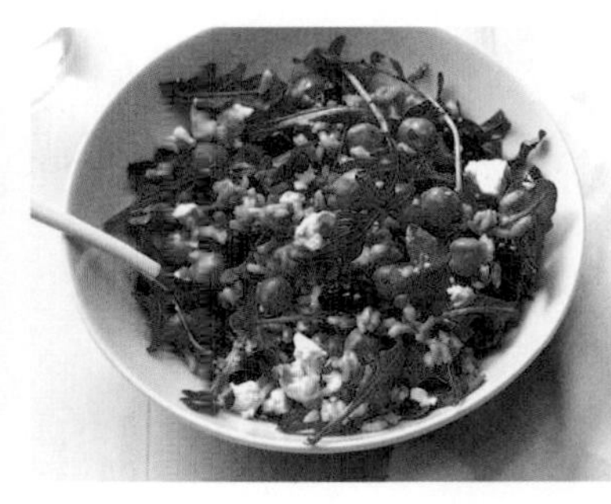

LUNCH
Arugula & Brown Rice Salad, *p. 116*

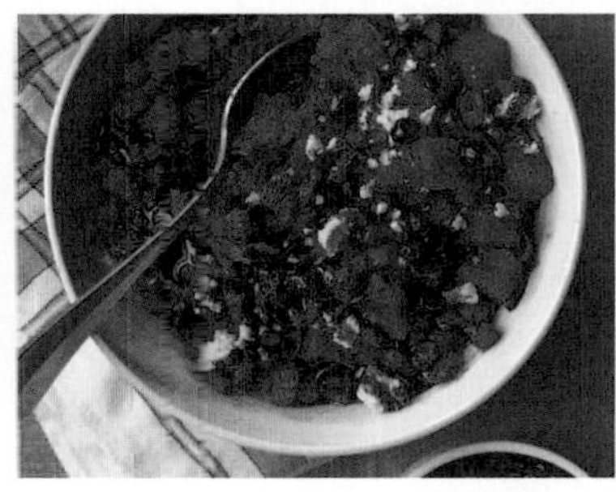

DINNER
Curry Pomegranate Protein Bowl, *p. 128*

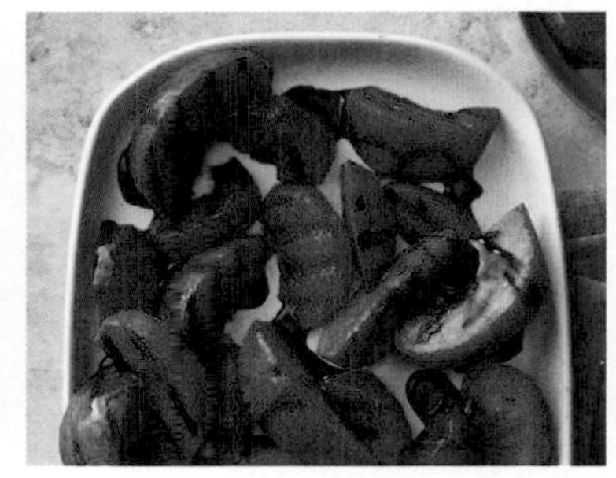

SNACK
Grilled Stone Fruits with Balsamic Syrup, *p. 288*

RECIPE INDEX

A

B

C

D

E

F